MEDICAL PEER REVIEW
theory and practice

MEDICAL PEER REVIEW
theory and practice

Edited by

PAUL Y. ERTEL, M.D., F.A.A.P.

Research Scientist, Health Services Research Center,
University of Michigan, Ann Arbor;
Formerly Professor of Pediatrics,
Ohio State University,
Columbus, Ohio

M. GENE ALDRIDGE, B.A., M.A.

President, M. Gene Aldridge and Associates, Inc.,
International Health Planning and Policy Research,
Denver, Colorado

with 60 illustrations

THE C. V. MOSBY COMPANY

SAINT LOUIS 1977

Printed in the United States of America

Distributed in Great Britain by Henry Kimpton, London

The C. V. Mosby Company
11830 Westline Industrial Drive, St. Louis, Missouri 63141

Library of Congress Cataloging in Publication Data

Main entry under title:

Medical peer review.

    Bibliography: p.
    Includes index.
    1. Medical care—Evaluation. 2. Medical care—
United States—Evaluation. 3. Professional standards
review organizations (Medicine)—United States.
I. Ertel, Paul Y., 1929- II. Aldridge, Melvin Gene
1940-
RA394.M42   362.1   77-23556
ISBN 0-8016-1533-X

GW/CB/B 9 8 7 6 5 4 3 2 1

Contributors

M. GENE ALDRIDGE, B.A., M.A., is President of M. Gene Aldridge and Associates, Inc., of Denver, Colorado. His firm is involved in education, research, and problem solving with various international and national health organizations. He is an educator and a social psychologist with applied research experience both in and out of the health care field. He assisted in the development of a medical peer review system in Colorado and served as Associate Director of that project for a number of years. He has assisted various allied health groups in designing and developing a statewide peer review system. During the past few years he has conducted numerous educational institutes on peer review, PSRO, and the problem-oriented medical record system. His international experiences have provided him with a working knowledge of various cultural diversities associated with health care delivery processes. His publications and research activities include issues surrounding quality care, cost reduction and educational influence, health planning and change, alternatives in caring for the aged, alternatives in primary health care, education for community health decision making, small group problem solving, and self-care.

GORDON C. BLACK, Col. USA, Ret., M.H.A., is currently serving as Deputy Commissioner Hospital Management, Division of Mental Health, in the Ohio Department of Mental Health and Mental Retardation. He was formerly Special Assistant to the Director of the Ohio Department of Mental Health and Mental Retardation for Quality Assurance, Planning and Management Information Systems. Mr. Black was Project Director under contract with the Bureau of Quality Assurance, U.S. Department of Health, Education, and Welfare, for development of a Model Utilization and Medical Care Assessment Program for State Mental Hospitals. His research and publications cover numerous areas including quality assurance, improved hospital management, health testing, and

emergency medical care services. His professional memberships include the American College of Hospital Administrators, American Hospital Association, and International Hospital Federation. He serves on the Board of Directors of the Society of Advanced Medical Systems (SAMS) and chairs the Society's Task Force on Emergency Medical Service.

MARSHA A. BREMER, B.S., is Project Director for the Quality Assurance Monitor package at the Commission on Professional and Hospital Activities (CPHA). In her four years at CPHA, Mrs. Bremer has served as a health record analyst in the Data Research and Statistics Department and in the Hospital Liaison Department. As an instructor in the Education Department she authored *JCAH Audit Using PAS—A Handbook for Health Record Analysts.* Since 1974 her primary responsibility has been the development of data tools to aid in medical care evaluation.

ROBERT H. BROOK, M.D., Sc.D., is a senior staff health services researcher at the Rand Corporation, Associate Professor of Medicine and Public Health at the UCLA Schools of Medicine and Public Health, and Director of the Robert Wood Johnson Foundation Clinical Scholars Program at the UCLA School of Medicine. Dr. Brook has been a leader in the use of process and outcome assessment to measure quality of care for the past five years. His concern with methods of evaluating the quality of medical care has led him to perform some of the very few studies that compared different approaches to evaluating quality of care given to the same groups of patients. In addition, he has recently completed an evaluation of the impact of the peer review system at the New Mexico Experimental Medical Care Review Organization during its first two years of operation. Dr. Brook has written extensively on both the practical and research issues relating to methods of evaluating the quality of medical care.

CLEMENT R. BROWN, Jr., M.D., currently is Director of Medical Education, South Chicago Community Hospital, and Associate Professor of Medical Education, Center for Educational Development, University of Illinois College of Medicine. Dr. Brown developed the Bi-Cycle concept relating continuing medical education directly to patient care in 1968 and designed and conducted workshops for over 300 hospitals helping to institutionalize the Bi-Cycle concept. He also designed and conducted the "Mandate Project," which institutionalized continuing medical education related to patient care in ten hospitals as an experimental program (reported in *Pediatrics,* May 1976). He was a consultant to the American Hospital Association (AHA), chairman of the panel that developed the AHA's Quality Assurance Program, and Director of Medical Affairs and Professional Services, American Hospital Association. He was a member of the National Professional Standards Review Council, U.S. Department of Health, Education, and Welfare from 1973 to 1976.

JAMES P. COONEY, Jr., Ph.D., is Chief Executive Officer of Rhode Island Health Services Research, Inc. (SEARCH). For more than five years Dr. Cooney has been involved in developing the use of patient-related data for purposes of quality assurance as well as developments related to collection and processing of health care data with special emphasis on those data related to patient care. Previously he was Associate Professor of Public Health and Associate Dean, School of Public Health, UCLA, and a professor in the Graduate School of Management, Northwestern University. Dr. Cooney has served as Director of Research for the American Hospital Association, Associate Director of Research, Blue Cross Association, and Director, Health Services Research Center, Chicago, Illinois. He is a member of the U.S. National Committee on Vital and Health Statistics.

ALLYSON DAVIES-AVERY, M.P.H., is a health services researcher at the Rand Corporation. Ms. Avery is actively involved in a study to develop short-term outcome measures for use in assessing the quality of medical care. She has coauthored several papers with Dr. Robert H. Brook, reviewing the history of quality assessment in the United States and discussing current issues in quality of care evaluation methodology.

AVEDIS DONABEDIAN, M.D., M.P.H., has devoted himself to research and teaching in preventive medicine and the organization of health services since 1961 when he joined the faculty of the School of Public Health, the University of Michigan, where he has held the post of Professor of Medical Care Organization since 1966. He received his medical training at the American University of Beirut, where he subsequently taught in the school of medicine and directed the health service plan for students and faculty. Dr. Donabedian has served as a member of the Governing Council of the American Public Health Association and is a member of the Institute of Medicine. His major publications include *A Guide to Medical Care Administration: Medical Care Appraisal—Quality and Utilization* (APHA); *Aspects of Medical Care Administration: Specifying Requirements for Health Care* (Harvard); and *Benefits in Medical Care Programs* (Harvard).

PAUL Y. ERTEL, M.D., F.A.A.P., is a senior research scientist at the Health Services Research Center, University of Michigan, where his primary activity is to investigate the delivery of health care and evaluate its quality and impact. Until recently he was Professor of Pediatrics at Ohio State University, where he was active for over ten years in research and development projects involving medical data systems and evaluation of health care. Beginning in 1972 he served as a co-principal investigator in a project to design and implement a computer-based peer review system. This cooperative project was initiated by the Ohio State Medical Association through its affiliate, the Medical Advances Institute, in which Dr. Ertel was Director of Clinical Systems. (The entire Medical Advances Institute criteria set and a description of its review methodology will soon be available in a book entitled *Quality Criteria for Automated Peer Review* published by The C. V. Mosby Co.) Dr. Ertel is a fellow of the American Academy of Pediatrics, a past president of the Association for Health Records, and currently is a member of the Technical Consultant Panel for the Uniform Discharge Data Set of the U.S. Department of Health, Education, and Welfare.

CARLOS J. M. MARTINI, M.D., M.P.H., M.Sc., is a senior lecturer in the Medical School, Department of Community Health, University of Nottingham, England. He previously served as Deputy Director of the Health Services Research Group in the Department of Community Health of the same university. Dr. Martini is also a member of the Faculty of Community Medicine at the Royal College of Physicians in the United Kingdom. He is responsible for several research projects in the areas of health measurements and primary medical care and is actively involved in the teaching of undergraduates and postgraduates in the Medical School.

ROSEMARY McCONKEY, M.S., is currently Special Assistant for Prevention, Control, and Education, Office of the Director, Division of Lung Diseases, National Heart, Lung, and Blood Institute, National Institutes of Health. Formerly an assistant director of medical education and on the staff for the Quality Assurance Program of the American Hospital Association, the coauthor of Chapter 13 has had extensive involvement in national workshop training of physicians, allied health professionals, hospital administrators, and trustees in the Bi-Cycle concept and in the implementation of the system in community hospitals.

IAN McDOWELL, B.A., is a lecturer in the Department of Community Health, Nottingham University Medical School, England. Mainly interested in evaluative methodology, he worked for three years in Uganda before going to Nottingham. In both posts his chief research interest has been in developing indices for use in health care evaluation.

ALAN R. NELSON, M.D., is Assistant Clinical Professor of Medicine at the University of Utah School of Medicine and is a practicing internist. His interest in peer review has focused on the application of combined utilization review and quality assurance methods on a statewide level. He is a past president of the Utah Professional Review Organization. He was elected a member of the Institute of Medicine, National Academy of Sciences, in 1975 and has served as a member of the National Professional Standards Review Council since 1973.

BEVERLY C. PAYNE, M.D., F.A.C.P., is currently Associate Professor of Internal Medicine and Postgraduate Medicine at the University of Michigan Medical School and Director of the Health Services Research Center at the University of Michigan. For 28 years after the completion of his training his primary activity was in the private practice of general internal medicine, first in Champaign, Illinois, and after 1952, in Ann Arbor, Michigan. His first health services research involvement was with Walter McNerney in a Michigan hospital and physician study (reported in *Hospital and Medical Economics,* 1961). He has since pioneered the development of the predetermined criteria evaluation of medical care quality and hospital utilization. The developing methodology has led to studies of the components and correlates of optimal medical care delivery in Nassau County, New York, and the states of Hawaii and Michigan. The emphasis has been on outcomes of care as well as the process measures in medical care delivery. He is presently a Michigan Governor for the American College of Physicians.

JAMES J. SCHUBERT, M.D., is currently Medical Director of the Medical Care Foundation and the Foundation Health Plan in Sacramento. He is in private practice as an orthopedic surgeon and is Associate Clinical Professor of Orthopedic Surgery, University of California at Davis Medical School. He is a former president of the Medical Care Foundation of Sacramento. He was active in de-

veloping the Certified Hospital Admissions Program (CHAP) in 1969 and has been on the Board of Directors or an officer of the Medical Care Foundation since that time. He also has been an officer of the American Association of Foundations for Medical Care and is a past president of the United Foundations for Medical Care (a California association). He has served on the Advisory Committee on PSRO of the American Medical Association, chaired the PSRO Task Force of the American Association of Foundations for Medical Care, was a delegate to the California Medical Association House of Delegates, and a member of the California Medical Association Medi-Cal Prepayment Committee.

VERGIL N. SLEE, M.D., F.A.C.P., is President of the Commission on Professional and Hospital Activities (CPHA), a nonprofit, nongovernmental education and research center dedicated to the improvement of medical care. He has been a pioneer in peer review methodology since 1950, when he became chairman of the committee of the Southwestern Michigan Hospital Council that developed the Professional Activity Study (PAS). PAS, the only computerized medical record information system designed especially to evaluate medical care, is now CPHA's principal program. Dr. Slee is a fellow of the American College of Physicians and an honorary fellow of the American College of Hospital Administrators. Dr. Slee's most recent articles on methods of peer review are "PSRO and the Hospital's Quality Control" (*Annals of Internal Medicine,* July 1974) and "Screening in Medical Care Assessment" (*ACS Bulletin,* June 1975).

JAMES E. SORENSEN, Ph.D., is Professor of Accounting at the University of Denver, Denver, Colorado. Dr. Sorensen has completed numerous research projects related to the application of behavioral sciences to accounting. He has written numerous articles in the past ten years on his research projects, on the theory and practice of accounting, and on accounting and management information systems. Some of the articles related to discussions in this book include the "Using and Understanding Cost-Outcome and Cost-Effectiveness in Program Evaluation," "Using Cost-Outcome and Cost-Effectiveness for Improved Human Service Program Management and Accountability," "Improved Cost-Finding Information for Rate-Setting and Managerial Uses," and "Cost-Quality Model for Delivery of Mental Health Services."

ALBERT C. STOLPER, B.S., is currently Executive Director of Vermont PSRO, Inc. Previously he served as Project Manager for the Criteria Development Project of the AMA, which developed sample sets of medical criteria to screen the appropriateness, necessity, and quality of medical service in hospitals through the coordinated effort of over thirty national medical specialty societies. Prior to that responsibility he was Administrative Assistant to the Executive Director of the American Academy of Pediatrics.

CLAUDE E. WELCH, A.B., M.A., M.D., D.Sc. (honorary), currently is Senior Surgeon, Massachusetts General Hospital, and Clinical Professor of Surgery, Emeritus, Harvard Medical School. He is President of the American Surgical Association and a past president of the American College of Surgeons. The American College of Surgeons has been particularly concerned with the improvement of care for the surgical patient, and he developed a great interest in this particular subject during his long term of service as an officer in this organization. He was the chairman of the AMA committee that developed the sample screening criteria described in Chapter 12.

Preface

Anthropology and the history of medicine reveal that the art, science, and technology associated with the practice of medicine have roots dating back more than 2000 years. It is the continuing obligation of the health professions to sort through this legacy in order to retain appropriate knowledge, concepts, and practices that are useful to both society and the health professions.

As the delivery of contemporary health care exposes the public to new technologies, the public increasingly demands the benefits of these new technologies. However, as the cost of the technology increases, it becomes evident that not all of this demand can be met. The theory of "rising expectations" developed in the political and social sciences is applicable to the current debate surrounding medical and health care delivery.

While medical science and technology are advancing, our ability to measure the effects of these advancements on the quality of health care has been less than systematically analyzed and applied. We have successfully met the problems associated with some major epidemics and have begun the technological process of transplanting organs, but we have not been able to systematically monitor the quality and the cost of more mundane clinical and health care matters. And despite all the technological advances, the health professions still need good practitioners who can translate the new technologies into effective and humane patient care.

Society, however, has not registered unbounded trust or satisfaction with American health professionals, as witnessed by the unprecedented malpractice actions, the medical fraud complaints, and the numerous laws and regulations focused on public accountability. There is a clear direction that would demythologize the "priestly role" that the medical practitioner has previously played.

There must be some reason why health professionals have not dealt as well with their declining social acceptance as they have with their ascending scientific progress. Perhaps the motivational philosophy behind health care, like its art, simply has not been able to keep up with the pace of its science. Health professionals would seem to modernize their professional philosophy with decreasing success and update their sense of social obligation with increasing reluctance. That reluctance appears directly proportional and parallel to the health professional's rising comfort with the rational appeal of medical technology. In dealing with patients, it is virtually irresistible to become dependent on all that technology and its attendant hardware. This includes the tools that permit health professionals to predictably manipulate organic systems and to apply reliable management principles based on the physical and social sciences. In the process, medicine would appear to many to be increasingly preoccupied with its own technology to the point that we have lost sight of both the art and humanism. This myopia has produced a health system wherein the health professional is becoming progressively alienated from those persons it serves. What else could explain the paradoxical change from a degree of pride, which reasonable men might be expected to hold for the successes of the medical profession, into the quite different attitude of bringing it to task?

Appropriate and effective action must be taken to evaluate health care. Accurate *planning, rate setting, reimbursement,* and *regulation* of health care systems cannot be established without more precise evaluation and feedback on the outcomes of the health system. The question is *how* do we evaluate the current delivery system? Many methods, concepts, and models have been proposed. However, they all hinge upon whether there is a professional commitment to address these issues forthrightly, in order that the health care professions can work toward a delivery system that meets both social and medical obligations. The implementation of an effective evaluation system for health and medical care is essential in order to correct any imbalances of care and contain runaway costs. This book proposes that the evaluation approach must be couched in an effective and systematic approach to peer review. Public trust must be earned. The public listens carefully to what is said and watches the actions of the health profession, measuring results from actions, however, not words.

Apparently either societal expectations have exceeded the medical profession's capacity to respond or it lacks awareness of the intensity and urgency of social demands. We believe it is essential now to deal with the complex and difficult problems that are vexing society with the same competence and priority with which technological problems have historically been addressed. Peer review provides a means of organizing the labyrinthian complexity and guiding the necessary corrective activity.

Physicians and other health professionals should be accountable to society for what they do, and not all social expectations are irrational or inimical to medical progress. Personal accountability is a concept wholly in keeping with professional ethics; now hopefully the health and medical professional can effectively demonstrate corporate accountability through the application of its own evaluation technology. Peer review offers a systematic means of achieving professional accountability.

From these fundamental rationales have emerged the objectives for this book. Past generations of physicians bequeathed the science and the skills to practice medicine effectively. Accompanying that capability is the obligation of physicians and the related health care disciplines to use their technology to proper ends and to practice medicine as professionals. We view medical peer review systems as serving the achievement of both ends.

In planning this book, our objective has been to provide a work of some enduring relevance. We wish to focus on those aspects of health care and its evaluation that will be as important tomorrow as they are today. Our design strategy, therefore, was to present valid principles of peer review and facts about operative review systems for interested health care personnel. We have presumed that our readers will be highly trained in the health or information science fields, will possess analytic capability, and will be interested in medical peer review. Such readers will want to compare and judge the concepts and applications described in this volume by relying on the common language of plain, spoken English in lieu of technical jargon. Moreover, we seek to protect our readers from those vocal "experts" who choose to dazzle with cybernetic mystique and nightmarish data systems. Instead we focus the reader's attention on those concepts and processes that are rationally substantive and fundamental to peer review.

In the absence of any single, unifying theory of peer review, we have sought to present our readers with generic information. It is equally important to minimize fragmentary information. Readers must not be left with the impression that a peer review system is merely a collection of evaluators' techniques. The final chapters show the convergent trends in peer review that lend coherence to seemingly divergent elements presented earlier in the book. The major concepts do articulate, and we have made every effort to help the reader recognize this.

Part one of the book traces the evolution of medical practice, social values, and attitudes toward health care from their separate origins to their recent impact point, the PSRO Act of 1972. This legislation will have far-reaching effects on medical practice. Thus physicians have an enormous stake in the development of evaluative systems. To familiarize our readers with the realm of possibilities, we have traced each major evaluation mode from its underlying concepts, through planning, design, and development, to implementation as a system applicable to health care. Part one then proceeds from an explanation of general theoretical concepts for health and medical evaluation to theoretical applications of these concepts.

In Part two the applications are particularized by describing operating review systems. Here the developers of a representative spectrum of nationally recognized evaluative systems are provided a forum for discussion of issues, description of technologies and methodologies, assessment of practice, and analysis of results in the medical community.

One final note is required. A specific frame of reference has been conveyed by the title of this book. We would be remiss if we did not explicitly share that frame of reference via specific definitions for each of the words utilized in the title. The following definitions are provided.

Medical is used in its broadest dictionary sense to connote that the given subject under discussion relates to or is concerned with "the practice of medicine." It is not intended that this term apply narrowly to physicians only unless it is obvious from the context.

Peer, in its usual dictionary sense, is used to refer to "one that is of equal standing with another." By this we mean that the peer of a physician is a physician, the peer of a nurse is a nurse, and so on, and that all health professionals who deliver clinical services directly to patients are included in general references to "peers" (again, unless otherwise specifically restricted by the context).

Review carries the dictionary definition "to go over or examine critically or deliberately."

Peer review, as used in the title of this book, refers to the broadest generic term that embraces the whole of this field. We fully recognize and wish to alert the reader also to the fact that others (notably Brown and McConkey in Chapter 17) utilize the term "quality assurance" in this generic sense. More for reasons of convenience and economy than any other, we opted to use the term "peer review" in the title because most contributing authors also used the term in this generic sense and for reasons of conceptual consistency. There is a parallel to the *assurance of quality care* which is the *assurance of efficient care* (resource utilization). Since "quality review" and "utilization review" are often contrasted with each other, "quality assurance" carries no literal connotation in regard to encompassing utilization. We therefore settled on "peer review" as it is a term that unequivocally embraces both concepts of quality review and utilization review.

The only form of peer review discussed in this book is a holistic, systematic, and integrated approach to the evaluation of care (as opposed to the more fragmented and informal or "traditional" form of peer review). It is fully recognized that at some point in the evaluation of health care, regardless of how the review is conducted, an implicit judgment must be rendered as to its efficacy and efficiency. The systematic approach to peer review so structures the review process as to create an environment wherein the often hidden (implicit) assumptions concerning optimal care are minimized and explicit or objective criteria for assessing care are maximized. The more systematic it is, the more each of the steps in the review process are seen to interact with all others, and the more any given step reflects the context and purpose in the evolution of the whole review process.

Theory and *practice,* the two major divisions of this book, are intended to be complementary from a structural viewpoint. There was, however, no constraint placed on any author to conform to ideas or concepts put forth by any other author. Rather the content boundaries of all chapters (and particularly so in the Theory Section) were reasonably well defined in advance simply to assure thoroughness in topical coverage and continuity while avoiding duplication. For reasons of economy, therefore, several authors cross-refer to segments in each other's chapters, but this practice is not to be interpreted necessarily as an endorsement of concepts unless so stated.

While we share with many a conviction that the whole field of health evaluation technology is currently in ferment, we also believe that in its present context, peer review is much too nascent to discuss co-herently without defining what is meant by some of the more essential and basic terms. Wherever this occurs, it is done to enhance an understanding of how such terms are used in this text and not to impose any general restrictions on concepts. It is in this spirit of enhancing communication that we offered the definitions above. We have also provided a glossary of terms and list of abbreviations common to peer review.

In this same sense we have defined medical peer review as follows:

Medical peer review is the investigational, managerial, and educational process for systematically monitoring medical and health care in which the judgments regarding provider performance and recommendations regarding corrective actions are based on a review of appropriate case data and are made by qualified professional peers who practice in the same community and who communicate the results of their efforts to the public.

Our common goal then is to describe the theory and practice of medical peer review as it is understood today. Admittedly this is an ambitious objective, perhaps even optimistic. Nevertheless the attempt has been made to incorporate into this one volume important theoretical considerations, topics of factual importance in the field, and insights derived from practical experiences with some of the peer review systems and tools in current use.

Paul Y. Ertel
M. Gene Aldridge

Acknowledgments

No text of this kind can be developed without the magnificent help of various human beings who are able to see the total worth of the effort. We wish to thank all of the authors who contributed their time and talents in guiding our thoughts and directions throughout the project. Each of the authors spent many hours refining and responding to our many notes and memos. We would also like to express our gratitude to Lee S. Hyde, M.D., for his willingness to permit us to quote from *A Discursive Dictionary of Health Care* (prepared for use of the Subcommittee on Health and the Environment of the Committee on Interstate and Foreign Commerce, U.S. House of Representatives) in the Glossary. In addition, the talents of Mrs. Virginia (Ginny) Wigfield and Susan M. Cockings have provided many hours of editing assistance, communication with the authors, and the grueling work associated with producing the manuscripts for publication. Special appreciation to Susan Cockings and Dee Nelson are also in order for the high-quality research support they provided for the project. Special thanks also to Rochelle Bock who was able to find the time to help us with our library fact-finding problems. Roy R. Miller, M.D., was the source of much of the initial impetus to launch this effort, and his original ideas contributed much to the ultimate result. A personal thank you is due R. James Ertel whose editorial assistance went far beyond the call of fraternal duty. Finally, we wish to thank our families and friends for the gentle encouragement that was appreciated throughout the project.

Paul Y. Ertel
M. Gene Aldridge

Contents

PART ONE **THEORY,** 1

SECTION I **Evolution of medical evaluation and peer review,** 5

1 Perspectives of medicine and society: evolution and role of peer review in medical practice, 7
PAUL Y. ERTEL

2 Evaluating the quality of medical care, 50
AVEDIS DONABEDIAN

3 A matrix for assessing health care quality, 76
AVEDIS DONABEDIAN

SECTION II **Critical issues of peer review,** 87

4 Functions of peer review, 89
M. GENE ALDRIDGE

5 Quality assessment: issues of definition and measurement, 111
ROBERT H. BROOK
ALLYSON DAVIES-AVERY

6 Measurement of outcomes: primary health care evaluation in the United Kingdom, 132
CARLOS J. M. MARTINI
IAN McDOWELL

SECTION III **Organizational issues of peer review,** 145

7 Organizational issues in systematic peer review, 147
GORDON C. BLACK
PAUL Y. ERTEL

8 An operational model of systematic peer review, 197
PAUL Y. ERTEL
GORDON C. BLACK

9 Design and content determinants of systematic peer review, 230
PAUL Y. ERTEL

10 Management information systems and the costs of systematic
peer review, 243
JAMES E. SORENSEN
PAUL Y. ERTEL

PART TWO **PRACTICE,** 271

SECTION I **Basic instruments for peer review,** 273

11 The AMA model screening criteria, 275
CLAUDE E. WELCH
ALBERT C. STOLPER

12 Information systems and peer review, 287
MARSHA A. BREMER
VERGIL N. SLEE

13 Assistance for hospital informational needs: the health data broker, 296
JAMES P. COONEY, Jr.

SECTION II **Functioning systems,** 305

14 The Medical Care Foundation of Sacramento, 307
JAMES J. SCHUBERT

15 Quality assessment and utilization review in a functioning peer
review system, 325
ALAN R. NELSON

16 Research in quality assessment and utilization review in hospital
and ambulatory settings, 335
BEVERLY C. PAYNE

17 The quality assurance system, 356
CLEMENT R. BROWN, Jr.
ROSEMARY McCONKEY

PART THREE **PRINCIPLES,** 379

18 Principles of peer review, 383
PAUL Y. ERTEL
M. GENE ALDRIDGE

Glossary, 393
Abbreviations, 405

MEDICAL PEER REVIEW
theory and practice

PART ONE

THEORY

There is nothing more difficult to take in hand, more
perilous to conduct, or more uncertain in its success, than
to take the lead in the introduction in a new order of
things.

Machiavelli (AD 1469-1527)

The Theory Part of this text is designed to bring together the various implicit and explicit formulations, principles, and general concepts about peer review. When viewed separately, a number of these concepts may seem to be in conflict. However, when viewed as part of an evolutionary change process, they are not. As Kaplan has stated, "Without a theory, however provisional or loosely formulated, there is only miscellany of observations, having no significance either in themselves or over against the plenum of fact from which they have been arbitrarily or accidentally selected."[1,p.268]

Whatever evolutionary focus peer review ultimately might have developed spontaneously is a matter for speculation; what is clear is that the PSRO law (Public Law 92-603, 1972) has created an unprecedented role for peer review as the mechanism for institutional and professional accountability in health care delivery. The accountability function is a most important variable in the peer review process. The accountability function provides for representatives of the public to participate in what was until 1972 singularly a professional activity. Regardless of the rationale for or against the enactment of this law, its very existence poses both problems and challenging opportunities for medical professionals. Society will now be watching closely to see how the problems and the opportunities are handled.

The opportunities, which the PSRO law has provided, are both derived from and contingent upon professional participation in the mechanism of public accountability plus adequate funding to develop a greatly strengthened, orderly, and efficient system of peer review. This, in turn, promises to become the feedback mechanism needed by the medical profession to develop a more effective and humane health care system. Thus, when peer review becomes the mechanism for the public accountability function in medical care, it also represents a tremendous potential for effecting desirable change in the health care

1

system. On the other hand, should this machinery become the monopoly of a single constituency, it could (and most probably would) become highly limited in use. There is little justification for allowing any single group to maintain full control over any of the evolutionary tools of society, and public accountability is no exception to the general rule.

The actual structure of our social, political, and economic tools may enhance or hinder the appropriate application of these tools by society. This principle, as applied to medicine, implies that the way we choose to structure the evaluation system for examining the process and output of our health system will determine not only how we view the review system but also how we use it as a resource. The use of peer review, its mechanics, and society's view of it, then, are interdependent issues that must be simultaneously addressed if a peer review system is to be thoroughly understood. In the Theory Part we have spelled out as clearly as possible the limitations and the problems as well as the potentials that exist in the structural and mechanical aspects of peer review. This is done out of respect for the criticism put forth by Ellul in his work *The Technological Society,* namely that any proposed technique tends to integrate the machine into society.[2] The machine (in this case, computers), when linked to a peer review system, could become antisocial in both character and function. It has the potential to alienate the very people it was designed to assist—the patient and the professional. Thus we have done our utmost to present a balanced account of the advantages and disadvantages of systematic peer review.

To maximize the value of a theory of peer review, it seems appropriate to review three major research needs that confront medicine as it seeks to establish workable public and professionally acceptable methods for achieving accountability:

1. The need to find an effective methodology in which to evaluate the delivery of medical care in a medical institution setting
2. The need to find a methodology to measure, validly and reliably, health status outcomes of medical care
3. The need to find a methodology that would measure the impact of medical care systems (illness intervention) and health care systems (preventive medicine) on the health status of populations served by those systems

Peer review methods have been evolving for decades in an attempt to better answer the first of the above needs. With the advent of PSRO this work has taken on a new impetus and importance. But the ultimate success of daily peer review operations in a community will most depend on whether local health professionals will adequately support and participate in peer review activities in their own hospital or place of practice. What will be required over the next few years is a professional investment that will apply the development of technological assessment strategies to review activities. Technology has been defined as the "systematic application of organized knowledge to practical activities, especially productive ones."[3] This means that the health professional and the public must see practical and worthwhile improvements in the cost and quality of care for patients as a direct result of the applied peer review systems.

But we can move realistically toward such an ultimate system of accountability only if we follow scientific concepts and move in a series of approximations. In this sense every piece of new data is provisional. Understanding and providing appropriate methods for peer review in the United States must move in much the same way. An attempt has therefore been made to organize the material in the Theory Part to provide the reader with benchmarks by which to gauge the extent of the progress of peer review applications and review methodologies as presented in the Practice Part of this book.

The Theory Part was organized to enable the reader to move from the historical and evolutionary roots of medicine, through the emergence of issues critical to peer review, on to some of the more applicable organizational concepts, and ultimately to some practical suggestions derived from a model of operational peer review systems. The views offered in this section obviously do not incorporate all the worthwhile thinking that could be presented on such a large topic as peer review. They do, however, represent the concerns and views that have been generally discussed in the literature over the last decade.

To maintain a consistent frame of reference, it was decided to focus much of the discussion in this Theory Part on peer review as performed in hospitals (where PSRO is initially focused). But most of the theory presented really is not specific to the hospital setting and can be applied to virtually any other health care environment (for example, nursing homes, mental health institutions, and statewide physical therapy, occupational therapy, and nursing systems of peer review).

Finally, most contributing authors have presented their discussions of medical peer review from the perspective of the contemporary, practicing health professional. There are at least two good reasons for doing so. First, it is the practicing health professional whose career and working conditions will be most affected by peer review and who therefore has most at stake. Second, maintaining a clinical context holds the best promise of showing the relevance of the theory and the growing body of scientific concepts that underlie the evaluation technology used in the assessment of medical care. And the function of scientific concepts, after all, is to create sets of ideas that will tell us more about the subject matter than any other sets of ideas.[1,p.52] To this end we share our investment in peer review.

M. Gene Aldridge

REFERENCES

1. Kaplan, A.: The conduct of inquiry, San Francisco, 1964, Chandler Publishing Co.
2. Ellul, J.: The technological society, New York, 1964, Vintage Books, p. 5.
3. Ayers, R. U.: Technological forecasting and long-range planning, New York, 1969, McGraw-Hill Book Co., p. 46.

Evolution of medical evaluation and peer review

1

Perspectives of medicine and society: evolution and role of peer review in medical practice

PAUL Y. ERTEL

The single overriding point to be made in this chapter is that we are experiencing an unprecedented moment in history in which competing forces are contesting for control of the decision-making processes that can affect medical practice in this country for generations to come.

What has brought about this critical turning point is the maturation of three evolutionary developments at one point in time: (1) care technology has evolved to the point where the capability exists to effectively influence the health outcome of a significant spectrum of human disorders; (2) society has escalated its demands that this capability be translated into an established reality for all, meaning that medical care be uniformly of the highest quality, available, affordable, and that medicine be held publicly accountable for all three; and (3) evaluation technology has evolved to the point where it is now technically feasible to carry out the mandate of public accountability and to channel the allocation of health manpower and resources toward almost any predetermined health care objective.

As long as medicine merely presided in sympathetic ceremonies to the inevitable (that is, officiated over the course of dis-

eases about which it could do little or nothing), it was virtually irrelevant to inquire whether physicians in general were doing a good job. It really did not matter. Now it does. Further, control over the profession has now become politically attractive, in part because of public demand for equity in the distribution of medical care and in part because medical costs have become so unreasonable that they invite governmental controls. And at just this precise time the technology is available to make the imposition and maintenance of external control feasible. There can be no serious doubt that an effort at control is being made.

Just where the federal government stands in regard to the control of medicine is a matter of record. The U.S. Department of Health, Education, and Welfare (HEW) has produced a "Forward Plan for Health FY 1977-81." In this plan HEW makes a declaration that government intends to share with medicine in the evaluation and management of medical practices:

It is the shared responsibility of health professionals and government to provide a reasonable basis for confidence that action will be taken both to assess whether services meet professionally recognized standards and to correct any deficiencies that may be found.[1]

From a dispassionate viewpoint the fact that the HEW plan was even conceived and that PSRO already exists probably means that the time has already passed when medicine can enjoy the luxury of developing systematic peer review simply because it is intellectually or scientifically the right thing to do. Medicine can now only react to issues made public by others in full knowledge of the consequences of any failure on its part to maintain credibility. The developers of peer review systems are thus obliged to recognize the potential harm that misguided or manipulated applications of their methodologies could inflict on the practice of medicine under the conditions of imposed external control in contrast to voluntary internal (hospital) control. But it is not for us to take advocacy positions in regard to the political machinations that swirl about peer review. Instead the focus is on the job to be done.

This book is about the role of peer review in assuring that the highest quality of care is available to everyone in general, that the care each patient receives is the best for him in particular, that patient care be provided within reasonable cost parameters, and that all these things be properly documented and convincingly demonstrated to the public.

With the worthiness of these goals assumed, the immediate task then is not to persuade but rather to clarify and to chart a clear course through the complexities of theory so that a sense of direction is maintained while avoiding distraction.

It is the aim of this chapter to seek guidance from historical perspectives that can tell us something about how medical care developed into what it is today and the direction in which things appear to be headed. Along the way we will also attempt to identify major problem areas and to flag those spots in which theory becomes dangerously thin, reasoning becomes uncomfortably rough, or where

portions of the conceptual foundation lie neglected and incomplete. As will be shown later, there is no good reason to expect finality concerning any of these topics, since they are dynamic and responsive to evolutionary forces. But it is reasonable to expect coherency in discussing the nature of the problems we face and the alternatives available in seeking solutions.

It is far easier to see the threads of continuity if they are held against an historical background that reflects how major influences have shaped medical practices in the past, which ones are still operating today, and which might shape the future course of medicine. From this perspective the potential impact of the concepts and technologies of peer review can be more fully appreciated.

While I lay no claim to a particular knowledge of the history of medicine, it is nevertheless necessary to the task at hand to explore the pages of history to discern the speed and direction of evolutionary trends in medicine with which peer review must keep pace. The historical perspective should help us appreciate to what extent current concepts and techniques in peer review can be expected to impel medicine in a direction that is desirable or one that would be better redirected in more appropriate ways.

If the reader will grant us the license to reduce some of the most fascinating history of man's creative energies to an interpretive summary, we will be swift in coming to grips with the real issues that confront all of us who are concerned about the status of medical care today and the status of the medical profession tomorrow.

A BRIEF SYNOPSIS OF MEDICAL HISTORY RELEVANT TO PEER REVIEW

It is not possible to pinpoint any one time when medicine, as we would define it today, can be said to have actually begun.[2,p.1] There is indisputable archeological evidence, however, that trephining of

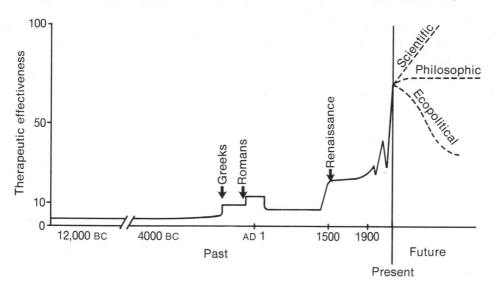

Fig. 1-1. Evolution of medical progress.

the skull (to let the demons out) was being performed in the Stone Age.[3] It is therefore reasonable to trace the evolutionary development of medical practices back to that period.

Fig. 1-1 portrays a hypothetical evolution of the therapeutic effectiveness of medicine (the degree to which it has succeeded in combating disease and improving health) and conveys three major points:

1. Medical progress, being the product of many impinging factors, has been uneven throughout history.
2. While medical progress in the twentieth century reflects the social upheavals of our time, it nevertheless has advanced on an unprecedented scale.
3. Future progress would probably continue at a rapid rate if allowed to reflect purely scientific capabilities; however, it could stagnate if troublesome moral and ethical issues are unresolved, or it could even decline if, through political or economic retrenchment, society refuses to continue its support of medical care at present levels.

We learn that during the Stone Age (12,000-4000 BC) major illnesses or injuries were resolved either by magic (with the aid of an empiric healer) or the patient was killed to eliminate a burden on the tribe.[4,p.561] This establishes an early origin of the concept of social intervention into health problems in the name of the public good and of healers acting in the role of protector of individuals.

A dualism was evident in the descriptions of archaic medicine in ancient Egypt and elsewhere (4000-1000 BC).[4,p.561] Magical or ritualistic medical practices were common among the masses since they were inexpensive. Empirical and rational medical practices, being more expensive, were reserved for the wealthy. To Osler, the nonreligious view of disease that evolved in this period represented the earliest impressions of man's moral awakening.[5] It would appear that the practice of medicine has maintained a dualism that now is shaped by the compassion and humanism of its art on the one side and the empiricism and technology of its science on the other.[6,p.10]

The ancient Greeks (786-285 BC) evolved rational thinking into the scientific spirit[2,p.22] and introduced the concept that diseases were natural afflictions.[7,8,p.13] The life, works, and oath of Hippocrates fused for all time the moral and ethical aspects of medical care with a devotion to service and a recognition of obligations to both patients and to the profession.[9,p.189] The public responded by accepting the physician as a necessary aid to living in human society.[10]

The Romans (285 BC-AD 476) not only refined and organized medical thought[11] but also applied medical thinking to the solution of vexing social problems. They promoted personal hygiene and constructed sanitary projects of considerable benefit to society.[6,p.21] Ironically the elevated social status and respect they accorded to physicians was at a time when the therapeutics of patient care were virtually limited to placebo effects, sympathy, and human understanding, since the ability to effectively intervene in pathologic processes was all but nonexistent.

With a loss of the attitude of inquiry the practice of medicine was marked by stagnation throughout the ensuing Middle Ages (AD 565-1453).[8,p.70,12] However, it was during this period that the stage was set for the evolution of modern medicine in the sense that the Middle Ages saw the development of the three essential institutions upon which the kind of medicine we know today would be later based. Hospitals, universities, and public health systems all began during this period,[4,p.564] even though personal medical services of the time were still little more than imitations of ancient exorcisms and nostrums.

The first real applications of the scientific method to medical thought occurred during the Renaissance[10] (1453-1610), which therefore dates the roots of modern medicine probably no further back than the fifteenth century. Thus the direct line to the origins of today's medical science and technology extends only 450 years or so,[2,p.16] while the origins of the art and ethics of medicine extend back at least 2500 years and probably more. But historical accounts generally become preoccupied with progress in medicine's science once it appeared on the scene, and historians have either paid less attention to

the evolution of the art of medicine or there has been no comparable progress in the medical arts.

While the systematists placed the patient at the center of both the study of disease and the teaching of physicians during the seventeenth century, this focus on the whole patient[4,p.567] was short lived in one sense. The eighteenth century witnessed the dawning of medical specialization.[4,p.569] It is of more than symbolic significance that the really great contribution of this century to modern medical practice, Jenner's vaccination for smallpox,[6,p.47] will probably soon be discontinued throughout the world. It is precisely because this technology has effectively done its job and virtually wiped out one of the major plagues of humankind that it is being abandoned. This points up the everpresent need to keep the practice of medicine current with the changing needs of society. To do that requires realistic feedback of what medicine's impact on society has been and is.

The nineteenth century saw the example set by Jenner become widely emulated. Systematic quests based on scientific experimentation were launched out of social consciousness[6,p.59] to discover the cures for other plaguing illnesses that were recognized as scourges on society. Paul Ehrlich was the first to succeed with the development of the arsenical salvarsan for the treatment of syphilis. With this achievement modern therapeutics was born,[4,p.571] although ancient remedies persisted and leeching remained widespread for many years to come.

The twentieth century has been marked by a completely unprecedented rate of technologic development that has vastly expanded medicine's capacity to intervene effectively in disease processes. The machines of the "machine age of medicine" finally arrived.[9,p.165] When it is realized that as this century began, physicians did not even have the electrocardiograph as a diagnostic tool and that there were still no antibiotics available until almost the century's midpoint, then it can be appreciated how broadly and how far the practice of medicine evolved in our own time. Even the major therapeutic contributions of this century are too extensive to list here. They range from tranquilizers to synthetic human hormones and from basic life-support systems to organ replacements.

Therapeutic potency engendered a growing need to monitor the patient's response to treatment, and a wide range of sophisticated and expensive physiologic monitoring equipment has been developed. The introduction of the computer a quarter century ago not only opened up a whole new field of diagnostics but also made it practical for the first time to undertake both research and patient-care activities that are dependent on the acquisition and processing of vast amounts of data. Subsequently there have been many breakthroughs that are heavily dependent on computer-based evaluation technology. It is probably safe to say that modern evaluation technology has only just begun to serve in its more needed applications and is only now beginning to have its most important impacts on medicine.

At no comparable time period in history has so much diagnostic and therapeutic effectiveness been made available to medicine as has occurred within the single career span of many physicians practicing today. So many effective medical and surgical therapies have been introduced in such a short period of time that the spectrum of disease to which man is now subject undergoes continual change while his overall survival continues to increase. While multiple factors (including nonmedical ones) are no doubt responsible for many of these changes, it is clear that the engineering approach to care (technology) has been successful. What is relevant to our present discussion is the fact that the medical needs of society are undergoing change at a time when the practice of medicine itself is changing more rapidly than at any other time in its his-

tory. For example, computers have assumed more than just monitoring or data storage functions for medicine, as they have been used to activate control loops that infuse medications into patients based on monitored physiologic parameters. This is a true innovation because it introduces artificial intelligence into the patient care equation.

There has also been a recognition of the need to deal with diseases that originate from without as well as those that arise from within the patient (the ecologic approach to medicine). But these two approaches to medical care tend to move medicine in different directions. The engineering approach, which is best suited to managing disease entities, tends to move medicine toward the care of sick individuals. The ecologic approach, which aims at discovering and eliminating the root causes of illness, tends to move medicine toward dealing with a patient's internal and external environment, to work toward disease prevention in populations and not just cures in individuals, and to be concerned for the quality of life and not just survival.

There is no convincing indication, however, that the humanistic aspects of care have undergone comparable changes or have kept pace with accelerated advances in either aspect of contemporary medicine. Surely there are no reports of dramatic breakthroughs in either the arts or the ethics of medicine in recent years. Nor does it appear that sufficient effort has been made to integrate the many individual technical advances of medicine into an efficient overall care delivery system capable of meeting the health needs of all citizens regardless of socioeconomic status or place of residence.

At this point in history an unprecedented surge of progress in evaluation technology has occurred, which is being successfully applied both in the care delivery process and in the conduct of peer review. The significance of this development will lie not only in identifying the solvable problems in health care delivery but also in how it is used to guide change in contemporary medicine and prepare it for its future. Thus we extend this discussion of medical history by projecting present trends just a bit into the future to reveal the direction that peer review itself must move to. solve the new set of problems confronting medicine today.

THE UNSOLVED PROBLEMS

It takes little more than a superficial reading of history to realize that the arrival of such a sudden and huge burst of expensive medical technology accompanied by unprecedented demands for medical services must spell trouble for somebody, and as Alan Norton so clearly demonstrated in his excellent book, *The New Dimensions of Medicine*,[13] that somebody is everybody.

Demand

The medical care delivery system in the United States is an example of runaway demands for medical services. A number of factors contribute to this demand, and we will cite a dozen of the more important ones beginning with the advance of medical science per se.

Scientific advances. As Norton sees it, the apparently unending march of medical science is accompanied by a limitless demand on the number of doctors wanted. He also sees this behavior on the part of the public to have a parallel in the demanding behavior of researchers. As long as there is money to pay for it, he sees no constraints on medical research either. As researchers develop more medical technology, this generates more demand for services, and the cycle thus repeats. The escalation of public demand has arisen, he concludes, not so much in response to expanding basic medical needs (meaning the care of obvious illnesses or ill health), but more because of the advance of medical science and the publicity that the mass media has given it.

Some of the factors responsible for causing this demand for services to rise so *sharply* are presented in the following discussion.

Increased survival. Reduced annual death rates continue to appear across a broad spectrum of diseases including those conditions among the leading causes of death,[14] and the prolongation of life in patients with chronic diseases means a prolongation of the demand for medical services.

Mandated screening programs. There are any number of health-screening and preventive-care programs that are not only sponsored by governmental agencies, such as the nationwide program under Medicaid, but also those actually required among certain populations by law. These are mostly statewide and include PKU tests in newborn, premarital serologies, preschool vision and hearing evaluation, immunization, and so on. While there may be some variance from state to state, the list continues to grow and to contribute to demand.

Voluntary screening programs. By their attendance and participation in voluntary screening programs and well-person examinations of all kinds, including automated health testing, a large segment of the public has given evidence of an increased consumer demand for medical services unrelated to the relief of symptoms or management of illness.

Early diagnosis and treatment. Another expansionary trend arises from the general notion that the earlier the diagnosis and treatment of subclinical or presymptomatic chronic disease states, the better the patient outcome. Physicians are seeking to diagnose and initiate therapy much earlier than was traditional in the past. The detection and early or expectant management of hypertension (while still asymptomatic) is a case in point. There are those who are convinced that a higher value is placed on these activities by the general public than is reflected in the level of professional acceptance.[15]

Comprehensive care. Symptoms or conditions that may have little clinical consequence other than to bring patients into the care system are often utilized by physicians to initiate comprehensive health assessments, which then may lead to the detection of more significant medical problems. The result is that many a physician finds himself uncovering real medical needs that accompany unnecessary demands.[13]

Distribution of services. Whatever is made available by technologic advances in metropolitan centers (sophisticated surgery, kidney machines, intensive care units, flying coronary units) will soon be demanded in the towns and villages, and in all fairness they can hardly be denied.

Elective services. Advances in many areas, especially in surgical subspecialties, have created whole new categories of optional services, including many operations that are clearly cosmetic. Increasing numbers of patients want their noses straightened, bumps removed, breasts enlarged, or sex changed, and increasing numbers of surgeons have been trained to perform such procedures. To the objective mind, some point must be reached where medical care ceases to be a necessity and becomes a luxury.[13]

Provider incentives. Existing payment mechanisms are said to give some economic incentive for providers to render services beyond those justified purely on the basis of medical necessity (for example, unnecessary hospitalization and surgery). Studies of Blue Cross and Blue Shield data apparently show a relationship between increased insurance coverage and increased utilization.[16]

Definition of need. In virtually all fields of medicine a wider definition of health needs has been developed by the public and professionals alike. This trend is very much in evidence in Norton's assessment, which concluded that "what appears to be an unjustified demand today becomes tomorrow's need."[13,p.271] This phenomenon is progressively being compounded by a blurring of the boundaries that separate truly medical problems from the social and economic difficulties experienced by patients.

General climate of demand. It can also be true that what may begin as a clear expression of need can be extended to unnecessary patient demands. This kind of demand may also arise from third-party payment mechanisms, whether public or private. The reasoning is that the beneficiary of the insurance policy or subsidized health benefit program comes to view medical services themselves rather than their reimbursement coverage as "something that is coming to them" and that they would therefore be foolish not to demand. Some are even willing to sue if they do not get it.[17] This is but one manifestation of a rather pervasive climate of rising demands of all kinds. On the front page of a recent edition of a midwestern newspaper were headlines proclaiming that welfare cost had recently risen 21%, that the courts had notified the county that it was illegal to withold welfare payments to nonworking employable single persons, and that the police had obtained an 18% pay raise in a strike settlement.[18] Such news stories are steady diet, and it would be stretching credulity to assume that none of this climate of demand spills over into the medical sector.

Medical egalitarianism. There is not much room for doubt that a specific demand for health services has a high priority in the public mind. Emerson expressed it this way: "The first wealth is health." Thus as huge numbers of people become aware of medicine's advances, not only do they demand its fruits, but it now appears that the right to health, insofar as medical science can ensure it, has gradually come to be regarded as a basic human freedom that Norton views as an extension of this century's pervasive egalitarianism.[13]

Summary. By no means do these dozen factors encompass all the sources and pressures that have swelled the contemporary demand for health services. However, the recognition that demand is the product of many and varied factors is sufficient to lead to the following observations:

1. Demands arise from the consumers and providers of health services individually and collectively and from government.

2. Demands reflecting a broad spectrum of legitimacy, from the highly defensible to the highly capricious, have arisen from all sources.

3. The impact of increased health services may or may not be expected to materially improve the health of patients or populations, depending on whether those services are directed at real (basic) health needs, are optional (luxuries), or are misdirected, as in unnecessary surgery or the attempt to treat symptoms (complaints) that have their true origin in the social or the economic distress of patients rather than in medical or emotional disorders per se.

4. Demands arising from technologic progress in the kind of health care that is beneficial to the health of patients are likely to continue at a brisk pace.

5. Since some demand factors arise externally to medicine, so must forces to control them. In other words, some demand factors may be responsive to peer review control mechanisms, but it is also clear that many are not because they lie outside the purview of clinical medicine.

Cost

Rising costs seem to follow rising demands[19] like night follows day. There are so many important aspects to the cost problem that only the points most relevant to the scope of peer review can be touched on here. For clarity we chose to organize related points into categories that deal with the sources of cost, the influence of payment mechanisms on cost, the magnitude of the cost problem, and the impact of rising costs on medicine and society.

Source. Technologic advances contribute both directly and indirectly to cost problems: complex machines and equipment, complicated surgery, a proliferation of medications, computers, and data processing—all generally cost more money than they save. There are few advances in the category of drug therapies for tuberculosis and mental disorders, which have shortened hospitalizations or avoided them altogether and therefore really have saved money, whereas the list of expensive innovations in medicine is virtually endless. In fact, it has been said that "Most of the new advances have led to a large increase in the cost of medicine."[13,p.274]

The PSRO legislation (Public Law 92-603) specifically singles out care and services provided in hospitals to be reviewed for the purpose of determining whether "(A) such services and items are or were medically necessary; (B) the quality of such services meets professional recognized standards of health care."[20]

It is hardly by chance that this legislation calls for an accounting of the cost of hospitalization, as this constitutes the largest single fraction of the total expenditure for medical care.[19] There are many factors responsible for this. Everything hospitals buy and use has risen in price, and catch-up increases in the wages of their employees (and house staff) who were underpaid for so many years have also contributed to recent increments in hospital costs. And of course expensive equipment is located and costly therapies, such as intensive care, are delivered in hospitals.

If one were to take a broad view of where medical costs originate, the bulk of them can always be traced to the pen of a physician[21] who has written a prescription, ordered diagnostic tests, or has admitted a patient to the hospital. But that amounts to focusing on the mechanics rather than the true source of costs. However, the personal income of physicians is a cost factor, and only objective data can end the conjecture concerning how much this factor contributes to the overall costs of medical care. Addressing this issue in his book *In Critical Condition*, Senator Edward Kennedy several years ago was of the opinion

Table 1-1. Prevailing charges

Fees	Number of items	Variability factor*
All (combined) charges	39	3×−10×
Medical visits (office, hospital)	4	3×−8×
Surgical procedures	18	3×−17×
Laboratory procedures	11	3×−18×
Radiology procedures	6	4×−8×

*Calculated as the maximum fee times the minimum fee.

that providers cannot be blamed for trying to make a good income, but he nevertheless posed these questions: "Does the provider's income-consciousness have to result in people's paying higher costs, getting less care, or being subject to harassment and bankruptcy? Is their income-consciousness a constructive or a destructive thing?"[22] It behooves us to take a close look at this cost source.

Fortuitously, during the preparation of this chapter, preliminary nationwide data concerning physicians' fees and other charges became available for the first time in this country. A report from the Office of the Assistant Secretary for Planning and Evaluation (HEW) published in the spring of 1976 provides a descriptive analysis of physician fee patterns under Medicare.[23] Reimbursement rates were analyzed for 39 medical procedures (charges) in 292 local Medicare areas. Prevailing charges were found to vary widely, and the degree of this variability was found to be a function of the type of services being billed (Table 1-1). It made a significant difference, for example, whether a medical visit was to a generalist or specialist, whether the visit took place in his office or at the hospital, and whether it was an initial or follow-up visit. On further inspection of the data pertaining to surgical procedures, the authors made the following observation: "The results . . . suggest that fees are a function of the technical complexity of the procedure."[23]

Such data could be interpreted as being contrary to some of the suppositions that have grown up in regard to physicians' fees over the years. For example, the supposed arbitrariness of physicians' charges is not borne out by data that reflect responsiveness to distribution factors, to supply and demand, and to the dissemination of information regarding prevailing fees.

One factor that has surely eclipsed physicians' fees (and perhaps every other expense associated with medical care in terms of its rate of rise) is the cost of malpractice insurance. According to a report prepared by the Secretary's Commission on Medical Malpractice (HEW): "The cost of a constant level of malpractice insurance coverage increased seven-fold for physicians, ten-fold for surgeons, and five-fold for hospitals between 1960 and 1972."[24,p.1] While the term *crisis* has probably been overused for years in describing various aspects of medical care, the intensification of malpractice charges probably has earned the title of crisis[25] if not disaster. Despite a disclaimer inserted in a footnote, a government report accurately predicted that the costs of insurance would be passed on to the consumers of health services: "Should insurance costs indeed rise to levels which are 'astronomical' by today's standards, the most likely course of events is that fees will be raised in an attempt to cover the increased costs."[24,p.25]

The insurance premium is but the most visible aspect of the total cost generated by the malpractice problem. Nobody seems to know for sure what fraction is involved, but even a visitor to our shores recognizes "that some of the cost [of medical care] is associated with the defensive medicine practices because of this fear of litigation."[26]

Payment mechanism. The law of supply

and demand has not been repealed, and it very much applies to the impact of third party payment mechanisms on the costs of care. "So long as a rise in cost of hospital care can be covered by a corresponding rise in insurance there seems to be no limit that can be placed on it. And the more the average person has to pay in insuring himself against the cost of hospital treatment, the more he is likely to demand such treatment."[13] This opinion is entirely consistent with the view that the type of insurance (that is, its coverage) and the cost of its premium are contributory to rising hospital costs. It has long been contended that one of the reasons why it does so is that traditional medical insurance does not appropriately cover the expenses of procedures that could be performed more cheaply on an ambulatory basis. It was further reasoned that many patients are consequently hospitalized, often at their own request, in order to have such services paid for by their insurance.

Lewis and Keairnes[19] undertook to test this theory in a controlled experiment where Blue Cross insurance benefits were randomly expanded to cover the costs of diagnostic and treatment services outside the hospitals. The results were mixed. Families with expanded coverage had fewer hospital days, but singles had more. The investigators were unable to prove in this study "the appealing and logical assumption" that increased outpatient coverage would diminish admissions. They interpreted their data as being more in line with what Andersen and Riedel[27] found in a nationwide probability sample, namely, that increased insurance coverage was associated with increased frequency of hospitalization. Whatever the cause, these findings signal the need for much clearer understanding of the ultimate consequences of any large-scale approach to financing the medical care delivery system.

The entry of government as a purchaser of health services has certainly affected demand.[28] In 1969, Cohen counted some 50 new federal health laws that had been inacted in a span of the preceding 8 years,

and of course this was but the beginning of a trend that has since escalated to embrace the concept of national health insurance. The programs of the 1950s and 1960s, in Cohen's words, "were designed to assure the right of every American to high-quality health care."[29] Whatever the intent, it is already clear that one of their undeniable results has been a sizable increase in expenditures for health care.

An apparent reason for this is that the supply of services has not been expanded to the same extent that these programs have increased demand. Lewis and Keairnes projected from the findings of their study that "Increasing the effective demand of the consumer by expansion of his insurance coverage, in the face of a fixed supply of resources, and given the lack of controls in the current medical-care system, results in rapid escalation of costs."[27]

It is not only the size of the expansion that has exerted upward pressures on cost but the speed of growth as well. As Abelson commented in a recent editorial in *Science:* "Until 1965 the government spent only nominal amounts for health care. With the advent of Medicare and Medicaid, the federal treasury became an engine of inflation of health costs. Federal expenditures rose rapidly to $34 billion in 1975, and led to enhanced costs for the private system also."[28]

Magnitude. In the short span of a quarter of a century the total of all funds spent for health care in this country rose from $12 billion in 1950 to an incredible $118.4 billion in 1975.[30]

This order of magnitude increase in the total bill the nation is paying for health is even more impressive when compared to the expenditures of other nations. In 1961-62 the United States was already near the top among industrialized nations with 5.8% of our gross national product (GNP) going to health care[13] even before the big federal expansion began in 1965 with Medicare and Medicaid. The most current available data is for the year 1975 and shows that the portion of our GNP expanded for health care has now risen to 8.3%, and HEW projects the 1977 costs for Medicare and Medicaid alone at $30.4 billion, which is an enormous single-year increase of $5.4 billion over 1976.[30] The cost problem, however, is by no means unique to the United States. Indeed, nations throughout the Western world are increasingly alarmed at the observation that these yearly increases in the cost of care outstrip the rate of their economic growth. This is more than enough evidence to expose the error of supposing that the devotion of ample resources to medicine would be a once-and-for-all investment that would lead in time to a fall in demand through improved health.

Management. On completing a comparative international survey of the mechanisms for financing medical care in a number of countries, Norton concluded that no country has solved the problem of how it should best be done. However, in his view the steepness in the rise in cost of Western medicine is overwhelming the voluntary insurance principle, which he regards the main bastion against the erosion of private medicine.[13] The half dozen years since he came to that conclusion have seen nothing but mounting evidence to support his thesis.

As long as the public financing of health costs in this country was on a basis best described by President Lyndon Johnson's phrase "guns and butter," the pinch was never really allowed to be felt in the public sector. But by now the costs of medical services have begun to compete with other public undertakings such as welfare, road construction, education, service projects to combat unemployment, and the like. Choosing among social alternatives that collectively require more funds than are available requires political decisions. Because of its huge cost, medicine is now in politics and in all likelihood will stay there.

Summary. Following are observations derived from examining the problem of cost:

1. The sources of rising costs are many, some of which relate to better care while others do not; some respond to laws of supply and demand while others may not. As new information has begun to reveal the source of the upward pressure on costs, a number of misconceptions have already been exposed; but not nearly enough is yet known about the origin and containment of costs, which is part of the problem. However, specific data needs have now been identified that, once obtained, should provide a clearer understanding of the cost picture in the near future.

2. The magnitude of present and projected cost for health care in this country is simply staggering and is no doubt intolerable for much longer. If relief of this upward spiral is not checked soon, there can be little doubt that public reaction in the form of massive governmental intervention will have to come.

3. Payment mechanisms alone may present some limited opportunity for cost control, but there is also ample evidence that subsidized (government) programs that encourage utilization without increasing the availability of services greatly contribute to cost pressures and particularly to hospital costs.

4. It is in the medical profession's best interest to take all measures possible through ethical internal peer review mechanisms to eliminate any unnecessary costs associated with medically inappropriate practices, unneeded services, and care practices of doubtful clinical validity.

Problems for patients

We have seen that there is virtually an unbridled increase in patient demand, but for what? What is it that the average patient really wants from the health profession? Norton has said it very well. As he sees it: "the more specialist [*sic*] the rest of the medical care gets the more necessary it is for the patient to have someone who, beside being a primary physician and an expert in diagnosis, can also give advice, allay fears and educate."[13,p.265] Is this kind of care universally available to all citizens? If not, why?

Ironically, much of the difficulty medicine faces today seems to start with an overdose of the very technology that has brought the capability to do so much for patients. The truth is that the technologies of medicine, sanitation, and public health have been successful in eradicating the major plagues, scourges, and acute illnesses that destroyed so many of mankind in the past. But success in eliminating acute diseases means a shift in the health needs of patients toward a prevalence of chronic illnesses. "Since 1967 . . . most of the deaths in the age range 10 to 70 either are due to degenerative diseases or are fatalities arising from accidents, suicide, or homicide. The big killers are coronary heart disease, cancer, and stroke."[28] In addition to these chronic medical conditions, there has been an ascendency of mental and behavioral disorders and environmentally related illnesses associated with an increasingly complex and stressful society. Stress is thought by Jackson to be the largest single factor responsible for bodily ills.[31] But the technology of contemporary medical practice is best suited to care for individuals who are physically sick, and it is not as conceptually well suited to meet the humanistic needs of socially estranged populations. "Let it all hang out with your friendly computer" just does not make it. What this means to the thoughtful observer is that "the technologic model of care becomes increasingly less relevant to the needs of the patient."[32]

The patient of course has been increasingly aware of this particular side effect of medical technology and for some time has been reacting symptomatically. He has proclaimed loudly that he wants a physician who will make housecalls and complains bitterly when he cannot even find a physician! This situation was acknowledged in 1962 by Somers, who described this "paradox of medical progress" in these words: "as medical science has increased in sophistication and as medical technology has offered greater possibili-

ties of practical application than ever before in history, discontent with medical care seems to have grown space."[33] The basis for this discontent, of course, must be in the unfulfilled expectation of the patient. And what does the patient expect?

Health care as a right. Once the average patient takes health care itself as a basic human need and right,[13] as was discussed earlier, a change in attitude occurs, and the patient becomes vitally interested not only in the availability of care but in its quality as well. Taking this a step further, if one thinks of the patient not as an individual consumer of health services but as part of a corporation, a union, or as a representative of some other consumer group that can bring political pressure to bear, then as Hanlon phrased it: "we may expect penetrating questions directed to the providers of medical services, not only about quality and availability, but particularly about cost."[17] For the evidence that such questions are indeed on the mark, we need examine only a few.

Well-person care. Modern medical practices now have physicians seeing well people in addition to the sick ones. The same patients who want their doctor to make housecalls when they are sick also expect, when they are well, that the same physician will be in his office at all hours to provide them with immunizations, hearing and vision screening tests for their children, pap smears and glaucoma tests for themselves, health education, child-rearing instruction, genetic advice, and many other services that have now come to be expected. Screening, health maintenance, and educational programs aimed at the well cannot help but take some physician time away from the bedside of the sick (at a minimum, time must be spent supervising clinical assistants and providing overall case planning and so on). Most want both health care and illness care and feel frustrated if access to either is blocked.

Personal attention. Should a patient be admitted to the hospital, he encounters another kind of frustration from all the negative aspects of an impersonal technology under the direction of a clinical staff from whom he feels isolated.[24,p.40]

The personal needs and desires of anxious patients for sympathy, civilities, explanations, and assurance have given no evidence of diminishing. On the other hand, the capacity of contemporary medicine to meet these wants and desires apparently has diminished. Increasing demands on the clinician's time and distractions arising from an emphasis on the technical aspects of care seem to have eroded into the time available for the humanistic aspect of personal care. There certainly has been no clear evidence that the art of medicine has been able to keep pace with the technology of medicine.[34]

To the patient the complexities of modern diagnostic tests and therapies are often bewildering. The difficult logistics of transporting him from one special facility to another for tests and treatments with all the resultant delays and uncertainties can only reinforce a growing belief that his care is devoid of personal consideration. The constant flow of busy technicians and erudite consultants (each of whom is responsible for only a small part of his care) means that the faces which appear at his bedside are constantly changing, and none of them seems willing or able to perceive the drift of his questions and to provide the assurance he seeks. Is it any wonder he feels alienated and seeks satisfaction for his grievances in such ways as malpractice actions? Sadly, it is often the small personal disappointments that mar his perception of what technically was excellent care.

Explanation and assurance. Where then is the grievance mechanism to which a patient can turn for explanations or for redress of slights and injustices, whether real or imagined?[24,p.40] Even if there is an effective internal peer review mechanism, how can the patient be assured that he did, after all, receive quality care if he is neither a party to the review process nor

informed of its results? Is it any wonder that he turns to litigation?

Satisfaction of complaints. It would be all too easy to claim that opportunistic attorneys are responsible for our present medical malpractice crisis, but as Annas (a lawyer) recently remarked: "Blaming lawyers and the legal system for the medical malpractice crisis and the practice of defensive medicine is like blaming firemen for forest fires."[35] He went on to cite the findings of HEW's Malpractice Commission that lawyers take only about one in every eight malpractice cases that clients bring to them. The factual data presented in this rebuttal, at least, must be taken as sobering evidence that a great many patients are clearly not happy with medical practices in general and with their physicians in particular.

Summary. An inquiry into the contemporary problems experienced by patients leads to the following observations:

1. The present emphasis on personal health care has not addressed adequately the problems of organization and distribution of facilities and services to the society as a whole. As perceived by the patient, this leads to the unavailability of health care of the kind he wants or where and when it is needed the most.

2. As technology provided the capacity to bring under control those acute diseases and accidents that formerly evoked more sympathy than effective management, medicine apparently began to supply less of the gratifying medical arts along with the technologic aspects of care. The present technologic or engineering model for health care that has proved so successful in dealing with acute organic (medical) problems has not been appropriately adaptive to meet humanistic needs associated with chronic diseases or to deal in any concrete way with disorders of the human condition. This and many other factors have led to growing patient dissatisfaction with the kind of services available.

3. Lacking any effective means to ad-

dress their grievances with the care system (that is, no established mechanism to deal with the system), patients seem to react negatively toward medical personnel and thus compound the estrangement between them.

4. An obstruction to dealing effectively with these problems is a failure to recognize them for what they are. Physicians need to be informed as to what problems are perceived by patients, and the public needs to understand what problems are perceived by physicians. Peer review must thus serve as an instrument of communication if it is to serve both patients and health professionals.

Problems for health professionals

With as much dissatisfaction with care delivery as would appear to exist among the public that is in some way attributable to technology, one can only wonder what sort of impact this same factor might have on the medical profession. Since evaluative technology is now in the process of being turned to making observations on what is really happening to the practice of medicine, we are in all likelihood about to find out. This is a remarkable prospect, because throughout its long history medicine as an institution has always lacked the information feedback not only to assess what its technology has meant to the health of a community or what it has accomplished as a social instrument, but even where its technology is taking it scientifically. How then could medicine possibly assimilate the magnitude of its own progress or recognize the magnitude of its unmet responsibilities? Many of our present problems and difficulties stem from this gap in essential feedback.

Information feedback. A starting place to understand why this lack of feedback is a fundamentally bad thing is the recognition that what limits scientific understanding is largely man's own ability to perceive the physical universe around him.[36] What this means is that the methods of empirical science which spawned modern medical technology depend on feedback from experience as the source of knowledge necessary to advance orderly progress. Without it, methodologic progress becomes stunted or technologic growth stops altogether.

Feedback is necessary to the orderly growth of medicine in much the same way it plays a role in neurologic development. Clark-Kennedy cited as an example that, with increasing differentiation (specialization) of the nervous system, there must be progressive integration to coordinate it. "But in medicine," he said, "we have not been particularly successful in effecting this necessary coordination to keep pace with our own modern discoveries which have broadened our front to an almost unmanageable extent."[34,p.43] The result is that the kind of technology which has been so effective in dealing with specific medical problems of patients on an individual basis has been found wanting in its ability to provide the integration needed to mount a successful health care program for the total population. In the absence of any demonstrable progress in this regard, medicine has opened itself to credibility problems that make it the target of virtually any criticism leveled at it, no matter how unfounded, such as the chronically festering suspicion that there must be a deliberate conspiracy to restrict the training of clinicians to maintain a high demand for their services and hence high fees.

Patient-physician relationship. The impact of technology has not left the cherished doctor-patient relationship unscathed either. The physician who used to station himself at the bedside of the sick person when he could do little else now must take the time necessary to tend his machines, monitor the results of lab tests, digest computer printouts, scanner tracings, charts, forms, and a tangle of red tape. Thus the personal satisfaction the physician cherishes in being close to his patient is often compromised to the demands of technology and regulations. Pressed into an ever-widening range of services on top of this, physicians begin to realize that they cannot be in two places at the same time. Consequently clinical tasks have been delegated, hesitatingly at first, but then increasingly so, to a burgeoning group of nurse practitioners, physician assistants, assorted technicians, and to automation.

Delegation of duties and authority. The extent to which delegation of duties and authority has been done now makes thoughtful observers uneasy that the pendulum in medical practice has swung all the way from a reluctance to share professional responsibilities to the point where too much of what a physician should do is being done by others or by machines. There are concerns that there be no delegation when the results of clinically important diagnostic tests need interpretation or when powerful drugs must be used with discretion. What such concerns as these amount to is that the basis of wise medicine remains a personal relationship and that no patient can relate either to a computer or to a clinician that acts only through assistants and rarely sees his patients. But the question is how close to mark is Norton's evaluation that "The march of science has made it almost impossible to combine the 'exclusive scientific life' with 'good warm contact with my neighbors' that physicians of only a generation or so ago enjoyed with their patients."[13,p.273] Hopefully this has not yet become the universal experience, and there is certainly no evidence that it represents a change that is welcomed by the profession.

Overdramatization of the professional role. Some wags have referred to the problem of overdramatization of the professional role truculently as the "Marcus Welby syndrome." Others such as Harrington see it as a more serious matter, reflecting a vestige of the "magical view of medical care," which leads to a distorted viewpoint that many patients seem to develop as a result of the way health care is delivered. Harrington sees the contemporary prac-

tice of medicine as "designed to distribute 'magical' solutions quickly and profitably, but less well designed for more time-consuming and involved tasks."[32] He further believes that a large number of patients have become conditioned to expect, and are willing to purchase, magical solutions to their difficulties.

There is always a price to be paid for distortion, and on the physician's side it may take the form of a displaced emphasis on establishing the diagnosis and prognosis as though these were themselves therapeutic. On the patient's side there appears to be a misguided tendency to confuse a pill or a surgical procedure with a long-range therapeutic program in which the patient himself should play an active role and assume participatory responsibility for the result. Unfortunately the consequences, which all too often occur when the implied magic doesn't work, is that patients feel cheated. Many conclude that their failure to obtain an easy cure could only be explained by inappropriate treatment, which must have been the physician's fault, and they wind up initiating a lawsuit.

Boundaries of professional responsibility. It would also appear that the public has developed some expectations that would require physicians to extend themselves beyond their training and traditional scope of duty. Medicine is now expected to spearhead drives to wipe out societal ills just as it wiped out polio and smallpox. Medical leadership is sought in combatting drug abuse, juvenile crime, child abuse, rape, automobile accidents, suicide, poverty, smoking, drinking, and many other examples of the "ecologic" health problems that beset society. Physicians along with other professionals often try to do what they can to help, but there has to be some limit or boundary to the responsibilities for which the individual medical practitioners should be held accountable.

As Donabedian pointed out in 1968, the focus of peer review in operational terms should be on those aspects of the medical care process that are significantly influenced by the actions of individual care providers.[37] It is therefore pointless to hold clinicians solely accountable at the periphery of social and environmental problems where the effects of their efforts are either attenuated or entangled with a host of other factors. Yet the criticism that the medical profession is failing to meet its social responsibilities is heard repeatedly. Perhaps our medical schools really should be teaching physicians how to recognize a broader definition of health and medical responsibility that is within the reach of their own professional careers to effect. But in any event, overextension is a common lot of health professionals.

Counter-productive health programs. When it comes to deciding what kind or what level of care is needed to deal with strictly medical problems, the physician of today discovers all too often that it isn't he who makes the critical determination. Too frequently some other decision maker reacting to a "crisis" proposes a program of action that cannot await adequate evaluative data to shape it. Instead the promotion of health programs is undertaken by advocates of change who are missionaries for whatever reasons, and who have found that an emotional appeal is frequently more effective than facts. As a public health advisor in the National Center for Health Services Research and Development (HEW) observed: "Most frequently the technique used is to create a demand for the program on the part of the general public, which then forces professional acceptance, often grudgingly."[38] Thus health professionals find themselves devoting precious manhours to some health scheme or other that promoters have been successful in funding but that may or may not command respect from the heart or mind of those who must carry them out.

Sacrifice of ethics. To many honest and competent physicians the PSRO amendments to the Social Security Act amounted to being held publicly accountable for justifying care and services to individual patients, which their professional judgment already held to be necessary. It was felt that this kind of accountability amounted to being considered guilty of fraud or deceit until proven innocent. The magnitude of the actual fraud problems in government-sponsored care programs is not at issue here, but it is relevant to point out, as did Lewis and Keairnes, that "Two to 3 percent of the physician population can create a 'leak' in the system through which an inordinate amount of dollars can pour without any improvement in the overall quality and quantity of health care rendered to society."[19] Yet there are also many physicians and other health professionals that have not forsaken professional integrity, nor have they forgotten that humanistic needs must also be served as they minister to physical needs of their patients. To men and women such as these, no PSRO performance profiles, norms, statistics, or computer printouts can in any way become satisfactory substitutes for their commitment to the ethics of medicine. PSRO can thus be viewed in their eyes as an unnecessary and even disheartening affront to the very foundation of a noble profession. Pretending that this is *not* the perception of many will not change the reality of it. It is something that must be faced in order to avoid alienating those who are among the most committed to improving medicine's service to society.

External dislocations. Over the past two or three decades the federal government's categorical health funding programs were accompanied by strings in the form of priorities that pulled and tugged medicine first one way then another—toward basic research, then toward applied research, or into educational thrusts or hospital construction, and into an assortment of care delivery initiatives. Currently called for is evaluation in the form of peer review, while the next tug is probably going to be in the direction of health care planning.[39]

Unquestionably, Cohen is right in pointing out that a considerable amount of the headway that has been made in removing the barriers of human want, ignorance, and illness were products of government funding and actions in a number of areas including medicine.[29] But it is also inevitable that, in manipulating the preoccupations of medicine, some of its natural evolutionary processes are being bypassed that took thousands of years to develop. These are the same evolutionary processes that can be credited with so many of the therapeutic and diagnostic capabilities we enjoy today, so that social value of their preservation is above question. The problem that arises from overly rapid shifts in the external manipulation of medical goals and objectives is that by the time medicine can get itself really geared for some new thrust sponsored by governments, foundations, regulatory agencies, or accrediting bodies, it often finds program priorities, requirements, and available funds have become earmarked to some other end. To what degree this causes dislocations in the overall course of medical evolution and what the long-term consequences of that might be is probably a matter for historians of another day to settle. Considering only the impact of fiscal infusions of the size that are involved today, it is difficult to believe that destabilizing forces of some magnitude have not been unleashed.

Lack of appreciation. What is implicit in the above discussion will be made explicit here. There is simply not sufficient incontrovertible evidence to clearly delineate the impact of society's perceived medical needs on the political process, or to understand the impact of governmental actions on medicine, or to evaluate the impact of medical progress on society. And as Schwartz points out: "one of the problems of public discussion today is the fact that this progress has been overlooked in consideration of public policy."[40] For example, he cites recent dramatic declines in death rates in this country not only generally but especially among the poor, minority groups, and infants, which he feels are not widely known let alone appreciated. But even if it were, it is *health* that is our pri-

mary concern, and, as this economist also points out, health is "obviously a multidimensional phenomenon and it cannot be measured by any one number." Thus, far more information is needed than can be revealed in mortality tables, and it is medicine that must recognize that it has the prime opportunity and thus the obligation to acquire it.

The lack of appreciation of what the true facts are in the state of our nation's health and what is happening to our health care system constitutes a burden for everyone to bear in or outside of medicine and contributes to the acuteness of many problems that confront medicine today. Perhaps a stabilizing sense of direction has never been more needed by medicine than now, and only time will tell whether peer review will be permitted to encourage those kinds of methodologic developments that can serve this constructive end.

Summary. A brief summary of the major problems confronting physicians at this time reveals the following:

1. Professional relationships with patients are being strained by an involuntary separation caused by time constraints placed on physicians, the distractions of technology to the delegation of duties and responsibilities to others, and by negative feelings engendered by unrealistic patient expectations.

2. This strain comes at a time when the boundaries of professional responsibility are being distended perhaps beyond reason. Physicians are being pressed between the ethics of their profession and the need to conform to governmental policies, regulations, and shifting program support. Medicine therefore finds itself in a dilemma of being caught between its desires to remain independent while at the same time recognizing no alternative to the continued financial support and concomitant evolutionary disruption that participation in public health programs so often brings.

3. In contrast to its development of precise physiologic monitors and complex data systems that reveal how an individual

patient is getting along clinically, medicine has been slow to develop comparable feedback mechanisms that can report on how the care delivery system is getting along and how society is responding to medical care. The seriousness of this lack of feedback for medicine lies in the fact that consequently there are no reliable means of distinguishing the difference between the perceived and the actual health care needs of society, when the two are incompatible, or even when those needs have been met.

4. Without valid performance feedback there has been no stimulus to develop integrative mechanisms for the coordination of services delivered to a community that are in any way comparable to what has been done to optimize the care of individuals. Health professionals are therefore handicapped in understanding their societal responsibilities and how to meet them so they can solve many of these problems.

Problems for government

Let us next consider some of the difficulties presented to public officials who share in the responsibility to carry out the legislated programs intended to promote the health and well-being of our nation's people.

Distribution of medical services. Is it not obvious that those who suffer the greatest deprivations in society—the urban and the rural poor—are also in the greatest need for health care as a class? Irving J. Lewis of HEW wrote in 1969 of the national imperative to improve the quality, effectiveness, and acceptability of health care for these people: "This 'other America' has the highest rates of infant and maternal mortality, the highest incidence of disease and the greatest number of disability days per year. The poor, who need care the most, receive it the least. What they need most urgently are simply the medical services that are proved and widely available to some of our people but somehow not to them."[41] From a manager's point of view, he sees the unavailability of care to the

poor as a symptom of the poor organization and coordination of the care delivery system itself.

Quality of care. When the managers who represent society's interests next turn their attention to the quality of care that is delivered to those who do receive it, what do they find? They find a gulf between the excellence of care that medical institutions claim to provide and what has so far been objectively documented by quantitative data. Even some physicians conclude from this lack of documentation that "self-acclaimed excellence is, in practice, a myth."[25] In the absence of direct evidence concerning the excellence of care, the planners and managers of legislated health-related programs have no option but to use what indirect evidence is available, namely, mortality rates and longevity data. While it is encouraging to note that life expectancy has risen from 54.1 years in 1920 to 71.3 in 1973, this increase still has been criticized on the grounds that it has not been anywhere near proportional to the increase in the amount of money spent on health care.[25] There is a countering argument, of course, which is that longevity is certainly no comprehensive indicator of beneficial care outcomes, nor can it continue to rise indefinitely in any event. Since there is this logical limit to the relevance of overall mortality statistics, infant death rates have been more widely used as an indicator of the level of health care in a given population. In 1920 the infant death rate in the United States was 85.8 per 1000 live births,[40] and by 1961 it was 25.3 per 1000,[42] which was quite an improvement yet still too high. An infant death rate of this magnitude has been repeatedly cited as a reproachful indictment against the whole health care delivery system in this country.[40] This characterized the general impression of health care in the United States until its infant death rate fell to the internationally comparable level of 16.5 per 1000 in 1974. This was "the lowest annual rate recorded in the United States and represents a decrease of 7 percent from the final rate of 17.1 for 1973."[14] If questions still persist as to the general quality of care in this country, then the value of infant mortality data as its measure must also be questioned. But planners and managers can hardly be blamed for having no better a statistical base to work with because it is not they but the medical professions that generate care-based medical data.

Health benefits. The plain truth is that it is difficult to measure outcome (health) benefits,[25] and that is why there is not much data available. It is probably also true that the medical profession until very recently really has not invested the effort needed to develop practical and efficient means to obtain such data. The result still is that society and its decision makers have not yet been presented with much hard evidence on which they can judge the true impact of quality medical care and how well the care system is working. To the lawmakers who have lavished so much money on health care, the continued absence of these data translates into the absence of any rational answer when the question is raised as to whether the public has benefited from the expenditure of its money.[43]

Proven value of services. When a public servant inquires whether the services that have been purchased with public monies are of proven value, again he encounters a lack of hard objective data about the sensitivity and specificity of some of the most basic diagnostic procedures or the efficacy of many of the most common treatment modalities.[44] Again there is a dearth of the simplest kind of data that are so necessary to sound management practices.

Why isn't the practice of clinical medicine on a more scientifically established basis? Why don't physicians utilize patient encounters for double-blind, randomized testing of the various candidate therapies to get some of the answers we need? Why can't all this be done? Law professor Charles Fried points out that "such a general scheme is largely impeded by what

we conceive as rights in medical care: patients expect an individualized judgment when they are treated. They expect to be told if they are being experimented on. They want to be told the risks, and they want to be able to participate in the choice between alternatives."[45] Also, of course, there are laws totally forbidding human experimentation of some kinds and regulations restricting many others.* Such constraints make the job of obtaining some useful data all that much harder or even impossible.

The intervention quandry. Meanwhile, legislators feeling responsive to the forces of change arising from obviously unmet health needs of society enact one program after another aimed at delivering medical care to the unserved sick and preventive care to the underserved well.[46] But one consequence of the steady rise in governmental funding of health care in this country has been "the explosive rise in medical costs" from $25.9 billion in 1960 to $118.4 billion in 1975.[30] This situation, coupled with a policy of curbing intervention in the private sector of medicine, has contributed to federal and state budget overruns and sharply higher private health insurance premiums,[46] both of which are capable of generating a whole net set of problems for government.

Summary. Government is confronted by demands that can only be described as insatiable and by medical costs that are plainly out of control. The lawmaker, the health planner, the manager, and the public servant all wish to know why health services cannot be more equitably distributed in this country, and they get no answer. When they then ask how good is the care provided those who are able to get it, again there is no answer. They cannot seem to find out whether all the public monies spent have made much of a difference to the health of the people one way or another, and few data exist to indicate

---

*Proposed policy for protection of human subjects (45 CFR 46), *Federal Register,* August 23, 1974.

whether the services that are being purchased are valid or efficacious. Without the facts, how can managers and planners reach rational decisions? The only thing of which the public servant can be certain is that he is expected to have all the answers for the questions he gets from Congress and the public. Is it any wonder that a society and a government are impatient with the medical profession?

An inquiry into the contemporary problems that penetrate to the public (governmental) level brings the following observations:

1. For whatever reasons, adequate medical care is not being evenly provided to the poor and to less populated areas.

2. A point has been reached wherein there no longer appears to be a direct relationship between the amount of money spent on health care and its demonstrable quality. (There has been no documentary evidence that increased costs have been matched by increased quality in the care delivered to the public.)

3. Methods for measuring health benefits and proving the value of services rendered remain undeveloped at a time when answers to basic questions of efficacy are at issue in deciding the future course of medicine in this country.

4. Government suffers from the same lack of vital information to aid in carrying out its responsibilities as does medicine.

The dilemma for society

The massive investment made by society in health care in this nation has had mixed results in that some people have been served very well, but it has not provided all the people access to quality health services, and therein lies the rub. It has been said that the primary moral imperative in making an economic decision is that of "distributive justice."[45] In a 1968 article entitled "The Tragedy of the Commons,"[46] Hardin characterized the overuse of resources with an analogy of a shared common meadow used for animal grazing by all the herdsmen in the area. Any single

herdsman who attempts to maximize his own gain, does so at the expense of the others (and eventually at his own as the meadow becomes destroyed by overgrazing). Hiatt used the same analogy in 1974 to describe the limit of resources any society can devote to health care.[44] Even as that limit is being approached, justice places additional demands to rectify inequities in the availability of care to large segments of the population who receive little or none. It is the insertion of these just demands on an already overextended health budget that has produced the major dilemma we face as a society.

The inequities that require immediate attention are clear enough: inaccessibility, fragmentation, and the high cost of health services combined with a lack of concern for the total well-being of the individual are legitimate grievances of many Americans.[29,41] Yet when the fiscal meadow is already overgrazed, the satisfaction of these grievances creates a conflict between the interests of the individual and those of society. It is a conflict that Hiatt believes can end only in tragedy unless society finds ways "to govern access to and control [of] the use of the medical commons."[44] And how might this be done? Norton is of the opinion that demand is so insatiable that resources have to be rationed, and in a free enterprise country he believes this will be effected through the purse.[13] There are other suggestions, however.

Those who favor governmental intervention call for a total reorganization in either the financing or in the delivery of medical care or both.[19] Proposed alternatives include a standardization of fees on a national basis, a nationalized health insurance scheme, the development of public-utility-like regional programs of health care, the promotion of prepaid, organized group practice, and the elimination of fee-for-service practice.

Those who side with the stand taken by organized medicine call for the preservation of private practice, fee-for-service, voluntary insurance, and free choice of physician, all of which are considered essential to the maintenance of high-quality care and a way of life that is compatible with the traditions and well-being of the United States.[13]

An alternative seldom mentioned as a conscious choice is to deliberately dilute care by offering a less comprehensive variety or by employing lesser trained personnel to provide it. Another alternative is to allow shortages to develop with resultant waiting lists for hospitalization and other major health services. Priorities can then be applied favoring the seriously ill. One alternative to be more seriously considered is a commitment to automate health care to the maximum degree that promotes efficiency. This is the one alternative that offers the hope that cost reduction can offset the expansion of services, but it is also the most depersonalized.

Is there really any way to know whether automation or any other alternative is in the long-term best interest of society? We cannot even be sure whether "high quality care and cost control may be mutually compatible."[47] In view of the prevailing uncertainty, we are advised that "We should avoid heavy investments in technology that automates or otherwise attempts to increase the efficiency with which we provide services of dubious efficacy."[43] It would appear then that there is no intellectually honest way to choose among the alternatives that are feasible until there is adequate scientifically based information on the efficacy and the efficiencies of present basic health services and care delivery mechanisms. The ever-present penalty for making wrong choices about overutilization can be underutilization and a degeneration of the quality of care.[47] The penalty of an unwise reorganization or redistribution of care is the dilution of quality.[13]

Clearly then care evaluation assumes prime importance as the necessary first step toward a rational plan for avoiding the tragedy of the commons. However, in the opinion of the National Academy of Sciences, "effective programs for quality-assurance in U.S. health care are not readily evident."[48] Fortunately at least a start had been made in this direction even before PSRO, so it is not a matter of starting from scratch. Some systematic peer review projects had been initiated within the private sector and others within the public sector via grant and contract mechanisms that have progressively grown in recent years. "A section on evaluation has become the *sine qua non* of every grant application for the support of projects for the development of health or medical care services."[38]

After adequate data have come in from all sources (including PSROs), the next step is one of interpreting those data properly.[49] It is here that the managers and lawmakers stand to benefit from the expertise and insights of the practicing professionals who are conversant with the intricacies of the care delivery process.[21] In the meantime the standard practice is to apply good sense in determining the best allocation of public resources, so that society's demand for health care is met at no higher a level than legitimate need requires. After all, is it not proper that the money spent on health care be subjected to the same budgetary constraints to which any other expenditures are subject?[19] But let us examine that closely. Is it really valid to equate health services with road building, urban renewal, or space probes? Not only can the quality of human existence be affected by medical care, but personal survival is at the bottom line of health care, and it is the "social product"[50] of the medical care effort that makes it deserving of special attention in the setting of priorities and allocation of resources.

But strident voices also call for priorities to improve housing or to do something about the jobless rate, and these things have come to directly affect the availability of resources to improve health.[51] Others have openly questioned how much a life is worth by pointing out that there are limits to what we will do to save lives.[44] It can only be assumed from arguments such as these "that life, far from having a value beyond price, has a quite determined, and even surprisingly, low value."[45]

All it takes to convert this kind of thinking into care policy is to create conditions where the decision-making process that controls the funding of health care is placed into the hands of a few managers who deal in large, impersonal statistics and fail to recognize their limitations.[52] The reason for concern derives from the coercive interpretation of statistics that overemphasizes the need for simplifying the planning and budgeting process at the expense of notions about long-term humanistic gains or losses. Remote from the bedside and having no personal contact with patients, managers would have little or no direct involvement in defending the rights of each individual patient on the issue of his right to personal care. Patients who are unseen and unheard can exert little real influence on the fiscal policy decisions that ultimately may deny them medical care.

Money managers probably would not see their budgetary decisions in that light, of course. They would likely see themselves only as limiting unrestrained spending and getting "a better distribution of quality care for the dollar."[29] After all, don't they leave it to the clinical experts to decide how available funds will be translated into medical service priorities (rationed) so that the most needy get the care? But no matter who does it, the inescapable effect would be the imposition of some sort of mandatory triage or sorting process that decides who receives health care services and who does not. Historically such measures have only been dictated by emergency conditions such as those of the battlefield or natural disasters, and no pretense to the contrary can alter the seriousness of placing fiscal or any other kind of restraints on the personal right to care in a democratic society.

Personal health care should not be defined either by statistics that pertain to the herd or by a social judgment of what constitutes equity and efficiency in the delivery of medical services. To limit one's definition to that is to succumb to what Fried calls "that fallacy of the lowest common denominator."[45] To go to the next step and dictate *routine medical triage* is a suspension of usual moral principles.[53] To quote Fried again, "It is when emergencies become usual that we are threatened with moral disintegration, dehumanization."[45]

An overview of the dilemma facing society leads to the following observations:

1. To provide appropriate quality medical care to those who are currently unserved or poorly served will inevitably increase demands on funding capabilities and medical resources that are already approaching the limit of tolerance.

2. The magnitude of resource demands for this purpose would appear to be attainable only at the expense of other established societal priorities of both medical and nonmedical service programs. Should that be done, the likely result will be a further increasing of cost pressures.

3. Those with legislative and managerial responsibilities lack some of the most basic performance data to evaluate existing health care programs in order to arrive at appropriate decisions whether they merit continued allocations of public resources. In the absence of detailed information, only the more obvious generalizations can be seen and dealt with superficially.

4. Oversimplification of the real problems that exist in care delivery in order to make them tractable to organizational solutions is dangerous. So is the imposition of patient triage or the rationing of health services. Both could lead to the degeneration and dehumanization of medicine.

The dilemma for medicine

Medicine finds itself in the dilemma of being caught between its own moral imperatives and those of society. Society expects nothing less than justice in the availability, cost, and distribution of medical care. But despite the fact that the medical practitioner generally concurs, he is nevertheless compelled to operate from a different moral imperative when dealing with the individual patient. In Donabedian's words: "This is because professional standards rest on the assumption that the best must be attempted for each patient."[37] It is the personal welfare of the individual that is the physician's primary professional responsibility and not a responsibility to an impersonal society.[34] But physicians, like all citizens, also have a responsibility to work for social justice. When the best interests of the individual do not happen to coincide with what is in the best interest of society, then medicine faces a dilemma. If it should occur that the only option open to those who actually deliver medical services is to extend care to the unserved by denying it to others, then this is a thing that physicians are sworn not to do. To impose this on each individual practitioner would be to force him into the ultimate professional dilemma, which would be unfair.[44]

The supreme ethic, the physician's obligation to the individual, holds that each and every patient has a right to medical care that goes beyond any legislated declaration of what constitutes his fair share. Objecting to an unrestricted right of the individual to personal health care on the grounds that it conflicts with social distributive justice simply argues against the easy assumption that a commitment to efficiency and equity in health care exhausts the entire moral universe;[45] there are other moral principles. What about a commitment to preserve life? Placing the value of an individual beyond price is an extension of this principle, and it argues against withholding any vital service from anyone on the basis of its cost—whatever that might be—just as it argues against the Stone Age practice of killing persons with fractures so they do not become "a burden to the tribe."[54]

The moral universe of medicine is of course founded on the Hippocratic oath, and since it plays a central role in this dilemma, it is only fitting to examine whether modern-day physicians are likely to hold anything more than sentimental attachment to their ancient oath and their ethical code.

It would very likely be impossible to find any circumstances in history where medicine was subjected to any more brutal dictation to act contrary to this oath than was directed against Dutch physicians under the Nazi occupation. Reminiscent of Stone Age morality, these physicians had been ordered to kill the infirm and sterilize the unfit. But they "refused to act against the spirit of the Hippocratic oath."[37,p.135] A hundred Dutch doctors were consequently sent to concentration camps, and their colleagues cared for their widows and orphans, but no Dutch medical men participated at any time in the amoral experiments and atrocities of their German counterparts. (NOTE: Even within Nazi Germany, of 90,000 doctors, only some 350 participated in medical crimes.) This particularly sorry footnote to state control over medicine was summarized by Abse in these words: "Conform or die was the dictate of the Nazi regime, an alternative that obtained then for Doctors eminent or otherwise, and that can become operative in any totalitarian country."[37,p.127] And he concludes that there is no justification for thinking that this lesson has been so soon forgotten by physicians anywhere.

To base actions on an assumption that somehow physicians will abandon their commitment to the individual in the name of the public good would be to risk a confrontation that would very likely unite the vast majority of physicians against whatever the threat to medical ethics might be, regardless of its source. This applies forcefully to the present dilemma in that there is little reason to expect that practitioners can or would condone any proposed triage system that would ration care, much less participate in it themselves. While some feel that medicine will accept society's constraints on eligibility for care,[44] if that is taken to mean physicians will be expected to rule on which of their patients are to be denied care so that others may receive it, the burden of moral discomfort that would entail every time such a choice was faced would make the professional existence intolerable. Professionals are therefore obliged to resist any movement in that direction. As Goodman stated it, "This is the sacred and final obligation of every professional . . . to do the work and to defend the condition under which the work can be done well."[55]

But attempting to wish away the problems of an inequitable distribution of health care and insufferable costs would accomplish nothing worthwhile either. Hiatt therefore believes the critical question confronting the medical profession today is not really whether society will find ways to control the use of the medical commons, but rather how physicians will participate "in the creation of control mechanisms in a manner that reflects both enlightened self-interest and the public interest."[44] Is it any wonder that physicians sometimes yearn for the "good old days" when there was no need for controls and when things were much simpler?[13]

To some it may seem like an almost unbearable irony to learn that some of the earliest written records of the "good old days" tell a different story. One of the most important relics from ancient Mesopotamia, a black stone inscribed with cuneiform writings, "represents the first historical attempt to legislate the professional practice of medicine."[54] Known as the "Code of Hammurabi," circa 1690 BC, its content portrays a society described in these words by Sir William Osler: "From the enactment of the code we gather that the medical profession must have been in a highly organized state, for not only was practice regulated in detail, but a scale of fees was laid down, and penalties extracted for malpraxis [sic]."[56] This latter feature is described by Osler as an application of the "lex talonis . . . an eye for an eye, bone for a bone and tooth for a tooth, which is a striking feature of the code." He was referring to such articles of the code as paragraph 218, which reads as follows: "If the doctor has treated a gentleman for a severe wound with a lancet of bronze and caused the gentleman to die, or has opened an abscess of the eye for a gentleman and has caused the loss of the gentleman's eye, one shall cut off his hands." Dr. Osler was prompted to remark of this code: "it is lucky we have these days escaped." But did we? Is medicine in this country regressing toward a modern variant of lex talonis, or do the signs portend revolutionary changes occurring that can avert such a fate?

The signs of impending major changes coming to medicine are everywhere. As Dunlap[57] has pointed out, these signs of turbulence are relatively recent, as the care system was in a relatively stable state until the late 1950s, when dislocating forces began to disturb the congruity of the parts and the stability of the whole. Hanlon[17] has identified four major dislocating factors: (1) billions of federal dollars pumped into research that increased knowledge and technology, (2) rising public expectations and demands, (3) new industrial and other third-party financing methods that developed concurrently, and (4) the flood of federal health legislation.

All of this happened at a time when large-scale dislocating forces beset our society as a whole: (1) the rebellion of the youth and disadvantaged minorities, (2) deference to the rising influence of consumerism in the formulation of policy decisions at all levels, (3) the assumption that health is a right rather than a privilege, and (4) the assumption that if the results of treatment are less than expected, then someone must pay for it.

These forces not only combine to press for social change but also "engender in legislative circles a disenchantment with professionalism and the value of research."[17] If there is no documentary evidence to indicate that either contribute toward solving the problems of society, then the legislature can only conclude that no alternatives exist other than to take effective action to change the care delivery system through the legislative process.

This potential for unilateral action is consistent with Bell's thinking. It is his view that the relationship of knowledge to power is "clearly a subservient one."[58] It is not the scientist who ultimately holds the power in his view, but the politician. What then can be learned from nations where politicians unequivocally do control medicine?

In reports from the British experience there is a mix of pluses and minuses. While cost containment has been much more effective in that country than in the United States, the British commentator Norton specifically cites discontent of the physicians as one of its prominent disadvantages.[13] Among other disadvantages are the overusage of services, undercapitalization, antiquated hospitals and facilities, counterproductive divisions between generalists and specialists, a divorce of preventive from curative medicine, and a lack of integrated planning among the professions. While the Russian experience is not sufficiently open for any reasonable evaluation, one indicator of a stagnation of its medical research is "fortified by the fact that no significant new drugs have been discovered in the USSR."[42]

It has been said that the strength of state control over medicine is the power over distribution, while the strength of free enterprise is the protection of the patient's personal right to health benefit.[21] There is no room for compromise on this latter position in a free society, since any denial of these benefits is a fundamental breech of faith between the physician and his patient.[45] The potential for harm in disrupting the understanding between patient and physician is so great that the consequences of purposefully abrogating that contract in any manner must be carefully weighed. As Fried put it: "The point is that our most exigent sense of rights and of the wrongs done in violating rights refers to harm done intentionally."[45] After

all, if the modern ethic is to be realized that patients should be brought more fully into participation in their own care, it can only be based on a relationship of earned faith as the patient's knowledge base is not equal to that of his physician. If the physician is forced to destroy that faith by involuntarily denying care to the patient, there is no basis left for a partnership.

Perhaps it is in an attempt to avoid even the appearance of intentionally violating the patient's right to personal care that this very issue has scarcely been raised as a part of the current public debate. In any case a greater threat to the independent practice of medicine may lie in the somewhat quieter erosive effects and external controls borne of administrative expediencies rendered in the absence of relevant data that reliably reflect the realities of medical practice.

Clinical management is usually a highly complex thing, and the care of a sick patient seldom can be made simple and be good. By contrast, as Harrington points out: "The patient and the physician both live in a culture which values specific solutions of complex problems."[32] It is the managerial tendency of simplifying medical problems to make them tractable to administrative solutions that inevitably produces imbalances and distortions in health care delivery. People are complex. Their health care is also typically complex, and their care needs are highly situational. There are no rules, no policies, no scientific formulae, and no generic criteria by which quality medical care can be directed for everyone through administrative fiat. The central dilemma for medicine is that society, through its managers and its government, appears to be striving to impose exactly that.

If this is an accurate description of the dilemma facing medicine at a time when its science and technology are racing ahead at dizzying speeds, then why hasn't the same science and technology come to the rescue of medicine? (This is a variant of the argument, "If we can put a man on the moon, why can't we . . . .") The answer to that can only come from an exploration into the fundamental nature of medicine itself. Is medicine a science or is it an art? Is it a pragmatic craft or a service in the cause of human morality? Is it, indeed, one profession with many helpers or many professions with one objective?

We submit that it is all of these things. Certainly science is at the basis of its research, its knowledge, and much of its teaching. Art is practiced at the bedside by all good physicians to aid them in explaining difficult concepts in terms that can be understood, in the enlistment of patient cooperation, in the allaying of fears, the building of hope, in presiding at moments of grief, and as an aid in meeting a multitude of other humanistic needs. Pragmatism must be there too, since the clinician is often presented with a choice between what he knows can be technically achieved and what the evidence would suggest is practical or legal. He must balance the likely risks of care against the possible benefits. He must also balance potential benefits against certain costs or pain. Unfortunately it is also too often that he must strike a balance between his better judgment of what ought to be done for the patient (or not done) against the odds of his getting sued, or the potential for violating some regulation, payment stipulation, or intrusion of law into the practice of medicine.

There also exists a great deal of confusion about just who is licensed by society to do what to which patients and whether our universities really train any of the growing list of health professions to perform as they actually wind up doing in practice. Indeed the whole concept of what constitutes a professional now has taken on undreamed of significance in the context of PSRO, for it determines who will sit in judgment of whom. This is a very serious matter for, as Enarson points out, if it leads to petty internecine squabbles at a time when momentous decisions are being made regarding medicine's future,

dismay will guide the decision making, and medicine will pay the price.[59]

To our way of thinking, the ultimate test of what medicine is all about and therefore what the professional destiny should be based on is what goes on in the middle of the night when lonely decisions of life and death are so often made. When the terminal cancer patient sinks into a coma because his kidneys have failed, the decision not to place him on the renal dialysis machine, for example, must be made by someone. In most cases (but not all) the best way to arrive at that decision is through the knowledgeable participation of patient, family, and physician. But note: whatever decision is made, it is a moral one, purely and simply.[34] All the science, technology, art, pragmatism, professionalism, and what have you, are swept before that ultimate moral decision.

We submit therefore that the practice of medicine should be operationally recognized as a fundamentally moral human enterprise. This would lead to a realization that the maldistribution of health services and their prohibitive costs are also moral issues that must then be addressed in moral terms and met with moral solutions whether statistically justifiable or not. Within this unifying concept, it then becomes proper to simultaneously apply all the instruments of science technology, art, pragmatism, government, and law, since all can then serve a common end rather than breed more conflict and more dilemmas.

In closing this discussion we wish to register the point that all parties to the issues discussed here would be well-served by disabusing themselves of any lingering notions that these moral dilemmas are either unique to medicine or that professionals in the health care fields are alone in finding themselves potentially in a contest with managers and government. Harvard sociologist Daniel Bell points to a similar dilemma confronted by science in general.[58] He believes that scientists likewise have a social responsibility for their own actions as do physicians and lawyers. He believes what sets the scientific commitment apart from direct service to society is that "science is a game against nature which is not the same thing as a game against persons," which of course is the essence of management, politics, and government. That brings Bell to the real problem, which he says is "How do you have a form of science that is responsive to social needs but also allows some degree of autonomy and breathing space?" This is probably the most burning question before medicine today as well.

An overview of the dilemma facing medicine leads to the following conclusions:

1. The individual physician is most equipped by his ethical orientation and formal training to deal with health problems that directly affect the individual patient and the relatively small group that comprises his own practice. On the other hand, what is in the best interest of the larger soceity may not be in the best interest of the individual patient or his own practice. In that event, it is the moral obligation of the physician both to protect the patient and to do what he can to minimize the negative consequences on society.

2. Societies, on the other hand, have felt free from time to time to call on the obligation of health professionals as citizens to request or demand that they act in the public interest in whatever way the government currently in power chooses to define that phrase. Such demands over recorded history have resulted in a range of impacts from highly beneficial to those that are counterproductive to both medicine and society and sometimes also those that have amounted to outright atrocities perpetrated "for the good of the tribe."

3. The ethical basis for medical practice is a moral one and has remained an unchanging constant over many centuries, whereas periodic declarations of the public good by governments are characteristically situational and changeable. This sets the stage for intermittent conflict between medicine and government. But there is no good reason to assume that this adversary relationship in itself need be either counterproductive or wrong, as there is no concrete evidence of a permanent state of conflict between medicine (or science in general) and the government of this or any other country.

4. In any legitimate conflict of purpose with government, medicine must always defend the interests of the individual patient. But to do this effectively, medicine is obliged to demonstrate that its independent course of action is ultimately of greater benefit to mankind than any proposed alternative. To be able to do this, in turn, it must first demonstrate the capability to effectively evaluate the efficacy of the health care it provides, the efficiency of its delivery system, and the benefits obtained by patients and society.

5. Once appraised of the status of its own care effectiveness, medicine must do more to exploit its art, technology, and available resources to successfully meet the moral challenges of securing distributive justice and bearable medical costs. That of course happens to be a public good.

6. But medicine can never change its practices at the expense of denying its own moral obligation to serve the patient first or it will be untrue to its origin and destiny to the end result that professionalism will lose its legitimacy. Similarly, government cannot and should not abandon its obligation to work for distributive justice that brings quality health care to all the people.

7. Both medicine and government should maintain the moral integrity of their respective positions but also build a structure for cooperation based on sound knowledge and a mutual respect for the moral obligations of the other. The alternative is a confrontation that could only add to the dilemmas faced by medicine, government, and society as a whole.

THE JOB TO BE DONE

In a recent work entitled *Change,* Watzlawick and associates[60] discussed concepts that bear forcefully on our discussion of what might be the most constructive way in which peer review might contribute to solving some of the problems facing medicine and society. They describe what is called first order change and second order change. To quote them directly: "If we accept this basic distinction between two theories, it follows that there are two different types of change; one that occurs within a given system which itself remains unchanged, and one whose occurrence changes the system itself."[60,pp.10–11] The example they use to illustrate their point is a person who is dreaming. The dreaming person might smile, laugh, cry, hit, push, shove, or scream, but none of the behaviors (changes) that occur within a dream will in itself stop the dream. This is an example of first order change. The kind of change required to actually stop the dream is the change from sleeping and dreaming to waking and alertness, or second order change. In the medical context, first order changes are typified by modifications in the techniques of delivering medical care, but *second order changes are modifications in the care delivery system itself.*

Sometimes merely by reframing a problem, its resolution through second order change can become a reality. King Christian X of Denmark faced a most perplexing problem with Nazi Germany during the war. The Nazis wanted to meet with him regarding a final solution to the Jewish problem in Denmark. On meeting with the Nazis the King replied, "We don't have a Jewish problem. We don't feel inferior [to them]."[60,p.107] That ended the discussion. But in the complexity of medical care, simple, single-stroke solutions are rare, and systematized programs for effecting change over time are needed instead. The very existence of mechanisms for effecting change within medicine has been challenged, and more specifically the peer review approach of the medical profession for controlling abuses or overutilization has not been considered effec-

tive.[19] But let us examine the reasons why that might be so.

If it is accepted that the recent surge in public demand for services has been of unprecedented intensity and of unforeseen speed, then it is not unreasonable to postulate that medicine's capability to respond was simply outstripped. A recognition of the need to devote adequate amounts of thought, energy, and money to prepare the solutions to broader-scale problems, such as how to assure a wider distribution of low-cost medical care, simply did not come soon enough to avoid the crunch. Medicine, it would seem, continued to rely too long on its one-at-a-time and nonsystematic approach to care delivery, which fails to deal in a direct way with broader care needs at the community or national level. It also clung largely to its personally based review mechanisms that are virtually preordained to fail as instruments of public accountability because of the traditional reluctance of physicians to interfere in each others' practice or to invoke the ill will of a colleague on whom one might depend for referrals or who later will trade places and become the reviewer.[37] The inevitable result for medicine as a whole has been some degree of forfeiture of the professional obligation to police itself. This is understandable no matter how lamentable because the critical evaluation of a colleague's performance is a difficult thing to do when it is placed on a personal basis.

The evidence of this failure was not lost on the U.S. Senate Finance Committee in preparing the report that accompanied the PSRO legislation, as it observed: "Where hospital beds are in short supply, utilization review is fully effective. Where there is no pressure on the hospital beds, utilization review is less intense and often token."[61]

Writing in the *AMA News* about the failure of self-policing in relationship to the malpractice crisis, Laurens White observed: "In considerable measure, we are to blame for this mess. We have put off doing anything about it until too late. We have, from sloth and loyalty, taken only token action against those physicians who practice negligent medicine."[62]

While it is undeniable that major changes in medical education, research, and care practices are basically dictated by the needs and wants of society,[63] it is still the option of the profession to choose between accepting change forced on it and attempting to guide the direction of change. Freymann suggests that "With so many brilliant men among its members the medical profession should not have to abandon direction of its destiny to outside focus."[63a] Donabédian is characteristically direct in citing a compelling reason why physicians should become involved: "Professional review of professional activities may, therefore, be properly viewed as a bulwark of autonomous, but responsible, professionalism rather than a negation of it."[37]

But involvement in what kind of professional review activity? If the aim is only to advance momentary preferences in care procedures, it will have little real impact on care practitioners and virtually none on the system of delivering care. If there is no commitment to evolve a mechanism for implementing recommendations for corrective actions when care deficiencies are revealed, then we simply remain confined to the first order changes of dreams or nightmares: flailing, kicking, and screaming from one behavior sequence to the next without evoking any significant improvements in the medical delivery system itself.

But just what are the prospects for accomplishing something of significance? What Cohen sees for the next decade and beyond is the potential for medical progress that will make achievements to date almost commonplace by comparison. "Yet," he says, "such progress will not occur without the full participation of the medical profession, the government, and the American people in taking up the great unfinished tasks."[29] And what are those

unfinished tasks? Again, Irving Lewis: "We can be proud in this country of the progress the health professions have made in expanding medical knowledge, perfecting medical technologies and building and operating medical institutions. We have done considerably less well, however, in the field of organization and delivery of health care."[41]

Contrast this assessment of care delivery in this country with an assessment of the status of its clinical research. After more than a year of study, the President's Biomedical Research Panel has just reported its findings, the first of which is cited here: "There do not appear to be any impenetrable, incomprehensible diseases.... What is needed now is some sort of settling down for the long haul. Most of all, the scientific enterprise needs stability and predictability [of funding]."[64]

Clearly there is far greater confidence in medicine's ability to discover new ways to improve care technology than to deliver it. However, it is essential to bear in mind that not all ill health is amenable to the scientific enterprise aspect of contemporary medical care. There are still so many diseases that the science of medicine alone cannot cure. There is abundant ill health that really does not even have a medical etiology in the usual sense but arises from stresses that are societal in origin.[31] The medical problems of these unfortunates are real enough, and medicine should do all it can to ameliorate their effects and relieve the symptoms, but ultimate cures must be found within society's province. As Wilcocks put it, the "troubles of urban life and poverty, and the industrial diseases, and the encouragement of standards of living which concur to good health, are more to be affected by administration action through social reform, economic advancement, housing and general sanitary measures ... than by action which could be regarded as purely medical."[52, p.263]

Then too the public would do well to temper its expectations of how much medicine should be expected to lower the cost of care by first recognizing that all individuals have an obligation to take better care of themselves than many do to reduce total medical needs. The costs of managing many of the leading causes of death in this country today must be laid directly at the feet of destructive personal habits and neglect,[28] as was so vividly revealed in the Framingham study.[65]

Physicians are not very successful in their efforts to get their patients to stop abuses such as smoking and excessive drinking or eating that have so seriously damaged their health in the first place, and there must be reasons why this is so. Societal acceptance, conditioned by the parading of these unhealthy habits and lifestyles in the public media, is probably no insignificant part of the reason they exist. This is a factor that obviously must be dealt with through cooperative efforts that extend beyond the physician's office.[52, p.263] But the nagging question remains whether some of the power to persuade has gone out of the art of medicine.

There is another group of patients with organic and emotional problems caused by occupational dislocations that in turn are produced by technology.[66] Illnesses produced by industrial pollution present yet another responsibility for medicine. Even an outright cure of the individual victim in either of these circumstances is but the beginning of the total management picture. The real job to be done is to clean up the environment and to alter the technology that brought harm, dislocation, or discomfort to people in the first place. It is therefore apparent that there are medical and technologic answers to some problems caused by technology and industry, but societal actions are clearly required to solve many others. In short, many of the diseases that patients develop are but the symptoms of deeper underlying disturbances with their true causes rooted in society. The outcome of medical care programs will consequently depend not only on the health services delivered but also on the economic level of the population, their health education, the physical environment, and the political climate.

Everything points to the notion that the scope of the total job to be done is much too large to be managed through any single cure-all type of technology, by the health professions acting alone, by governmental actions alone, or by any piecemeal approach. There must be a driving force that is at once unifying, powerful, and workable over the long haul if medicine is to become realistically accountable and if our nation is to avoid the tragedy of the commons. The question to be addressed then is, What should be the role of peer review in all of this?

Kerr White and his associates make the forceful argument that peer review appears to be essential if hospitals individually and collectively are to tackle the central issues of use, cost, quality, and efficiency. He then suggests how it might be of help: "Parsemonious collection of a minimal data set, through uniform hospital patient discharge abstracts and claim forms that relate persons, health problems and hospital charges to populations and institutions, has more power to influence medical care costs, hospital utilization, standards of care, and health services planning than any other health-information system likely to be available in the forseeable future."[43] This well-informed opinion points to the kind of technologic assessment strategy needed to get the job done. It is one that provides the information feedback essential to intelligent decision making.

What seems clear in retrospect is that the problem-solving mechanisms that characterized peer review in the past have employed first order change strategies that have focused on *care technology* without implementing the vital system component that might be called *feedback-evaluation technology.* That error has prevented medical practitioners from creating a decision matrix that can provide the second order changes so necessary to the well-being of both medicine and society. That then is the essential first step in approaching the job that is to be done.

But there are also risks associated with the implementation of second order changes, especially when coupled to a program for public accountability. The potential for a misuse of data always exists, as does the breech of confidentiality and arbitrariness in the setting of care standards and so on. The list of potential abuses is a long one, but the single point to be made here is that establishing firm assurances that such abuses will not occur is a very important aspect of the job that is to be done.

An overview of the job to be done leads to the following observations:

1. Some of the most compelling unfinished tasks before medicine are concerned with the organization, delivery, and integration of health care services.

2. It is selective second order change that is needed to evolve a more equitable care delivery system and to develop solutions to the problems related to that end.

3. Evolutionary forces of change need to be creatively shaped by a unity of purpose shared by medicine, government, and society at large. This requires access to accurate and relevant information feedback to guide the change process.

4. Obtaining information of this nature calls for the development of a feedback mechanism that can identify the kinds of second order changes that are needed to upgrade the care process.

5. There are risks associated with making second order changes that must be anticipated and realistically managed for successful and permanent improvements in care delivery to occur.

The basic instruments of peer review and the role of PSRO in their development

As we have seen, governmental reactions to public demands and dissatisfactions have taken the form of a whole series of legislated service and regulatory programs. Among them is PSRO, of course, which is a specific kind of evaluative tool mandated by Congress and which has been described by its implementors as a "landmark"[67] in that it relies on the mechanics of the peer review process for carrying it out. Before discussing PSRO, however, we wish to develop a broader perspective that encompasses a whole range of new evaluative technologies (including PSRO) that have begun to exert progressively larger impacts on medicine.

There is abundant evidence that care technology, when utilized prudently and appropriately, has contributed to the solution of many problems in the management of diseases. Unquestionably, care technology could contribute further to the management of disease problems and also address some of the organizational problems of care delivery if there were an unlimited supply of resources available to do it. But modern care technologies are expensive, and there is every likelihood that the setting of priorities will restrict the allocation of medical resources (in some manner) in the coming years. What we do not need under these circumstances is a continuation of an unguided, uncritical, and unlimited use of care technologies that produce only first order changes in the delivery of health services. What is needed instead is the application of evaluation technology that can lead to second order changes by helping health professionals to critically assess the relative merits of medical services and procedures now in place or under development. Medicine urgently needs a reliable means to select which technologic methods and innovations should be applied to medical and health service systems, not because these methods are available and feasible, but because they materially assist in meeting the needs of people.

But in view of past inaction, is it realistic to expect medicine to make the internal organizational changes needed to objectively appraise cherished care practices or to initiate innovative solutions to unsolved problems in health care distribution and cost containment and so on? We submit that it is because the present time seems particularly favorable to change. There are signs to suggest that medicine is currently caught up in the tide of a scientific revolution independent of PSRO or any other governmental action. Kuhn expressed it this way: "Professional insecurity is the result of a breakdown in the traditional way of doing business, and social pressure for reform builds up because existing institutions have ceased to meet adequately the problems posed by society. Under the conditions of scientific revolution an environment is created that is favorable for seeking new solutions to old problems."[68] But if order is to be maintained in the midst of change, there must be a professionally acceptable means to assess what is happening and to guide evolutionary forces into constructive channels. That is where peer review comes in.

Peer review is the tangible manifestation of the professional obligation of self-assessment, so it should be acceptable to professionals as a vehicle for advancing the kind of assessment technology that can lead to new solutions to refractory old problems. Ayres has defined technologic assessment as the "systematic application of organized knowledge to (operational) practical activities, especially productive ones."[69] While this definition does encompass automation as the hardware of assessment, it is not linked to just computerization. Included in this idea are software, review methods, procedures, and all the other techniques for developing complete feedback systems that allow for a systematic evaluation of medical care. To best appreciate the importance of the term *systematic* in the context of evaluating medical care, we must first explore what it means to the delivery of care.

Systematic approach to delivery of care. To set a frame of reference, let us first consider a simplified model of typical non-systematized care encounter. A patient becomes ill and develops symptoms for which he seeks medical help. The physician then investigates the patient's history, performs a physical examination, and obtains some laboratory data to establish a diagnosis on which he will base the therapy. He will also attend to those personal needs of the patient that work for the best patient outcome. The patient's disease is seen as a disruption of his bodily processes, and a cure is seen as the restoration of bodily and social functions. Throughout, the focus is on the patient as a person, meaning as a unique and independent entity.

But a general systems approach places the individual in a perspective that recognizes much broader concepts. These concepts may be paraphrased as follows:

1. The components and bodily processes of man are organized into discrete hierarchical levels (from organ systems down to the subcellular and even the molecular level).

2. Homeostasis depends not only on each level being intact and functioning but also that each must be in balance (homeostasis) with the physiologic characteristics of all other levels.

3. There must be a functioning feedback system between all levels to continuously direct the adjustment processes that maintain each level in dynamic balance with all the others.

4. Man himself (the patient) is a component (level) within even broader (external) hierarchies we refer to as the family, the community, and the human race.

Immediately this expanded conceptual base frees us from the confinement of traditional thinking, which holds no better definition of health than the absence of disease. Working from Laszlo's analysis of living things as natural systems,[70] Brody proposes the following definition of health: "The harmonious interactions of all hierarchical components."[71] Implicit in this definition is the notion that man and all his parts are components of a larger system (nature). In this broader context then the system encompasses hierarchical levels both within and external to man himself. Health, defined in this way, can therefore pertain to the individual, to his liver and its enzymes, to his family as a unit, and even to his community, because the concept of health in a natural system applies equally to all levels within it.

With this single unifying concept to guide us, it is possible to acquire a correspondingly broader understanding of what the total ramifications of diseases really are and how initial disruptions at one level are communicated through feedback mechanisms to become manifested as disruptions at other levels within the patient or his environment. The recognition that feedback exists between the hierarchical levels leads to a sorting out of secondary and accommodating disruptions (symptoms) at the person level from primary or etiologic perturbations (causes) that may have occurred at some more basic level within the individual, such as a specific organ, or that may have arisen from the external environment, such as air pollution. This in turn can lead to more rational care plans that identify and deal with the real underlying causes of diseases, thereby eliminating the unnecessary human and financial costs of treating the symptoms of diseases that can be prevented from developing in the first place.

Similarly a clearer understanding of how nonpreventable chronic or catastrophic diseases cause disruptions in a family or burden a community can engender a better appreciation of how and why community resources should be mobilized to deal with them more effectively. Along with a heightened realization that health care must extend beyond the context of the individual patient into his community comes the realization that the delivery of care must also extend beyond the office of the individual practitioner and into the community he serves.

Given the time for evolutionary processes to fully absorb systems concepts into the practice of medicine, it would soon become apparent that systematic care delivery is just as dependent on accurate feedback to maintain itself in ho-

meostatic balance as is an endocrine gland in controlling its activity. The first order of business would then be to develop and energize the informational feedback loops essential to maintain homeostatic balances both within the health professions themselves and between society's perceived care needs and the care delivery system as a whole. Reliable feedback of this magnitude would of course require the application of mature evaluation technology.

Evaluation technology in delivery of care. All this brings us to the question as to whether the evaluation technology (as opposed to care technology) is now available and functioning at a level that makes it useful to clinical medicine. There is ample evidence that the application of evaluative technology to case management is evolving rapidly. This becomes apparent in the attention being paid to it in the contemporary medical literature. For example, within a single recent issue of the *New England Journal of Medicine* devoted to medical decision making were articles that dealt with the critical evaluation of diagnostic procedures and their costs in terms of both money and health,[72] cost-effectiveness calculations dealing with a specific disease entity,[73] the value of case finding (triage) and its cost-benefit equation,[74] and even an approach to cost-benefit analysis that can be applied either to an individual patient or to a population.[75]

Projections of human costs as well as dollar costs are becoming available to temper selections of diagnostic and treatment modalities by helping the health professional to balance the probable risks against possible gains in given clinical conditions. Techniques are also becoming available to help in dealing with the more complex clinical management problems such as a decision tree that describes in comprehensible terms the alternative clinical courses of actions available and the consequences of each. Thus the newer evaluation techniques do hold considerable promise for making care delivery more manageable by directing medicine toward attainable solutions to those problems that were created by or left over from (unsolved by) its care technology. That is a pretty good general description of the kind of basic instruments peer review needs.

It is time therefore to broaden our horizon of what evaluation technology is all about and not to color our view of its future by our view of its past applications, for example, to cost control.

The following chapters amply testify to the range and extent of progress in evaluation technology as applied to peer review. But before looking into the "how" of conducting peer review, we pause to examine the conceptual origins of PSRO, its intended scope, and the overall role it is likely to play in the further evolution of peer review in its broader context as an evaluation technology.

PSRO in the evolution of peer review. We submit that it could be most fortuitous that at precisely this moment in history along comes the legal requirement and financial support to set up PSROs throughout the country because this is the equivalent of mandating and funding the development of a nationwide prototype health data feedback mechanism. While its scope is so far limited, it nevertheless does aim at assessing the interactions of the health care delivery system with society at large, how major health needs are being met (at least in hospitals), and the costs attendant on doing so. That is a significant start toward a nationwide information feedback system that has been slow in developing because local solutions to local problems, which characterized so many efforts in the past, do little to stimulate the development of sophisticated evaluation technologies.

Thus what really seems to be happening here is an inverted evolutionary process. We find that medicine's needed information feedback mechanism has been mandated (in part) by law rather than naturally evolving out of its own professional commitment to the systematic approach to medical care. It can only be hoped that evolutionary motion can now proceed in a retrograde fashion from the mechanics to the concept; that is, that the information actually derived from PSRO and other forms of peer review can direct evolutionary processes toward the development of a truly systematic approach to health care delivery. Therein lies the hope of making the second order changes that can eliminate the inequities and cost burdens of our existing health care institutions without either destroying their foundations of creating new inequities in patient care in the process of redressing existing ones.

One of the reasons that there is currently a greater chance than ever before that evaluation technology can be applied in such a manner is that an enlightened PSRO program could move developments in precisely that direction. Perhaps even more importantly, PSRO is even now providing a sense of urgency and an awareness of common purpose that links many concerned persons together. In this regard it has been the indirect stimulus to provide such forums as this book to share some of those thoughts.

But PSRO is also a program with a mission, and to understand that mission it is necessary to understand the conceptual roots of PSRO in the legislative process.

Origins and mission of PSRO. The Committee on Finance of the United States Senate, which introduced the amendments to the Social Security Act[20] (informally known as the PSRO legislation), spelled out in an accompanying committee report what they intended it to accomplish and how they expected this to be done. Among the critical points made in this 1972 document[61] are the following (cited by page number):

1. Both Medicare and Medicaid costs are "rising at precipitous rates" (p. 254).

2. "Witnesses testified that a significant proportion of the health services provided under Medicare and Medicaid are probably not medically necessary," (p. 254).

3. "Unnecessary hospitalization and un-

necessary surgery are not consistent with proper health care" (p. 254).

4. "That utilization controls are particularly important was extensively revealed in hearings conducted by the subcommittee on Medicare and Medicaid" (p. 254).

5. "The committee is particularly concerned that the utilization and review function is carried out in a manner which protects the patients while at the same time making certain that they remain in the hospital only so long as is necessary, and that every effort be made to move them from the hospital to other facilities which can provide less expensive but equal care to meet their current medical needs" (p. 255).

6. The report gets quite specific (as does the law itself[20]) in saying how the legislators expect utilization procedures to be conducted as, for example, in the certification of a length of stay once an admission has been approved. "It is expected that such certification would generally be required not later than the point where 50 percent of patients with similar diagnoses and in the same age groups have usually been discharged" (p. 263).

7. Such review procedures were clearly not intended to interfere with sound medical care: "This professionally determined time of certification of need for continued care is a logical checkpoint for the attending physician and is not to be construed as a barrier to further necessary care. Neither should the use of norms as checkpoints nor any other activity of the PSRO, be used to stifle innovative medical practice or procedures" (p. 263).

8. In contrast to such specific directive regarding resource utilization, a general statement is also made: "Emphasis should be placed on assuring high quality of performance and on discovering and preventing unsatisfactory performance" (p. 256). However, there is no discussion as to what this emphasis means, how it should be accomplished, or any comment on how this function would be funded once implemented.

9. There is no ambiguity, however, regarding who should be performing the review: "The committee believes that the review process should be based upon the premise that only physicians are, in general, qualified to judge whether services ordered by other physicians are necessary" (p. 256).

To summarize the original concept of PSRO as articulated by its creators, it was viewed essentially as a tool to restrain unnecessary hospitalization and surgery and at the same time to protect patients from unnecessary care. It utilizes norms, standards, and criteria that define appropriate admissions and lengths of stay. The review process is to be conducted locally with the active participation of practicing physicians. The role this best describes for PSRO is a form of utilization review carried out by a peer review mechanism.

The PSRO legislation was challenged by an organization representing a group of physicians in the courts, and on May 8, 1975, a ruling was handed down by a United States District Court in Illinois. Of relevance to this discussion are the opinions of record of federal judges regarding the purpose of this piece of federal legislation.[76] A few of the more salient points (also identified by page number) are as follows:

1. "In order to avoid overutilization of health care services and to achieve more effective control over the costs of those services Congress has enacted the 'Professional Standards Review' legislation" (p. 8).

2. "The statute, however, does not bar physicians from practicing their profession but only 'provides standards for the dispensation of Federal funds.'" (p. 8).

3. The plaintiffs in this suit argued that the norms of diagnosis, treatment, and care are inherently incapable of reduction to specific language. The reply of the Court was as follows: "The Court is cognizant of the difficulties encountered in drafting norms with sufficient specificity to afford meaningful notice to the practi-

tioner and with adequate flexibility to reach a multitude of individual medical cases. However, the task is not an impossible one" (p. 11).

4. In response to the argument of PSRO's interference with medical progress, the Court said: "Neither should the use of norms as checkpoints nor any other activity of the PSRO be used to stifle innovative medical practices or procedures" (p. 11).

5. In regard to the constitutionality of the limitations of liability, the Court said: "The norms which are to be established and which the plaintiffs must comply with are, by definition, typical medical practices within the region where the physician practices" (p. 15).

6. The final opinion to be cited here has to do with confidentiality: "The Professional Standards Review legislation contains provisions that properly balance the plaintiff's [physicians] right of privacy with the Government's interest in maintaining proper health in an economical matter" (p. 13).

To summarize this court opinion: as the largest health insurer in the United States, the federal government enacted the PSRO legislation to avoid overutilization of health care services and to control costs. Also the statute calls for the establishment of care standards that are defined by the typical medical practices within local regions.

By the time of this writing the staff of the Bureau of Quality Assurance has had experience with PSRO operations and the opportunity to provide a more definitive and updated description of what a PSRO hospital review system is all about.[67] There has also been a reflection of PSRO program policy as approved by the National Professional Standards Review Council,[77] so there is no need to examine the program in any detail here. What is germane is to take note of those major characteristics of the PSRO program that will shape the design requirements of any peer review system that is intended to be compatible with it. From the first of the above

communications[67] we learn the following:

1. Peer review is accepted as an effective means of public accountability for health services provided under third-party financing. Thus external reporting to the public is a required feature of compatible peer review systems.

2. It is also now seen as involving the function of quality assurance "encompassing all facets of the health care delivery system." Obviously this calls for review procedures that are comprehensive in scope.

3. Local, community-based organizations are required to demonstrate that their peer review systems are effective. This means that the review system itself must be evaluated.

4. The peer review organization must be sponsored externally to the hospital. This means that the system must prepare and direct managerial reports for external review.

From the second of these communications[77] we note the following:

5. The peer review process is expected not only to detect problems but to analyze the causes of care deficiencies and to develop, implement, and evaluate corrective programs. The implications of the latter means that the review process must be backed by a support program to change care policies and procedures or provider behaviors.

6. PSROs are expected to advance community-wide patient care that is integrated with continuing medical education. This means that neither the performance data nor performance-based educational initiatives are to be restricted to in-house activities.

Appropriate planning and designs for peer review systems would reflect each of the above six facets at a minimum.

The fact that the PSRO legislation was legally challenged is indicative of significant resistance to it. A lawyer's assessment of PSRO (as of February 1975)[78] raises a number of points about the law's inherent deficiencies that are therefore worthy of consideration. He cited the essentially uncontrolled central authority to direct PSRO activities, that the contracting process becomes the exclusive vehicle for policy making and implementation, that the process of administration through letter directives has already begun, and finally that: "At a point in time when methods of sophisticated peer review already exist, PSRO for lack of time to meet what is perceived to be the will of Congress, is becoming a hastily contrived structure that threatens to pay little attention to lessons already learned."

In fairness to all, it should be pointed out that reports of concrete achievement in systematic peer review methodologies have been somewhat scattered. This inevitably has hindered recognition of the real progress made in this field. Indeed, one of the purposes of this book is precisely to present side-by-side comparisons of the evaluation technology that has been applied to peer review systems, and another is to provide the platform to allow the developers of these systems to inform us of the lessons learned from their collective experiences.

If it is conceded that the problems besetting the delivery of health care in this country today are now severe enough that prudent change in the care system itself seems indicated, then it makes sense to look to systematic peer review as the feedback mechanism that can guide an evolutionary process of second order change to a better and more equitable health care system. Could what we propose be worse than the current distributive inequities, burdensome cost, uneven quality, and fragmentations in medical care that exist now or perhaps the total external control of medical practice that could come at any time? You will have to judge for yourself, but frankly we doubt it.

A systems overview of the kind of changes needed in the health care delivery system and the role of peer review (including PSRO) in evolving the neces-

sary tools to bring such changes about leads to the following conclusions:

1. A broad systems view of medical care would advance a broader and a better understanding of how man relates to discrete levels of his internal and external environments in the unifying context of an overall system.

2. A fuller understanding of the functional relationships between all levels in the system would help delineate the true causes of diseases from their overt manifestations and therefore help direct medical management more appropriately toward their causes rather than to treat their symptoms.

3. The vital importance of information feedback between the levels can also be better understood, and the role of evaluation technology in helping to guide and control care technology can be better appreciated, in the context of the systems approach.

4. While the tools of information feedback (evaluation technology) would more naturally evolve from an applied systematic approach to health care, the PSRO legislation has mandated that these tools be developed first. The consequences of their development without the guidance of a previously developed conceptual base are unknown.

5. While PSRO is presently of limited scope, it is nevertheless hoped that it can stimulate the development of broader scope systematic peer review methodologies on the one hand and the systematic delivery of effective and efficient health care on the other.

How to fail and how to succeed

A moment's reflection on the issues of cost and distribution of services reveals that solutions to managerial problems are now primarily needed[52,p.263] rather than solutions to clinical problems as in the past. This is a situation with profound implications in which pressures build for the participation of managers in decision-making processes that affect care availability.

Heretofore, decisions concerning who received what care were exercised almost exclusively by health professionals (especially physicians).[21] Thus conditions are now ripe either for an unprecedented era of cooperation[29] or for confrontation[19] between managers and clinicians, depending chiefly on the degree of understanding between them. The managers most likely to become directly involved in resource allocations include those working within health-related governmental agencies, those functioning as administrators of hospitals, those involved in various sponsored-care programs, in health departments, and in health-planning agencies. Perhaps also an enlarging managerial role may be in the offing for licensure authorities, semigovernmental accrediting commissions, for burgeoning data-processing organizations of various kinds, for the standards-setting machinery of professional societies, for organized consumer representation groups, and especially for the newest arrivals on the scene, the administrators of PSRO organizations (which could evolve into a managerial force in its own right). The relevant question is not who might contest with health professionals for the control of medicine[79] but how clinical practitioners can help to "guide the direction of change,"[46] so that the public is equitably served while clinical freedom to serve the individual patient is also preserved. But medical professionals traditionally have resisted external controls, in part because of their attachment to professional independence[21] and in part because of their apprehensions that the practice of medical care will suffer as managers place concerns for cost and administrative trivia above concerns for quality.[45,47]

If there is to be a confrontation between clinicians on the one side and managers who represent any of the power coalitions on the other side,[17] there will be no great mystery about what will be in contention. Given the circumstances that some kind of confrontation is inevitable, managers would logically attempt to exert a maximum of preemptive control over how care is delivered, and practitioners would logically attempt to insulate medicine from external control. A confrontation of this sort would be unfortunate because it would detract from the cooperation that is necessary to effectively come to grips with problems of the nature and magnitude described earlier.

As for myself, I have no preference for either the managerial or the professional route to the same disaster, so I hope neither course is actually being followed now. Nor can I accept as an inevitability that a polarization of opposing forces must occur in an attempt to insulate medicine on the one hand or to usurp control over it on the other. But I must reluctantly conclude that virtually the same erosive effects on both health care delivery and the integrity of the profession could result from a failure to appreciate the seriousness of purpose and the basic validity of positions taken by those who stand on opposite sides of the major issues confronting medicine today.

For cooperation to replace confrontation and for issues to be dealt with effectively, it is first necessary to see them for what they really are. This is why solutions of the unsolved problems in health care today await the information feedback that will allow us to go about this intelligently[80] by identifying realistically solvable problems,[81] establishing rational priorities for determining which problems need to be attacked first, and then establishing which attempts to improve the delivery of care prove to be effective. A large first step in this direction can be taken through cooperation between health care providers and all those managers who are in a position to advance the effectiveness and efficiency of a broadly based system for medical peer review.

A relevant question in this regard is, Where does the government and PSRO stand on the critical issues? Dr. Henry E. Simmons, speaking for HEW in 1975, addressed the issues of quality, cost, accountability, and responsibility with these words:[82]

The quality of medical care and the appropriate utilization of resources are of the utmost importance to American people. Congress has called upon physicians and, indeed, all health-care providers, to give an accounting of that quality.

The responsibility for providing that accounting is where it belongs on the local practicing physician. PSRO is their program.

Thus, the role of the Secretary [that is, the role of HEW] is limited to providing an administrative framework for the PSRO mechanism.

If the above describes a working relationship between government and medicine, which is forming and will operate in the foreseeable future, then there is every reason for optimism that the opportunity will arise for managers and clinicians to combine their thinking and skills in a complementary way to hasten the maturation of peer review as an effective instrument of public accountability. To make this a practical reality, some evaluation strategies and mechanisms are needed that have largely been confined to research because they are too expensive or too time-consuming to be applied to routine care surveillance. Peer review mechanisms with the capability to overcome these obstacles would in turn promote cost-effective health care and the kinds of second order changes in the care delivery system that would go a long way toward the development of responsible solutions to the moral and political issues confronting medicine, government, and society today. In the process, medicine will be meeting its social obligations for service and restoring public confidence in a profession that is accountable for what it does.

SUMMARY AND CONCLUSIONS

The history of medicine reveals that periodic tensions have arisen over the centuries between the technology of medicine and its own art, between society's expectations and medicine's capacity to fulfill them, and between the practitioners of medicine and the managers of society (government) for control of the medical destiny. When the creative balance between any of these critical internal and external variables is upset in any direction, it can be expected that the profession is likely to suffer consequences of some seriousness, but it is virtually inevitable that the patient will bear the brunt of it.

Some naturally occurring tension can be almost taken for granted as a product of the varying perceptions of what constitutes our most vital health needs as seen by government, medicine, and society, and their respective preferences for the direction the evolution of care delivery should take. The intensity of current imbalances in the distribution and costs of medical care now exerts tremendous (and probably irresistible) pressures on the patient, the physician, the government, and society at large to take effective steps in dealing with prevailing inequities and unresolved dilemmas. This chapter suggests some of the major failings or pitfalls that might make matters worse by forcing further imbalances between the art and the science (or technology) of medicine, and between medicine and government. It also raises some interesting questions about health policy decisions and resource allocations that cannot be properly resolved without relevant and appropriate feedback information to direct changes that reflect a strong commitment to moral principles on the part of both medicine and government.

A brief description of PSRO is presented to place it in perspective with some of the broader issues that relate to the role of peer review as an instrument for effecting second order changes within the medical care system. In one sense PSRO becomes an interesting experiment in that it tests the practicality of legally imposing the requirement on a profession that it utilize its own internal peer review mechanism for external (public) accountability.

Regardless of how that particular experiment turns out, systematic peer review itself can provide an effective feedback loop through which wiser decisions can be made concerning care delivery than have been possible in the past. It can do even more. It can become the communication channel through which factual information about legitimate needs of patients, society, and health professionals can be made known to all.

But peer review must be properly applied or there will be little hope for success in bringing about needed changes in health care delivery that will mutually benefit all concerned. Without the peer there is no such thing as peer review, without the patient there will be little understanding of what is relevant in patient care. Without public disclosure there can be no trusted accountability to society and the government. Without maintenance of the delicate balances between the rights of the individual, the demands of society, and legitimate professional prerogatives, we may be inviting the dehumanization of medical care. Statistics, regulations, or uninspired technology cannot, must not, be substituted for compassion.

Should it happen that you do not agree that coercive external control over the practice of medicine is a bad thing, then consider its most negative potential impact from an entirely personal viewpoint. Suppose you should find yourself as the coronary patient who is denied care so that someone else might have it. What would be your recourse if some panel determined that your care had a low priority, and how can such decrees be prevented once medical decisions made by practicing clinicians are compromised? Is it really your desire to see major decisions concerning your personal care removed from the hands of a personal physician who is obligated to place your right to care above everything else? Would you find much comfort in the knowledge of how much money was saved when the coronary unit was closed to you because you did not meet economic criteria or social priorities for

admission to it? Would you exhalt in the planner's wisdom for not squandering funds on a standby cardiac monitor you did not get to use? How much confidence do you think you would have in a care system in which the allocation of resources for your personal medical needs came out of a government-appointed committee of strangers, or worse, out of a computer?

Science fiction? We wish it were. This scenario is a direct and logical extension of the following set of feasible conclusions:

1. Society can or will no longer expend unlimited funds for medical services.

2. Demands for health services are likely to continue to rise despite a fiscal limit. This will effectively impose a service limit at some point below demand.

3. The moral obligation of patient advocacy widely felt on the part of health professionals precludes their active participation in routine triage activities that distribute health care services to some individuals while denying services to others on the basis of economics or social priorities.

4. The moral obligation of government to work toward distributive justice in the absence of a professional willingness to ration medical services will be interpreted as a mandate for government to set up a coercive body to effectively do just that in some form or another.

There is an alternative, but only one we can think of. A better and more economical way must be devised to deliver medical services more equitably than exists now. But there is no way anyone can learn how to do that in the absence of a wholly adequate feedback mechanism that can reliably tell us what medicine is doing now that is not working well and what are the valid alternatives to reduce the costs for delivering care of optimal quality. Only when such feedback information becomes available in sufficient scope and volume can medicine and government come to see what rationally needs to be done to change things for the better and how to go about doing it. Systematic medical peer review is the best candidate to become that needed feedback mechanism. And this brings us, of course, to the question of just how good peer review is or is likely to become, and that is the subject of the rest of this book.

We conclude this chapter as we began it—with a statement of belief that unprecedented pressures for change in the health care system have come at the same time that the availability of both the care technology and the evaluation technology have made it possible to purposefully shape the future evolution of medicine. What greater challenge or opportunity has medicine ever faced?

REFERENCES

1. U.S. Dept. of Health, Education, and Welfare, Public Health Service: Forward plan for health FY 1977-81, publ. no. (OS)-76-50024, August 1975, p. 143.
2. Singer, C., and Underwood, E. A.: A short history of medicine, ed. 2, New York, 1962, Oxford University Press.
3. Major, R. H.: A history of medicine, Springfield, Ill., 1954, Charles C Thomas, Publisher, p. 5.
4. Martí-Ibáñez, F.: History of medicine. In Encyclopedia Americana, New York, 1965, Americana Corporation, vol. 18.
5. Osler, W.: The evolution of modern medicine, Sillman Foundation Lectures at Yale in April 1913, New Haven, Conn., 1921, Yale University Press, p. 7.
6. Davidson, G. R.: Medicine through the ages, London, 1968, Methuen & Co.
7. Wilcocks, C.: Medical advance, public health, and social evolution, Oxford, 1965, Pergamon Press, p. 16.
8. Camac, C. N. B.: Imnhotep to Harvey: backgrounds of medical history, New York, 1931, Paul B. Hoeber.
9. Davis, N. S.: History of medicine with the code of medical ethics. Chicago, 1907. Cleveland Press.
10. Clark-Kennedy, A. E.: The art of medicine in relation to the progress of thought, Cambridge, Mass., 1945, The Macmillan Co., p. 14.
11. Buck, A. H.: The growth of medicine from the earliest times to about 1800, New Haven, Conn., 1917, Yale University Press, p. 132.
12. Fishbein, M.: Frontiers of medicine, New York, 1933, Century Co., p. 27.
13. Norton, A.: The new dimensions of medicine, London, 1969, Hodder and Stoughton.
14. U.S. Dept. of Health, Education, and Welfare, Public Health Service: Monthly vital statistics report, annual summary for the United States, 1974.
15. Thorner, R. M.: Health program evaluation in relation to health programming, Techn. Rep. **86:**525-532, 1971.
16. Solomon, M., and Ferber, B.: Patterns of repeated hospital admissions: Blue Cross and Blue Shield federal employees program: July 1960-December 1965, Blue Cross Rep. **6:**1-11, 1968.
17. Hanlon, C. R.: Shattuck lecture—the physician and organized medicine, N. Engl. J. Med. **284:** 1131-1134, 1971.
18. The Columbus Dispatch, Columbus, Ohio, vol. 105, no. 287, April 12, 1976.
19. Lewis, C. E., and Keairnes, H. W.: Controlling costs of medical care by expanding insurance coverage, N. Engl. J. Med. **282:**1405-1414, 1970.
20. Public Law 92-603, section 249F, Title II, 1972 amendments, Social Security Act, p. 105.
21. Curtis, P.: Problems in primary care, Update Int., pp. 296-298, 1974.
22. Kennedy, E. M.: In critical condition, the crisis in America's health care, New York, 1972, Simon & Schuster, p. 181.
23. Schieber, G. J., Burney, I. L., Golden, J. B., and Knaus, W. A.: Physician fee patterns under Medicare: a descriptive analysis, N. Engl. J. Med. **294:**1089-1093, 1976.
24. Kendall, M., and Haldi, J.: The medical malpractice insurance market, report no. SCMM-NP-IM (summary), Rockville, Md., 1972, U.S. Dept. of Health, Education, and Welfare.
25. Holman, H. R.: The "excellence" deception in medicine, Hosp. Prac., pp. 11-21, 1976.
26. Davidson, G. R.: Medicine through the ages, London, 1968, Methuen & Co., p. 59.
27. Andersen, R., and Riedel, D. C.: Comparisons of the uninsured, those with one policy, and those with multiple coverage, Blue Cross Rep. **5:**1-8, 1967.
28. Abelson, P. H.: Cost-effective health care, Science **192:**620, 1976.
29. Cohen, W. J.: Current problems in health care, N. Engl. J. Med. **281:**193-198, 1969.
30. Iglehart, J. K.: Health report: explosive rise in medical costs puts government in quandary. Natl. J., pp. 1319-1328, 1975.
31. Jackson, D. D.: Play, paradox, and people: comprehensive medicine, Med. Op. Rev., pp. 84-90, 1967.
32. Harrington, E. D.: A major pitfall: inadequate assessment of the patient's needs resulting in inappropriate treatment, Pediatr. Clin. North Am. **12:**141-173, 1965.
33. Somers, H. M., and Somers, A. R.: The paradox of medical progress, N. Engl. J. Med. **266:**1253, 1962.
34. Clark-Kennedy, A. E.: The art of medicine in relation to the progress of thought, Cambridge, Mass., 1945, The Macmillan Co.

35. Annas, G. J.: Don't blame lawyers for malpractice mess, Am. Med. News, March 3, 1975, p. 8.
36. Murdy, W. H.: Anthropocentrism: a modern version, Science **187:**1168-1172, 1975.
37. Donabedian, A.: Promoting quality through evaluating the process of patient care, Med. Care **6:**181-202, 1968.
38. Thorner, R. M.: Health program evaluation in relation to health programming, Techn. Rep. **86:**525-532, 1971.
39. Johnson, A. T.: Health planning law: what it means to you, Am. Acad. Pediatr. News, pp. 9-12, June 1976.
40. Schwartz, A.: A half century of health progress, Ohio State University Med. J., pp. 58-59, 1975.
41. Lewis, I. J.: Science and health care—the political problem, N. Engl. J. Med. **281:**888-896, 1969.
42. Abse, D.: Medicine on trial, New York, 1969, Crown Publishers.
43. White, K. L., Murnaghan, J. H., and Gaus, C. R.: Technology and health care, N. Engl. J. Med. **287:**1223-1226, 1972.
44. Hiatt, H. H.: Protecting the medical commons: who is responsible? N. Engl. J. Med. **293:**235-241, 1975.
45. Fried, C.: Rights and health care—beyond equity and efficiency, N. Engl. J. Med. **293:**241-245, 1975.
46. Hardin, G.: The tragedy of the commons, Science **163:**1243-1248, 1968.
47. Welch, C. E.: PSRO—pros and cons, N. Engl. J. Med. **290:**1319-1324, 1974.
48. National Academy of Sciences: Health care: there are problems in quality-assurance programs, News Rep. **27:**1-8, 1977.
49. Osborne, C. E., and Thompson, H. C.: Criteria for evaluation of ambulatory health care by chart audit: developing and testing of a methodology (final report of the Joint Committee on Quality Assurance of Ambulatory Health Care for Children and Youth), Pediatrics **56**(suppl.): 625-692, 1975.
50. Donabedian, A.: Evaluating the quality of medical care, Milbank Mem. Fund Q. **44**(166):208, 1966.
51. Mitchel, B. M., and Schwartz, W. B.: The financing of national health insurance, Science **192:** 621-630, 1976.
52. Wilcocks, C.: Medical advance, public health, and social evolution, Oxford, England, 1965, Pergamon Press, p. 258.
53. Williams, B.: A critique of utilitarianism—for and against. Ed. by Smart, J. J. C., and Williams, B., Cambridge, England, 1973, Cambridge University Press, pp. 75-155.
54. Martí-Ibáñez, F.: History of medicine. In Encyclopedia Americana, New York, 1965, vol. 18, p. 561.
55. Goodman, P.: Growing up absurd, New York, 1956, Vintage Books, p. 246.
56. Osler, W.: The evolution of modern medicine, Sillmand Foundation lectures at Yale in April 1913, New Haven, Conn., 1921, Yale University Press.
57. Dunlap, J. T.: Public-private partnership: problems and opportunities, Bull. N.Y. Acad. Med. **45:**1140-1147, 1969.
58. Bell, D.: Science as the imago of the future society, Science **188:**35-38, 1975.
59. Enarson, H. L.: Sobering thoughts about the health professions, Am. Med. News, vol. 19, no. 30, 1976.
60. Watzlawick, P., Weakland, J., and Fisch, R.: Change, New York, 1974, W. W. Norton & Co.
61. Report of the U.S. Senate Committee on Finance, Social Security amendments of 1972, Washington, D.C., 1972, U.S. Government Printing Office, pp. 254-268.
62. White, L. P.: MDs share malpractice fault for not expelling inept doctors, Am. Med. News, p. 8, March 3, 1975.
63. Churchill, E. D.: Medical wants and needs in mature and developing nations, Med. Times **89:** 1169-1176, 1961.
63a. Freymann, J. G.: Leadership in American medicine, N. Engl. J. Med. **270:**710-720, 1964.
64. Culliton, B. J.: Biomedical panel report says the enterprise is basically sound, Science **192:**762, 1976.
65. Kannel, W. B.: The disease of living, Nutr. Today **6:**1-11, 1971.
66. Rushmer, R. F., and Huntman, L. L.: Biomedical engineering, Science **167:**840-844, 1970.
67. Goran, M. J., Roberts, J. S., Kellogg, M. A., Fielding, J., and Jessee, W.: The PSRO hospital review system, Med. Care **13**(suppl.):1-32, 1975.
68. Kuhn, T. S.: The structure of scientific revolutions, ed. 2, Chicago, 1970, University of Chicago Press, p. 92.
69. Ayers, R. U.: Technological forecasting and long-range planning, New York, 1969, McGraw-Hill Book Co.
70. Laszlo, E.: The systems view of the world, New York, 1972, George Braziller.
71. Brody, H.: The systems view of man: implications for medicine, science and ethics, Perspect. Biol. Med., pp. 71-92, Autumn 1973.
72. McNeil, B. J., Keeler, E., and Adelstein, S. J.: Primer on certain elements of medical decision making, N. Engl. J. Med. **293:**211-215, 1975.
73. McNeil, B. J., Varady, P. D., Burrows, B. A., and Adelstein, S. J.: Cost-effectiveness calculations in the diagnosis and treatment of hypertensive renovascular disease, N. Engl. J. Med. **293:**217-221, 1975.
74. McNeil, B. J., and Adelstein, S. J.: The value of case finding in hypertensive renovascular disease, N. Engl. J. Med. **293:**221-226, 1975.
75. Pauker, S. G., and Kassirer, J. P.: Therapeutic

decision making: a cost-benefit analysis, N. Engl. J. Med. **293:**229-234, 1975.

76. Memorandum of the federal court decision concerning constitutionality of professional standards review legislation, Washington, D.C., 1975, U.S. Government Printing Office, pp. 1-17.

77. Jessee, W. F., Munier, W. B., Fielding, J. E., and Goran, M. J.: PSRO an educational force for improving quality care, N. Engl. J. Med. **292:**668-676, 1975.

78. Willett, J. D.: PSRO today: a lawyer's assessment, N. Engl. J. Med. **292:**340-343, 1975.

79. Wallis, W. A.: Will tomorrow's health care be controlled by lawyers? Res. Staff Phys., pp. 43-44, August 1975.

80. Brody, E. B.: The freedom of medical information, ASM News **41:**477-485, 1975.

81. Elsom, K. O.: Elements of the medical process, J.A.M.A. **217:**1226-1232, 1971.

82. Simmons, H. E.: PSRO today: the program's viewpoint, N. Engl. J. Med. **292:**365-366, 1975.

2

Evaluating the quality of medical care

AVEDIS DONABEDIAN

This chapter attempts to describe and evaluate current methods for assessing the quality of medical care and to suggest some directions for further study. It is concerned with methods rather than findings, and with an evaluation of methodology in general rather than a detailed critique of methods in specific studies.

This is not an exhaustive review of the pertinent literature. Certain key studies, of course, have been included. Other studies have been selected only as illustrative examples. Those omitted are not, for that reason, less worthy of note.

This chapter deals almost exclusively with the evaluation of the medical care process at the level of physician-patient interaction. It excludes, therefore, processes primarily related to the effective delivery of medical care at the community level. Moreover, this chapter is not concerned with the administrative aspects of quality control. Many of the studies reviewed here have arisen from the urgent need to evaluate and control the quality of care in organized programs of medical care. Nevertheless these studies will be discussed only in terms of their contribution to methods of assessment and not in terms of their broader social goals. The author

Reprinted with modifications from the *Milbank Memorial Fund Quarterly* **44**(part 2):166-206, 1966. Used by permission of the Milbank Memorial Fund.

has remained, by and large, in the familiar territory of care provided by physicians and has avoided incursions into other types of health care. Also, consideration of the difficult problem of economic efficiency as a measurable dimension of quality has been excluded.

Three general discussions of the evaluation of quality have been very helpful in preparing this review. The first is a classic paper by Mindel Sheps, which includes an excellent discussion of methods.[1] A more recent paper by Peterson provides a valuable appraisal of the field.[2] The paper by Lerner and Riedel[3] discusses one recent study of quality and raises several questions of general importance.

DEFINITION OF QUALITY

The assessment of quality must rest on a conceptual and operationalized definition of what the "quality of medical care" means. Many problems are present at this fundamental level, for the quality of care is a remarkably difficult notion to define. Perhaps the best-known definition is that offered by Lee and Jones[4] in the form of eight "articles of faith," some stated as attributes or properties of the process of care and others as goals or objectives of that process. These articles convey vividly the impression that the criteria of quality are nothing more than value judgments that are applied to several aspects, properties, ingredients, or dimensions of a process called medical care. As such, the definition of quality may be almost anything anyone wishes it to be, although it is ordinarily a reflection of values and goals current in the medical care system and in the larger society of which it is a part.

Few empirical studies delve into what the relevant dimensions and values are at any given time in a given setting. Klein and co-workers[5] found that 24 administrative officials, among them, gave 80 criteria for evaluating patient care. They conclude that patient care, like morale, cannot be considered as a unitary concept and "it seems likely that there will never be a single comprehensive criterion by which to measure the quality of patient care."

Which of a multitude of possible dimensions and criteria are selected to define quality will of course have profound influence on the approaches and methods one employs in the assessment of medical care.

APPROACHES TO ASSESSMENT:
WHAT TO ASSESS
Outcome

The outcome of medical care in terms of recovery, restoration of function, and survival has been frequently used as an indicator of the quality of medical care. Examples are studies of perinatal mortality,[6,7] surgical fatality rates,[8] and social restoration of patients discharged from psychiatric hospitals.[9]

Many advantages are gained by using outcome as the criterion of quality in medical care. The validity of outcome as a dimension of quality is seldom questioned. Nor does any doubt exist as to the stability and validity of the values of recovery, restoration, and survival in most situations and in most cultures, though perhaps not in all. Moreover, outcome tends to be fairly concrete and, as such, seemingly amenable to more precise measurement.

However, a number of considerations limit the use of outcome as a measure of the quality of care. The first of these is

whether the outcome of care is, in fact, the relevant measure. This is because outcome reflects both the power of medical science to achieve certain results under any given set of conditions and the degree to which scientific medicine, as currently conceived, has been applied in the instances under study. But the object may be precisely to separate these two effects. Sometimes a particular outcome may be irrelevant, as when survival is chosen as a criterion of success in a situation that is not fatal but is likely to produce suboptimal health or crippling.[10]

Even in situations where outcome is relevant and the relevant outcome has been chosen as a criterion, limitations must be reckoned with. Many factors other than medical care may influence outcome, and precautions must be taken to hold all significant factors other than medical care constant if valid conclusions are to be drawn. In some cases long periods of time, perhaps decades, must elapse before relevant outcomes are manifest. In such cases the results are not available when needed for appraisal, and the problems of maintaining comparability are greatly magnified. Also, medical technology is not fully effective, and the measure of success that can be expected in a particular situation is often not precisely known. For this reason comparative studies of outcome, under controlled situations, must be used.

Although some outcomes are generally unmistakable and easy to measure (death, for example), other outcomes not so clearly defined can be difficult to measure. These include patient attitudes and satisfactions, social restoration, and physical disability and rehabilitation.[11] Even the face validity that outcomes generally have as a criterion of success or failure is not absolute. One may debate, for example, whether the prolongation of life under certain circumstances is evidence of good medical care. McDermott and associates have shown that although fixing a congenitally dislocated hip joint in a given position is considered "good medicine for the white man," it can prove crippling for the Navajo Indian who spends much time seated on the floor or in the saddle.[12] Finally, although outcomes might indicate good or bad care in the aggregate, they do not give an insight into the nature and location of the deficiencies or strengths to which the outcomes might be attributed.

These limitations to the use of outcomes as criteria of medical care are presented not to demonstrate that outcomes are inappropriate indicators of quality but to emphasize that they must be used with discrimination. Outcomes, by and large, remain the ultimate validators of the effectiveness and quality of medical care.

Process

Another approach to assessment is to examine the process of care itself rather than its outcomes. This is justified by the assumption that one is interested not in the power of medical technology to achieve results but in whether what is now known to be good medical care has been applied. Judgments are based on considerations such as the appropriateness, completeness, and redundancy of information obtained through clinical history, physical examination, and diagnostic tests; justification of diagnosis and therapeutic procedures, including surgery; evidence of preventive management in health and illness; coordination and continuity of care; acceptability of care to the recipient, and so on. This approach requires that a great deal of attention be given to specifying the relevant dimensions, values, and standards to be used in assessment. The estimates of quality one obtains are less stable and less final than those that derive from the measurement of outcomes. They may, however, be more relevant to the question at hand: whether medicine is properly practiced.

This discussion of process and outcome may seem to imply a simple separation between means and ends. Perhaps more correctly one may think of an unbroken chain of antecedent means followed by intermediate ends, which are themselves the means to still further ends.[13] Health itself may be a means to a further objective. Several authors have pointed out that this formulation provides a useful approach to evaluation.[14,15] It may be designated as the measurement of procedural end points and included under the general heading of "process" because it rests on similar considerations with respect to values, standards, and validation.

Structure

A third approach to assessment is to study not the process of care itself but the settings in which it takes place and the instrumentalities of which it is the product. This may be roughly designated as the assessment of structure, although it may include administrative and related processes that support and direct the provision of care. It is concerned with such things as the adequacy of facilities and equipment, the qualifications of medical staff and their organization, the administrative structure and operations of programs and institutions providing care, fiscal organization, and the like.[16,17] The assumption is made that given the proper settings and instrumentalities, good medical care will follow. This approach offers the advantage of dealing, at least in part, with fairly concrete and accessible information. It has the major limitation that the relationship between structure and process or structure and outcome is often not well established.

Sources and methods of obtaining information

The approach adopted for the appraisal of quality determines in large measure the methods used for collecting the requisite information. Since these range the gamut of social science methods, no attempt will be made to describe them all. Four, however, deserve special attention.

Clinical records are the source documents for most studies of the medical care process. In using them one must be aware of their several limitations. Since the private office practice of most physicians is not readily accessible to the researcher, and the records of such practice are generally disappointingly sketchy, the use of records has been restricted to the assessment of care in hospitals, outpatient departments of hospitals, and prepaid group practice. Both Peterson[18] and Clute[19] have reported the prevailing inadequacies of recording in general practice. In addition, Clute has pointed out that in general practice "the lack of adequate records is not incompatible with practice of a good, or even an excellent quality." On the other hand, a recent study of the office practice of a sample of members of the New York Society of Internal Medicine[20] suggests that abstracts of office records can be used to obtain reproducible judgments concerning the quality of care. But to generalize from this finding is difficult. It concerns a particular group of physicians who are more likely to keep good records than the average. Moreover, for one reason or another the original sample drawn for this study suffered a 61% attrition rate.

Assuming the record to be available and reasonably adequate, two further issues to be settled are the veracity and the completeness of the record. Lembcke[10] has questioned whether key statements in the record can be accepted at face value. He has questioned not only the statements of physicians about patients and their management but also the validity of the reports of diagnostic services. The first is verified by seeking in the record, including the nurses' notes, what appears to be the most valid evidence of the true state of affairs. The second is verified by having competent judges reexamine the evidence (films, tracings, slides) on which diagnostic reports are made. Observer error tends to be a problem under the best of circumstances.[21] But nothing can remove the incredulity from the finding by Lembcke, in one hospital, that the true incidence of uterine hyperplasia was between 5% and 8% rather than 60% to 65% of uterine curettages, as reported by the hospital pathologist. In any case the implications of verification as part of the assessment of quality must be carefully considered. Errors in diagnostic reports no doubt reflect particularly on the quality of diagnostic service and on the care provided by the hospital in general. But physicians may be judged to perform well irrespective of whether the data they work with are valid. This is so when the object of interest is the logic that governs physicians' activities rather than the absolute validity of these activities.

Much discussion has centered on the question of the completeness of clinical records and whether, in assessing the quality of care based on what appears in the record, one is rating the record or the care provided. What confuses the issue is that recording is itself a separate and legitimate dimension of the quality of practice, as well as a medium of information for the evaluation of most other dimensions. These two aspects can be separated when an alternative source of information about the process of care is available, such as the direct observation of practice.[18,19] In most instances, however, they are confounded. Rosenfeld[22] handled the problem of separating recording from care by examining the reasons for downrating the quality of care in each patient record examined. He demonstrated that the quality of care was rated down partly because of what could have been poor recording (presumptive evidence) and partly for reasons that could not have been a matter of recording (substantial evidence). He also found that hospitals tended to rank high or low on both types of errors, showing that these errors were correlated. Since routine recording is more likely to be complete in the wards, comparison of ward and private services in each hospital by type of reason for downrating might have provided further information on this important question. Other investigators have tried to allow for incompleteness in the record by supplementing it with interviews with the attending physician and making appropriate amendments.[23-25] Unfortunately only one of these studies (length of stay in Michigan hospitals) contains a report of what difference this additional step made. In this study "the additional medical information elicited by means of personal interviews with attending physicians was of sufficient importance in 12.6 per cent of the total number of cases studied to warrant a reclassification of the evaluation of necessity for admission and/or the appropriateness of length of stay."[3,25] When information obtained by interview is used to amend or supplement the patient record, the assumption may have to be made that this additional information has equal or superior validity. Morehead, who has had extensive experience with this method, said: "many of the surveyors engaged in the present study employed the technique of physician interview in earlier studies without fruitful results . . . The surveyor was . . . left in the uncomfortable position of having to choose between taking at face value statements that medical care was indeed optimal, or concluding that statements presented were untrue."[26] Even in an earlier study where supplementation by interview is reported to have been used,[24] verbal information was discarded unless it was further corroborated by the course of action or by concrete evidence.[27]

Another question of method is whether the entire record or abstracted digests of it should be used as a basis for evaluation. The question arises because summaries and abstracts can presumably be prepared by less skilled persons allowing the hard-to-get expert to concentrate on the actual task of evaluation. Abstracting, however, seemingly involves the exercise of judgment as to relevance and importance. For that reason it has been used as a first step in the evaluation of quality only in those studies that use specific and detailed standards.[10] Even then little information is available about how reliable the process of abstracting is, or how valid it is when compared with a more expert reading of the chart. The study of New York internists demonstrated a high level of agreement between physicians and highly trained nonphysicians abstracting the same office record.[20]

While the controversy about the record as a source of information continues, some have attempted to reduce dependence on physicians' recording habits by choosing for evaluation diagnostic categories that are likely to be supported by recorded evidence additional to the physicians' entries.[28] This explains, in part, the frequent use of surgical operations as material for studies of quality.

In general practice, patient records are inadequate to serve as a basis for evaluation. The alternative is direct observation of physicians' activities by well-qualified colleagues.[18,19] The major limitation of this method would seem to be the changes likely to occur in the usual practice of physicians who know they are being observed. This has been countered by assurances that physicians often are unaware of the true purpose of the study, become rapidly accustomed to the presence of the observer, and are unable to change confirmed habits of practice. Even if changes do occur, they would tend to result in an overestimate of quality rather than the reverse. These assurances notwithstanding, measuring the effect of observation on practice remains an unsolved problem.

Those who have used the method of direct observation have been aware that the problem of completeness is not obviated. Practicing physicians often know a great deal about their patients from previous contacts, hence the need to select for observation new cases and situations that require a thorough examination irrespective of the patient's previous experience. Moreover, not all of the managing physicians' activities are explicit. Some dimensions of care not subject to direct observation must be excluded from the scheme of assessment. Selective perception by the observer may be an additional problem. The observer is not likely to be first a neutral recorder of events and then a judge of these same events. His knowledge and criteria are likely to influence what he perceives and thus to introduce a certain distortion into perception.

An indirect method of obtaining information is to study behaviors and opinions from which inferences may be drawn concerning quality. A sociometric approach has been reported by Maloney et al.,[29] which assumes that physicians, in seeking care for themselves and their families, exhibit critical and valid judgments concerning the capacity of their colleagues to provide high quality care. Such choices were shown to identify classes of physicians presumed to be more highly qualified than others. But both sensitivity and specificity, using as criterion more rigorous estimates of the quality of care, lack validation. Georgopoulos and Mann[30] used what might be called an "autoreputational"* approach in assessing the quality of care in selected community hospitals. This grew out of previous studies showing that people are pretty shrewd judges of the effectiveness of the organizations in which they work.[31] The hospitals were rated and ranked concerning the quality of medical care and other characteristics using opinions held by managerial, professional, and technical persons working in or connected with each hospital, as well as by knowledgeable persons in the community. The responses were sufficiently consistent and discriminating to permit the hospitals to be ranked with an apparently satisfactory degree of reliability despite the generally self-congratulatory nature of the responses that classified the quality of medical care in the hospitals as very good, excellent, or outstanding in 89% of cases and poor in almost none. The authors provide much evidence that the several opinions, severally held, were intercorrelated to a high degree. But little evidence supports the validity of the judgments by using truly external criteria of the quality of care.

SAMPLING AND SELECTION

The first issue in sampling is to specify precisely the universe to be sampled, which

*One of my students, Arnold D. Kaluzny, helped me coin this word.

in turn depends on the nature of the generalizations one wishes to make. Studies of quality are ordinarily concerned with one of three objects: (1) the actual care provided by a specified category of providers of care, (2) the actual care received by a specified group of people, and (3) the capacity of a specified group of providers to provide care. In the first two instances representative samples of potential providers or recipients are required, as well as representative samples of care provided or received. In the third instance a representative sample of providers is needed, but not necessarily a representative sample of care. A more important aspect is to select, uniformly of course, significant dimensions of care. Perhaps performance should be studied in certain clinical situations that are particularly stressful and therefore more revealing of latent capacities or weaknesses in performance. Hypothetical test situations may even be set up to assess the capacity to perform in selected dimensions of care.[32-34]

The distinctions made above, and especially those between the assessment of actual care provided and of the capacity to provide care, are useful in evaluating the sampling procedures used in the major studies of quality. By these criteria some studies belong in one category or another, but some seem to combine features of several in such a way that generalization becomes difficult. For example, in the first study of the quality of care received by Teamster families the findings are meant to apply only to the management of specific categories of hospitalized illness in a specified population group.[28] In the second study of this series somewhat greater generalizability is achieved by obtaining a representative sample (exclusive of seasonal variation) of all hospitalized illness in the same population group.[26] Neither study is meant to provide information about all the care provided by a representative sample of physicians.

The degree of homogeneity in the universe to be sampled is of course important in any scheme of sampling or selection. The question that must be asked is to what extent the care provided by physicians maintains a consistent level. Do specific diagnostic categories, levels of difficulty, or dimensions of care exist in which physicians perform better than in others? Can one find, in fact, an "overall capacity for goodness in medical care,"[18] or is one dealing with a bundle of fairly disparate strands of performance? One might similarly ask whether the care provided by all subdivisions of an institution are at the same level in absolute terms or in relation to performance in comparable institutions. Makover, for example, makes an explicit assumption of homogeneity when he writes: "No attempt was made to relate the number of records to be studied to the size of enrollment of the medical groups. The medical care provided to one or another individual is valid evidence of quality and there should be little or no chance variation which is affected by adjusting the size of the sample."[23] Rosenfeld began his study with the hypothesis "that there is a correspondence in standards of care in the several specialties and for various categories of illness in an institution."[22]

The empirical evidence concerning homogeneity is not extensive. Both the Peterson and Clute studies of general practice[18,19] showed a high degree of correlation between performance of physicians in different components or dimensions of care (history, physical examination, treatment). Rosenfeld demonstrated that the differences in quality ratings among several diagnoses selected within each area of practice (medicine, surgery, and obstetrics-gynecology) were not large. Although the differences among hospitals by area of practice appeared by inspection to be larger, they were not large enough to alter the rankings of the three hospitals studied.

The two studies of care received by Teamster families[26,28] arrived at almost identical proportions of optimal and less than optimal care for the entire populations studied. This must have been coin-cidental, since the percentage of optimal care in the second study varied greatly by diagnostic category from 31% for medicine to 100% for ophthalmology (nine cases only). If such variability exists, the "diagnostic mix" of the sample of care must be a matter of considerable importance in assessment. In the two Teamster studies, differences in "diagnostic mix" were thought to have resulted in lower ratings for medicine and higher ratings for obstetrics-gynecology in the second study than in the first. That the same factor may produce effects in two opposite directions is an indication of the complex interactions the researcher must consider. "The most probable explanation for the ratings in medicine being lower in the present [second] study is the nature of the cases reviewed." The factor responsible is less ability to handle illness "which did not fall into a well recognized pattern." For obstetrics and gynecology the finding of the second study "differed in one major respect from the earlier study where serious questions were raised about the management of far more patients. The earlier study consisted primarily of major abdominal surgery, whereas this randomly selected group contained few such cases and had more patients with minor conditions."[26] In studies such as these where the care received by total or partial populations is under study, the variations noted stem partly from differences in diagnostic content and partly from institutionalized patterns of practice associated with diagnostic content. For example, all nine cases of eye disease received optimal care because "this is a highly specialized area, where physicians not trained in this field rarely venture to perform procedures."[26]

Sampling and selection influence and are influenced by a number of considerations in addition to generalization and homogeneity. The specific dimensions of care that interest one (preventive management or surgical technique, to mention two different examples) may dictate the selection of medical care situations for evaluation. The situations chosen are also related to the nature of the criteria and standards used and of the rating and scoring system adopted. Attempts to sample problem situations, rather than traditional diagnoses or operations, can be difficult because of the manner in which clinical records are filed and indexed. This is unfortunate because a review of operations or established diagnoses gives an insight into the bases on which the diagnosis was made or the operation performed. It leaves unexplored a complementary segment of practice, namely the situations in which a similar diagnosis or treatment may have been indicated but not made or performed.

Measurement standards

Measurement depends on the development of standards. In the assessment of quality, standards derive from two sources.

Empirical standards are derived from actual practice and are generally used to compare medical care in one setting with that in another, or with statistical averages and ranges obtained from a large number of similar settings. The Professional Activities Study is based in part on this approach.[35]

Empirical standards rest on demonstrably attainable levels of care and for that reason enjoy a certain degree of credibility and acceptability. Moreover, without clear normative standards, empirical observations in selected settings must be made to serve the purpose. An interesting example is provided by Furstenberg et al.,[36] who used patterns of prescribing in medical care clinics and outpatient hospitals as the standard to judge private practice.

In using empirical standards one needs some assurance that the clinical material in the settings being compared is similar. The Professional Activities Study makes some allowance for this by reporting patterns of care for hospitals grouped by size. The major shortcoming, however, is that care may appear to be adequate in comparison to that in other situations and yet fall short of what is attainable through the full application of current medical knowledge.

Normative standards derive in principle from the sources that legitimately set the standards of knowledge and practice in the dominant medical care system. In practice they are set by standard textbooks or publications,[10] panels of physicians,[25] highly qualified practitioners who serve as judges,[26] or a research staff in consultation with qualified practitioners.[22] Normative standards can be put very high and represent the best medical care that can be provided, or they can be set at a more modest level signifying acceptable or adequate care. In any event their distinctive characteristic is that they stem from a body of legitimate knowledge and values rather than from specific examples of actual practice. As such, they depend for their validity on the extent of agreement concerning facts and values within the profession or at least among its leadership. Where equally legitimate sources differ in their views, judgments concerning quality become correspondingly ambiguous.

The relevance of certain normative standards developed by one group to the field of practice of another group has been questioned. For example, Peterson and Barsamian report that although spermatic fluid examination of the husband should precede surgery for the Stein-Leventhal syndrome, not one instance of such examination was noted and that this requirement was dropped from the criteria for assessment.[37] Dissatisfaction has also been voiced concerning the application to general practice of standards and criteria elaborated by specialists who practice in academic settings. The major studies of general practice have made allowances for this. Little is known, however, about the strategies of good general practice and the extent to which they are similar to or different from the strategies of specialized practice in academic settings.

Some researchers have used both normative and empirical standards in the assessment of care. Rosenfeld used normative standards but included in his design a comparison between university-affiliated and community hospitals. "Use of the teaching hospital as a control provides the element of flexibility needed to adjust to the constantly changing scientific basis of the practice of medicine. No written standards, no matter how carefully drawn, would be adequate in five years."[22] Lembcke used experience in the best hospitals to derive a corrective factor that softens the excessive rigidity of his normative standards. This factor, expressed in terms of an acceptable percentage of compliance with the standard, was designed to take account of contingencies not foreseen in the standards themselves. It does, however, have the effect of being more realistically permissive as well. This is because the correction factor is likely to be made up partly of acceptable departures from the norm and partly of deviations that might be unacceptable.

Standards can also be differentiated by the extent of their specificity and directiveness. At one extreme the assessing physician may be simply instructed as follows: "You will use as a yardstick in relation to the quality of care rendered, whether you would have treated this particular patient in this particular fashion during this specific hospital admission."[26] At the other extreme a virtually watertight logic system may be constructed that specifies all the decision rules that are acceptable to justify diagnosis and treatment.[37,38] Most cases fall somewhere in between.

Highly precise and directive standards are associated with the selection of specific diagnostic categories for assessment. When a representative sample of all the care provided is to be assessed, little more than general guides can be given to the assessor. Lembcke, who has stressed the need for specific criteria, has had to develop a correspondingly detailed diagnostic classification of pelvic surgery, for example.[10] In addition to diagnostic specificity, highly directive standards are associated with the preselection of specific dimensions of care for evaluation. Certain diagnoses, such as surgical operations, lend themselves more readily to this approach. This is evident in Lembcke's attempt to extend his system of audits to nonsurgical diagnoses.[39] The clear, almost rule-of-thumb judgments of adequacy become blurred. The data abstracted under each diagnostic rubric are more like descriptions of patterns of management with insufficient normative criteria for decisive evaluation. The alternative adopted is comparison with a criterion institution.

Obviously the more general and nondirective the standards are, the more one must depend on the interpretations and norms of the person entrusted with the actual assessment of care. With greater specificity the research team is able, collectively, to exercise much greater control over what dimensions of care require emphasis and what the acceptable standards are. A great deal appears in common between the standards used in structured and unstructured situations as shown by the degree of agreement between intuitive ratings and directed ratings in the Rosenfeld study[22] and between the qualitative and quantitative ratings in the study by Peterson et al.[18] Indeed, standards used in qualitative and quantitative ratings were so similar that they could be used interchangeably.

When standards are not specific and the assessor must exercise personal judgment in arriving at an evaluation, expert and careful judges must be used. Lembcke claims that a more precise and directive system such as his does not require expert judges. "It is said that with a cookbook, anyone who can read can cook. The same is true, and to about the same extent, of the medical audit using objective criteria; anyone who knows enough medical terminology to understand the definitions and criteria can prepare the case abstracts and tables for the medical audit. However, the final acceptance, interpretation and application of the findings must be the responsibility of a physician or group of physicians."[40] The "logic system" developed by Peterson and Barsamian appears well suited for rating by computer once the basic facts have been assembled, presumably by a record abstractor.[37, 38]

The dimensions of care and the values one uses to judge them are of course embodied in the criteria and standards used to assess care.* These standards can therefore be differentiated by their selectivity and inclusiveness in the choice of dimensions to be assessed. The dimensions selected and the value judgments attached to them constitute the operationalized definition of quality in each study.

The preselection of dimensions makes possible, as already pointed out, the development of precise procedures, standards, and criteria. Lembcke[10] has stressed the need for selecting a few specific dimensions of care within specified diagnostic categories rather than attempting general evaluations of unspecified dimensions that, he feels, lack precision. He uses dimensions such as the following: confirmation of clinical diagnosis, justification of treatment (including surgery), and completeness of the surgical procedure. Within each dimension, and for each diagnostic category, one or more previously defined activities are often used to characterize performance for that dimension as a whole. Examples are the compatibility of the diagnosis of pancreatitis with serum amylase levels or of liver cirrhosis with biopsy findings, the performance of sensitivity tests prior to antibiotic therapy in acute bronchitis, and the control of blood sugar levels in diabetes.

In addition to the extent to which preselection of dimensions takes place, assessments of quality differ with respect to the number of dimensions used and the exhaustiveness with which performance in each dimension is explored. For example, Peterson et al.[18] and Rosenfeld[22] use a

large number of dimensions. Peterson and Barsamian,[37, 38] on the other hand, concentrate on two basic dimensions, justification of diagnosis and of therapy, but require complete proof of justification. A more simplified approach is illustrated by Huntley et al.,[41] who evaluate outpatient care using two criteria only: the percentage of work-ups (not including certain routine procedures) and the percentage of abnormalities found that were not followed up.

Judgments of quality are incomplete when only a few dimensions are used and decisions about each dimension are made on the basis of partial evidence. Some dimensions, such as preventive care or the psychological and social management of health and illness, are often excluded from the definition of quality and the standards and criteria that make it operational. Examples are the intentional exclusion of psychiatric care from the Peterson study[18] and the planned exclusion of the patient-physician relationship and the attitudes of physicians in studies of the quality of care in the Health Insurance Plan of Greater New York.[27] Rosenfeld[22] made a special point of including the performance of specified screening measures among the criteria of superior care, but care was labeled good in the absence of these measures. In the absence of specific instructions to the judges, the study by Morehead et al.[26] includes histories of cases considered to have received optimal care in which failure of preventive management could have resulted in serious consequences to the patient.

Another characteristic of measurement is the level at which the standard is set. Standards can be so strict that none can comply with them, or so permissive that all are rated good. For example, in the study of general practice reported by Clute,[19] blood pressure examinations, measurement of body temperature, otoscopy, and performance of immunizations did not categorize physicians because all physicians performed them well.

---

*The dimensionality of the set of variables incorporating these standards remains to be determined.

Measurement scales

The ability to discriminate different levels of performance depends on the scale of measurement used. Many studies of quality use a small number of divisions to classify care, seen as a whole, into categories such as excellent, good, fair, or poor. A person's relative position in a set can then be further specified by computing the percentage of cases in each scale category. Other studies assign scores to performance of specified components of care and cumulate these to obtain a numerical index usually ranging from 0 to 100. These practices raise questions relative to scales of measurement and legitimate operations on these scales. Some of these are described below.

Those who adhere to the first practice point out that any greater degree of precision is not possible with present methods. Some have even reduced the categories to only two: optimal and less than optimal. Clute[19] uses three, of which the middle one is acknowledged to be doubtful or indeterminate. Also, medical care has an all-or-none aspect that the usual numerical scores do not reflect. Care can be good in many of its parts and be disastrously inadequate in the aggregate due to a vital error in one component. Of course this is less often a problem if it is demonstrated that performance on different components of care is highly intercorrelated.

Those who have used numerical scores have pointed out that there is much loss of information in the use of overall judgments[37] and that numerical scores, cumulated from specified subscores, give a picture not only of the whole but also of the evaluation of individual parts. Rosenfeld[22] has handled this problem by using a system of assigning qualitative scores to component parts of care and an overall qualitative score based on arbitrary rules of combination that allow for the all-or-none attribute of the quality of medical care. As already pointed out, a high degree of agreement was found between intuitive and structured ratings in the Rosenfeld study[22] and between qualitative and quantitative ratings in the study by Peterson et al.[18]

A major problem yet unsolved in the construction of numerical scores is the manner in which the different components are to be weighted in the process of arriving at the total. At present this is an arbitrary matter. Peterson et al.,[18] for example, arrive at the following scale: clinical history, 30; physical examination, 34; use of laboratory aids, 26; therapy, 9; preventive medicine, 6; clinical records, 2; total, 107. Daily and Morehead[24] assign different weights as follows: records, 30; diagnostic work-up, 40; treatment and follow-up, 30; total, 100. Peterson et al. say: "Greatest importance is attached to the process of arriving at a diagnosis since, without a diagnosis, therapy cannot be rational. Furthermore, therapy is in the process of constant change, while the form of history and physical examination has changed very little over the years."[18] Daily and Morehead offer no justification for their weightings, but equally persuasive arguments could probably be made on their behalf. The problem of seeking external confirmation remains.*

The problem of weights is related to the more general problem of value of items of information or of procedures in the medical care process. Rimoldi et al.[33] used the frequency with which specified items of information were used in the solution of a test problem as a measure of the value of that item. Williamson had experts classify specified procedures, in a specified diagnostic test setting, on a scale ranging from very helpful to very harmful. Individual performance in the test was then rated using quantitative indices of efficiency, proficiency, and overall competence, depending on the frequency and nature of the procedures used.[34]

---

*Peterson et al.[18] attempted to get some confirmation of weightings through the procedure of factor analysis. The mathematically sophisticated are referred to the footnote on pp. 14-15 in their text.

A problem in the interpretation of numerical scores is the meaning of the numerical interval between points on the scale. Numerical scores derived for the assessment of quality are not likely to have the property of equal intervals, and they should not be used as if they had.

Reliability

The reliability of assessments is a major consideration in studies of quality, where so much depends on judgment even when the directive types of standards are used. Several studies have given some attention to agreement between judges. The impression gained is that this is considered to be at an acceptable level. Peterson et al.,[18] on the basis of 14 observer revisits, judged agreement to be sufficiently high to permit all the observations to be pooled together after adjustment for observer bias in one of the six major divisions of care. In the study by Daily and Morehead "several cross-checks were made between the two interviewing internists by having them interview the same physicians. The differences in the scores of the family physicians based on these separate ratings did not exceed 7 per cent."[24] Rosenfeld[22] paid considerable attention to testing reliability and devised mathematical indices of agreement and dispersion to measure it. These indicate a fair amount of agreement, but a precise evaluation is difficult, since no other investigator is known to have used these same measures. Morehead et al.,[26] in the second study of medical care received by Teamster families, report initial agreement between two judges in assigning care to one of two classes in 78% of cases. This was raised to 92% following reevaluation of disagreements by the two judges.

By contrast to between-judge reliability, little has been reported about the reliability of repeated judgments of quality made by the same person. To test within-observer variation, Peterson et al.[18] asked each of two observers to revisit four of his own previously visited physicians. The level of agreement was lower within observers than between observers, partly because revisits lasted a shorter period of time and related, therefore, to a smaller sample of practice.

The major mechanism for achieving higher levels of reliability is the detailed specification of criteria, standards, and procedures used for the assessment of care. Striving for reproducibility was, in fact, a major impetus in the development of the more rigorous rating systems by Lembcke and by Peterson and Barsamian. Unfortunately no comparative studies of reliability exist using highly directive versus nondirective methods of assessment. Rosenfeld's raw data might permit a comparison of reliability of intuitive judgments and the reliability of structured judgments by the same two assessors. Unreported data by Morehead et al.[26] could be analyzed in the same way as those of Rosenfeld[22] to give useful information about the relationship between degree of reliability and method of assessment. The partial data that have been published suggest that the postreview reliability achieved by Morehead et al., using the most nondirective of approaches, is comparable with that achieved by Rosenfeld who used a more directive technique.

Morehead et al. raised the important question of whether the reliability obtained through the detailed specification of standards and criteria may not be gained at the cost of reduced validity. "Frequently, such criteria force into a rigid framework similar actions or factors which may not be appropriate in a given situation due to the infinite variations in the reaction of the human body to illness. . . . The study group rejects the assumption that such criteria are necessary to evaluate the quality of medical care. It is their unanimous opinion that it is as important for the surveyors to have flexibility in the judgment of an individual case as it is for a competent physician when confronting a clinical problem in a given patient."[26]

The reasons for disagreement between judges throw some light on the problems of evaluation and the prospects of achieving greater reliability. Rosenfeld found "that almost half the differences were attributable to situations not covered adequately by standards, or in which the standards were ambiguous. In another quarter differences developed around questions of fact, because one consultant missed a significant item of information in the record. It would therefore appear that with revised standards, and improved methods of orienting consultants, a substantially higher degree of agreement could be achieved."[22] Less than a quarter of the disagreements contain differences of opinion with regard to the requirements of management. This is a function of ambiguity in the medical care system and sets an upper limit of reproducibility. Morehead et al. report that in about half the cases of initial disagreement "there was agreement on the most serious aspect of the patient's care, but one surveyor later agreed that he had not taken into account corollary aspects of patient care".[26] Other reasons for disagreement were difficulty in adhering to the rating categories or failure to note all the facts. Of the small number of unresolved disagreements (8% of all admissions and 36% of initial disagreements), more than half were due to honest differences of opinion regarding the clinical handling of the problem. The remainder arose out of differences in interpreting inadequate records or out of the technical problems of where to assess unsatisfactory care in a series of admissions.[27]

A final aspect of reliability is the occasional breakdown in the performance of an assessor, as so dramatically demonstrated in the Rosenfeld study.[22] The question of what the investigator does when a well-defined segment of his results are so completely aberrant will be raised here without any attempt to provide an answer.

Bias

When several observers or judges describe and evaluate the process of medical care, one of them may consistently employ more rigid standards than another or interpret predetermined standards more strictly. Peterson et al.[18] discovered that one of their observers generally awarded higher ratings than the other in the assessment of performance of physical examination but not in the other areas of care. Rosenfeld[22] showed that, of two assessors, one regularly awarded lower ratings to the same cases assessed by both. An examination of individual cases of disagreement in the study by Morehead et al.[26] reveals that in the medical category the same assessor rated the care at a lower level in 11 out of 12 instances of disagreement. For surgical cases one surveyor rated the care lower than the other in all eight instances of disagreement. The impression is gained from examining the reasons for disagreement on medical cases that one of the judges had a special interest in cardiology and was more demanding of clarity and certainty in the management of cardiac cases.

The clear indication of these findings is that bias must be accepted as the rule rather than the exception and that studies of quality must be designed with this in mind. In the Rosenfeld study,[22] for example, either of the two raters used for each area of practice would have ranked the several hospitals in the same order, even though one was consistently more generous than the other. The Clute study of general practice in Canada,[19] on the other hand, has been criticized for comparing the quality of care in two geographic areas, even though different observers examined the care in the two areas in question.[42] The author was aware of this problem and devised methods for comparing the performance of the observers in the two geographic areas, but the basic weakness remains.

Predetermined order or regularity in

the process of study may be associated with bias. Therefore some carefully planned procedures may have to be introduced into the research design for randomization. The study by Peterson et al.[18] appears to be one of the few to have paid attention to this factor. Another important source of bias is knowledge, by the assessor, of the identity of the physician who provided the care or of the hospital in which the care was given. The question of removing identifying features from charts under review has been raised,[3] but little is known about the feasibility of this procedure and its effects on the ratings assigned. Still another type of bias may result from parochial standards and criteria of practice that may develop in and around certain institutions or schools of medical practice. To the extent that this is or is suspected to be true, appropriate precautions need to be taken in the recruitment and allocation of judges.

Validity

The effectiveness of care in achieving or producing health and satisfaction, as defined for its individual members by a particular society or subculture, is the ultimate validator of the quality of care. The validity of all other phenomena as indicators of quality depends utlimately on the relationship between these phenomena and the achievement of health and satisfaction. Nevertheless, conformity of practice to accepted standards has a kind of conditional or interim validity that may be more relevant to the purposes of assessment in specific instances.

The validation of the details of medical practice by their effect on health is the particular concern of the clinical sciences. In the clinical literature one seeks data on whether penicillin promotes recovery in certain types of pneumonia, anticoagulants in coronary thrombosis, or corticosteroids in rheumatic carditis, what certain tests indicate about the function of the liver, and whether simple or radical mastectomy is the more life-prolonging procedure in given types of breast cancer. From the general body of knowledge concerning such relationships arise the standards of practice, more or less fully validated, by which the medical care process is ordinarily judged.

Intermediate or procedural end points often represent larger bundles of care. Their relationship to outcome has attracted the attention of both the clinical investigator and the student of medical care organization. Some examples of the latter are studies of relationships between prenatal care and the health of mothers and infants[43, 44] and the relationship between multiple screening examinations and subsequent health.[45] An interesting example of the study of the relationship between one procedural end point and another is the attempt to demonstrate a positive relationship between the performance of rectal and vaginal examinations by the physician and the pathologic confirmation of appendicitis in primary appendectomies, as reported by the Professional Activities Study.[46]

Many studies reviewed[18, 19, 23, 26, 28] attempt to study the relationship between structural properties and the assessment of the process of care. Several of these studies have shown, for example, a relationship between the training and qualifications of physicians and the quality of care they provide. The relationship is, however, a complex one, and is influenced by the type of training, its duration, and the type of hospital within which it was obtained. The two studies of general practice[18, 19] have shown additional positive relationships between quality and better office facilities for practice, the presence or availability of laboratory equipment, and the institution of an appointment system. No relationship was shown between quality and membership of professional associations, the income of the physician, or the presence of x-ray equipment in the office. The two studies do not agree fully on the nature of the relationship between quality of practice and whether the physician obtained his training in a teaching hospital or not, the number of hours worked, or the nature of the physician's hospital affiliation. Hospital accreditation, presumably a mark of quality conferred mainly for compliance with a wide range of organizational standards, does not appear, in and of itself, to be related to the quality of care, at least in New York City.[26]

Although structure and process are no doubt related, the few examples cited above indicate clearly the complexity and ambiguity of these relationships. This is the result partly of the many factors involved and partly of the poorly understood interactions among these factors. For example, one could reasonably propose, based on several findings,[26, 37] that both hospital factors and physician factors influence the quality of care rendered in the hospital, but that differences between physicians are obliterated in the best and worst hospital and express themselves in varying degrees in hospitals of intermediate quality.

An approach particularly favored by students of medical care organization is to examine relations between structure and outcome without reference to the complex processes that tie them together. Some examples of such studies already have been cited.[6-9] Others include studies of the effects of reorganizing the outpatient clinic on health status,[47] the effects of intensive hospital care on recovery,[48] the effects of home care on survival,[49] and the effect of a rehabilitation program on the physical status of nursing home patients.[50]* The lack of relationship to outcome in the latter two studies suggests that current opinions about how care should be set up are sometimes less than well established.

This brief review indicates the kinds of evidence pertaining to the validity of the various approaches to the evaluation of quality of care. Clearly the relationships between process and outcome and between structure and both process and outcome are not fully understood. With regard to this the requirements of validation are best expressed by the concept, already referred to, of a chain of events in which each event is an end to the one that comes before it and a necessary condition to the one that follows. This indicates that the means-end relationship between each adjacent pair requires validation in any chain of hypothetical or real events.[51] This is of course a laborious process. More commonly, as has been shown, the intervening links are ignored. The result is that causal inferences become attenuated in proportion to the distance separating the two events on the chain.

Unfortunately, little information is available on actual assessments of quality using more than one method of evaluation concurrently. Makover has studied specifically the relationships between multifactorial assessments of structure and of process in the same medical groups. "It was found that the medical groups that achieved higher quality ratings by the method used in this study were those that, in general, adhered more closely to HIP's Minimum Medical Standards. However, the exceptions were sufficiently marked, both in number and degree, to induce one to question the reliability* of one or the other rating method when applied to any one medical group. It would seem that further comparison of these two methods of rating is clearly indicated."[23]

Since a multidimensional assessment of medical care is a costly and laborious undertaking, the search continues for dis-

---

*These studies also include data on the relationships between structural features and procedural end points. Examples are the effect of clinic structure on the number of outpatient visits[47] and the effect of a home care program on hospital admissions.[49]

---

*Assuming the direct evaluation of process to be the criterion, the issue becomes one of the implications of reliability measures for validity.

crete, readily measurable data that can provide information about the quality of medical care. The data used may be about aspects of structure, process, or outcome. The chief requirement is that they be easily, sometimes routinely, measurable and valid. Among the studies of quality using this approach are those of the Professional Activities Study,[35] Ciocco et al.,[52] and Furstenberg et al.[36]

Such indices have the advantage of convenience, but the inferences drawn from them may be of doubtful validity. Myers has pointed out the many limitations of the traditional indices of the quality of hospital care, including rates of total and postoperative mortality, complications, postoperative infection, cesarean section, consultation, and removal of normal tissue at operation.[53] The accuracy and completeness of the basic information may be open to question. More important still, serious questions may be raised about what each index means, since so many factors are involved in producing the phenomenon it measures. Eislee has pointed out, on the other hand, that at least certain indices can be helpful if used with care.[35]

The search for easy ways to measure a highly complex phenomenon such as medical care may be pursuing a will-o-'the-wisp. The use of simple indices in lieu of more complex measures may be justified by demonstrating high correlations among them.[1] But in the absence of demonstrated causal links this may be an unsure foundation on which to build. On the other hand, each index can be a measure of a dimension or ingredient of care. Judiciously selected multiple indices may therefore constitute the equivalent of borings in a geologic survey that yield sufficient information about the parts to permit reconstruction of the whole. The validity of inferences about the whole will depend of course on the extent of internal continuities in the individual or institutional practice of medicine.

Some problems of assessing ambulatory care

Some of the special difficulties in assessing the quality of ambulatory care have already been mentioned. These include the paucity of recorded information and the prior knowledge by the managing physician of the patient's medical and social history. The first of these problems has led to the use of trained observers and the second to the observation of cases for which prior knowledge is not a factor in current management. The degree of relevance to general practice of standards and strategies of care developed by hospital-centered and academically oriented physicians also has been questioned.

Another problem is the difficulty of defining the segment of care that may be properly the object of evaluation in ambulatory care. For hospital care a single admission is usually the appropriate unit.* In office or clinic practice a sequence of care may cover an indeterminate number of visits, so that identification of the appropriate unit is open to question. Usually the answer has been to choose an arbitrary time period to define the relevant episode of care. Ciocco et al.[52] defined this as the first visit plus 14 days of follow-up. Huntley et al.[41] use a 4-week period after the initial work-up.

CONCLUSIONS AND PROPOSALS

This review has attempted to give an impression of the various approaches and methods that have been used for evaluating the quality of medical care and to point out certain issues and problems these approaches and methods bring up for consideration.

The methods used may easily be said to have been of doubtful value and more frequently lacking in rigor and precision. But how precise do estimates of quality have to be? At least the better methods

---

*Even for hospital care the appropriate unit may include care before and after admission as well as several hospital admissions. (See also reference 3.)

have been adequate for the administrative and social policy purposes that have brought them into being. The search for perfection should not blind one to the fact that present techniques of evaluating quality, crude as they are, have revealed a range of quality from outstanding to deplorable. Tools are now available for making broad judgments of this kind with considerable assurance. This degree of assurance is supported by findings, already referred to, that suggest acceptable levels of homogeneity in individual practice and of reproducibility of qualitative judgments based on a minimally structured approach to evaluation. This is not to say that a great deal does not remain to be accomplished in developing the greater precision necessary for certain other purposes.

One might begin a catalog of needed refinements by considering the nature of the information, which is the basis for judgments of quality. More must be known about the effect of the observer on the practice being observed, as well as about the process of observation itself—its reliability and validity. Comparisons need to be made between direct observation and recorded information both with and without supplementation by interview with the managing physician. Recording agreement or disagreement is not sufficient. More detailed study is needed of the nature of and reasons for discrepancy in various settings. Similarly, using abstracts of records needs to be tested against using the records themselves.

The process of evaluation itself requires further study. A great deal of effort goes into the development of criteria and standards that are presumed to lend stability and uniformity to judgments of quality; and yet this presumed effect has not been empirically demonstrated. How far explicit standardization must go before appreciable gains in reliability are realized is not known. One must also consider whether with increasing standardization so much loss of the ability to account for

unforeseen elements in the clinical situation occurs that one obtains reliability at the cost of validity. Assessments of the same set of records using progressively more structured standards and criteria should yield valuable information on these points. The contention that less well-trained assessors using exhaustive criteria can come up with reliable and valid judgments can also be tested in this way.

Attention has already been drawn in the body of the review to the little that is known about reliability and bias when two or more judges are compared and about the reliability of repeated judgments of the same items of care by the same assessor. Similarly, little is known about the effects on reliability and validity of certain characteristics of judges including experience, areas of special interest, and personality factors. Much may be learned concerning these and related matters by making explicit the process of judging and subjecting it to careful study. This should reveal the dimensions and values used by the various judges and show how differences are resolved when two or more judges discuss their points of view. Some doubt now exists about the validity of group reconciliations in which one point of view may dominate, not necessarily because it is more valid.[1] The effect of masking the identity of the hospital or the physician providing care can be studied in the same way. What is proposed here is not only to demonstrate differences or similarities in overall judgments but to attempt, by making explicit the thought processes of the judges, to determine how the differences and similarities arise and how differences are resolved.

In addition to defects in method, most studies of quality suffer from having adopted too narrow a definition of quality. In general they concern themselves with the technical management of illness and pay little attention to prevention, rehabilitation, coordination of continuity of care, or handling the patient-physician relationship. Presumably the reason for this is that the technical requirements of management are more widely recognized and better standardized. Therefore more complete conceptual and empirical exploration of the definition of quality is needed.

What is meant by "conceptual exploration" may be illustrated by considering the dimension of efficiency that is often ignored in studies of quality. Two types of efficiency might be distinguished: logical and economic. Logical efficiency concerns the use of information to arrive at decisions. Here the issue might be whether the information obtained by the physician is relevant or irrelevant to the clinical business to be transacted. If relevant, one might consider the degree of replication or duplication in information obtained and the extent to which it exceeds the requirements of decision making in a given situation. If parsimony is a value in medical care, the identification of redundancy becomes an element in the evaluation of care.

Economic efficiency deals with the relationships between inputs and outputs and asks whether a given output is produced at least cost. It is, of course, influenced by logical efficiency, since the accumulation of unnecessary or unused information is a costly procedure that yields no benefit. Typically it goes beyond the individual and is concerned with the social product of medical care effort. It considers the possibility that the best medical care for the individual may not be the best for the community. Peterson et al. cite an example that epitomizes the issue: "Two physicians had delegated supervision of routine prenatal visits to office nurses, and the doctor saw the patient only if she had specific complaints."[18] In one sense this may have been less than the best care for each expectant mother. In another sense it may have been brilliant strategy in terms of making available to the largest number of women the combined skills of a medical care team. Cordero, in a thought-provoking paper, has documented the thesis that

when resources are limited, optimal medical care for the community may require less than the best care for its individual members.[54]

In addition to conceptual exploration of the meaning of quality in terms of dimensions of care and the values attached to them, empirical studies are needed of what are the prevailing dimensions and values in relevant population groups.[5] Little is known, for example, about how physicians define quality, nor is the relationship known between the physician's practice and his own definition of quality. This is an area of research significant to medical education as well as quality. Empirical studies of the medical care process should also contribute greatly to the identification of dimensions and values to be incorporated into the definition of quality.

A review of the studies of quality shows a certain discouraging repetitiousness in basic concepts, approaches, and methods. Further substantive progress, beyond refinements in methodology, is likely to come from a program of research in the medical care process itself rather than from frontal attacks on the problem of quality. This is believed to be so because before one can make judgments about quality, one needs to understand how patients and physicians interact and how physicians function in the process of providing care. Once the elements of process and their interrelationships are understood, one can attach value judgments to them in terms of their contributions to intermediate and ultimate goals. Assume, for example, that authoritarianism-permissiveness is one dimension of the patient-physician relationship. An empirical study may show that physicians are in fact differentiated by this attribute. One might then ask whether authoritarianism or permissiveness should be the criterion of quality. The answer could be derived from the general values of society that may endorse one or the other as the more desirable attribute in social interactions.

This is one form of quality judgment and is perfectly valid, provided its rationale and bases are explicit. The study of the medical care process itself may, however, offer an alternative and more pragmatic approach. Assume, for the time being, that compliance with the recommendations of the physician is a goal and value in the medical care system. The value of authoritarianism or permissiveness can be determined in part by its contribution to compliance. Compliance is itself subject to validation by the higher order criterion of health outcomes. The true state of affairs is likely to be more complex than the hypothetical example given. The criterion of quality may prove to be congruence with patient expectations or a more complex adaptation to specific clinical and social situations rather than authoritarianism or permissiveness as a predominant mode. Also, certain goals in the medical care process may not be compatible with other goals, and one may not speak of quality in global terms but of quality in specified dimensions and for specified purposes. Assessments of quality will not, therefore, result in a summary judgment but in a complex profile, as Sheps has suggested.[1]

A large portion of research in the medical care process will, of course, deal with the manner in which physicians gather clinically relevant information and arrive at diagnostic and therapeutic decisions. This is not the place to present a conceptual framework for research in this portion of the medical care process. Certain specific studies may, however, be mentioned and some directions for further research indicated.

Research on information gathering includes studies of the perception and interpretation of physical signs.[55, 56] Evans and Bybee have shown, for example, that in the interpretation of heart sounds, errors of perception (of rhythm and timing) occurred along with additional errors of interpretation of what was perceived. Faulty diagnosis, as judged by comparison with a criterion, was the result of these two errors.[56] This points to the need for including in estimates of quality information about the reliability and validity of the sensory data on which management in part rests.

The work of Peterson and Barsamian[37, 38] represents the nearest approach to a rigorous evaluation of diagnostic and therapeutic decision making. As such, it is possibly the most significant recent advance in the methods of quality assessment. But this method is based on record reviews and is almost exclusively preoccupied with the justification of diagnosis and therapy. As a result, many important dimensions of care are not included in the evaluation. Some of these are considerations of efficiency and of styles and strategies in problem solving.

Styles and strategies in problem solving can be studied through actual observation of practice, as was done so effectively by Peterson et al. in their study of general practice.[18] A great deal that remains unobserved can be made explicit by asking the physician to say aloud what he is doing and why. This method of *réflexion parlée* has been used in studies of problem solving even though it may in itself alter behavior.[57] Another approach is to set up test situations, such as those used by Rimoldi et al.[33] and by Williamson,[34] to observe the decision-making process. Although such test situations have certain limitations arising out of their artificiality,[58] the greater simplicity and control they provide can be helpful.

At first sight the student of medical care might expect to be helped by knowledge and skill developed in the general field of research in problem solving. Unfortunately no well-developed theoretic base is available that can be exploited readily in studies of medical care. Some of the empiric studies in problem solving might, however, suggest methods and ideas applicable to medical care situations.[57-61] Some of the studies of troubleshooting in electronic equipment in particular show intriguing similarities to the process of medical diagnosis and treatment. These and similar studies have identified behavioral characteristics that can be used to categorize styles in clinical management. They include amount of information collected, rate of seeking information, value of items of information sought as modified by place in a sequence and by interaction with other items of information, several types of redundancy, stereotypy, search patterns in relation to the part known to be defective, tendencies to act prior to amassing sufficient information or to seek information beyond the point of reasonable assurance about the solution, error distance, degrees of success in achieving a solution, and so on.

Decision-making theory may also offer conceptual tools of research in the medical care process. Ledley and Lusted,[62, 63] among others, have attempted to apply models based on conditional probabilities to the process of diagnosis and therapy. Peterson and Barsamian[37, 38] decided against using probabilities in their logic systems for the very good reason that the necessary data (the independent probabilities of diseases and of symptoms and the probabilities of specified symptoms in specified diseases) were not available. But Edwards et al.[64] point out that one can still test efficiency in decision making by substituting subjective probabilities (those of the decision maker himself or of selected experts) for the statistical data one would prefer to have.

A basic question that has arisen frequently in this review is the degree to which performance in medical care is a homogeneous or heterogeneous phenomenon. This was seen, for example, to be relevant to sampling, the use of indices in place of multidimensional measurements, and the construction of scales that purport to judge total performance. When this question is raised with respect to individual physicians, the object of study is the integration of various kinds of knowledge and skills in the personality and behavior of the physician. When it is raised with respect to institutions and social systems, the factors are completely different. Here one is concerned with the formal and informal mechanisms for organizing, influencing, and directing human effort in general and the practice of medicine in particular. Research in all these areas is expected to contribute to greater sophistication in the measurement of quality.

Some of the conventions accepted in this review are in themselves obstacles to more meaningful study of quality. Physicians' services are not, in the real world, separated from the services of other health professionals, nor from the services of a variety of supportive personnel. The separation of hospital and ambulatory care is also largely artificial. The units of care that are the proper objects of study include the contributions of many persons during a sequence that may include care in a variety of settings. The manner in which these sequences are defined and identified has implications for sampling, methods of obtaining information, and standards and criteria of evaluation.

A final comment concerns the frame of mind with which studies of quality are approached. The social imperatives that give rise to assessments of quality have already been referred to. Often associated with these are the zeal and values of the social reformer. Greater neutrality and detachment are needed in studies of quality. More often one needs to ask, "What goes on here?" rather than, "What is wrong, and how can it be made better?" This does not mean that the researcher disowns his own values or social objectives. It does mean, however, that the distinction between values and elements of structure, process, or outcome is recognized and maintained and that both are subjected to equally critical study. Partly to achieve this kind of orientation emphasis must be shifted from preoccupation with evaluating quality to concentration on understanding the medical care process itself.

REFERENCES

1. Sheps, M. C.: Approaches to the quality of hospital care, Public Health Rep. **70:**877-886, 1955.

   This paper represents an unusually successful crystallization of thinking concerning the evaluation of quality. It contains brief but remarkably complete discussions of the purposes of evaluation, problems of definition, criteria and standards, various approaches to measurement, the reliability of qualitative judgments, and indices of quality. The bibliography is excellent.

2. Peterson, L.: Evaluation of the quality of medical care, N. Engl. J. Med. **269:**1238-1245, 1963.

3. Lerner, M., and Riedel, D. C.: The teamster study and the quality of medical care, Inquiry **1:**69-80, 1964.

   The major value of this paper is that it raises questions concerning methods of assessment, including the sampling of populations and diagnostic categories, the use of records and the need for supplementation by interview, the value of detailed standards, the need for understanding the auditing process, the definition of terms and concepts (of "unnecessary admission," for example), and the problems of defining the relevant episode of care.

4. Lee, R. I., and Jones, L. W.: The fundamentals of good medical care, Chicago, 1933, University of Chicago Press.

5. Klein, M. W., et al.: Problems of measuring patient care in the outpatient department, J. Health Hum. Behav. **2:**138-144, 1961.

6. Kohl, S. G.: Perinatal mortality in New York City: responsible factors, Cambridge, Mass., 1955, Harvard University Press.

   This study, sponsored by the New York Academy of Medicine, was an examination by an expert committee of records pertaining to a representative sample of perinatal deaths in New York City. Preventable deaths were recognized and responsibility factors identified, including errors in medical judgment and technique. The incidence of both of these was further related to type of hospital service, type of professional service, and type of hospital, indicating relationships between structure and outcome as modified by the characteristics of the population served.

7. Shapiro, S., et al.: Further observations on prematurity and perinatal mortality in a general population and in the population of a prepaid group practice medical care plan, Am. J. Public Health **50:**1304, 1317, 1960.

8. Lipworth, L., Lee, J. A. H., and Morris, J. N.: Case fatality in teaching and nonteaching hospitals, 1956-1959, Med. Care **1:**71-76, 1963.

9. Rice, C. E., Berger, D. G., Sewall, L. G., and Lemkau, P. V.: Measuring social restoration performance of public psychiatric hospitals, Public Health Rep. **76:**437-446, 1961.

10. Lembcke, P. A.: Medical auditing by scientific methods, J.A.M.A. **162:**646-655, 1956. (Appendices A and B supplied by author.)

    This is perhaps the single best paper that describes the underlying concepts as well as the methods of the highly structured approach developed by Lembcke to audit hospital records. Also included is an example of the remarkable effect that an external audit of this kind can have on surgical practice in a hospital.

11. Kelman, H. R., and Willner, A.: Problems in measurement and evaluation of rehabilitation, Arch. Phys. Med. Rehabil. **43:**172-181, 1962.

12. McDermott, W., et al.: Introducing modern medicine in a Navajo community, Science **131:** 197-205, 280-287, 1960.

13. Simon, H. A.: Administrative behavior, New York, 1961, The Macmillan Co., pp. 62-66.

14. Hutchinson, G. B.: Evaluation of preventive services, J. Chronic Dis. **11:**497-508, 1960.

15. James, G.: Evaluation of public health, Report of the second national conference on evaluation in public health, Ann Arbor, Mich., 1960, The University of Michigan School of Public Health, pp. 7-17.

16. Weinerman, E. R.: Appraisal of medical care programs, Am. J. Public Health **40:**1129-1134, 1950.

17. Goldmann, F., and Graham, E. A.: The quality of medical care provided at the Labor Health Institute, St. Louis, Missouri, St. Louis, 1954, The Labor Health Institute.

    This is a good example of an approach to evaluation based on structural characteristics. In this instance these included the layout and equipment of physical facilities, the competence and stability of medical staff, provisions made for continuity of service centering around a family physician, the scheduling and duration of clinic visits, the content of the initial examination, the degree of emphasis on preventive medicine, and the adequacy of the medical records.

18. Peterson, O. L., et al.: An analytical study of North Carolina general practice: 1953-1954, J. Med. Educ. **31**(pt. 2):1-165, 1956.

    Already a classic, this study is distinguished by more than ordinary attention to methods and rather exhaustive exploration of the relationship between quality ratings and characteristics of physicians, including education training and methods of practice. The findings of this study, and others that have used the same method, raise basic questions about traditional general practice in this and other countries.

19. Clute, K. F.: The general practitioner: a study of medical education and practice in Ontario and Nova Scotia, Toronto, 1963, University of Toronto Press, chap. 1, 2, 16, 17, and 18.

    Since this study uses the method developed by Peterson et al.,[18] it offers an excellent opportunity to examine the generality of relationships between physician characteristics and quality ratings. In addition the reader of this elegantly written volume gets a richly detailed view of general practice in the two areas studied.

20. Kroeger, H. H., Altman, I., Clark, D. A., et al.: The office practice of internists. I. The feasibility of evaluating quality of care, J.A.M.A. **193:** 371-376, 1965.

This is the first of a series of papers based on a study of the practice of members of the New York Society of Internal Medicine. This paper reports findings concerning the completeness of office records, their suitability for judging quality, and the degree of agreement between abstracts of records prepared by physicians and by highly trained nonphysicians. Judgments concerning the quality of care provided are not given. Other papers in this series currently appearing in *The Journal of the American Medical Association* concern patient load (August 23, 1965), characteristics of patients (September 13, 1965), professional activities other than care of private patients (October 11, 1965), and background and form of practice (November 1, 1965).

21. Kilpatrick, G. S.: Observer error in medicine, J. Med. Educ. **38:**38-43, 1963. For a useful bibliography on observer error see Witts, L. H., editor: Medical surveys and clinical trials, London, 1959, Oxford University Press, pp. 39-44.

22. Rosenfeld, L. S.: Quality of medical care in hospitals, Am. J. Public Health **47:**856-865, 1957.

This carefully designed comparative study of the quality of care in four hospitals addresses itself to the problems of methods in the assessment of quality. Here one finds important information about the use of normative and empirical standards, reliability and bias in judgments based on chart review, the correlation between defects in recording and defects in practice, and homogeneity in quality ratings within and between diagnostic categories.

23. Makover, H. B.: The quality of medical care: methodological survey of the medical groups associated with the Health Insurance Plan of New York, Am. J. Public Health **41:**824-832, 1951.

This is possibly the first published report concerning an administratively instituted but research-oriented program of studies of the quality of care in medical groups contracting with the Health Insurance Plan of Greater New York. Unfortunately much of this work remains unpublished. A particular feature of this paper is that it describes and presents the findings of simultaneous evaluation of structure (policies, organization, administration, finances, and professional activities) and process (evaluation of a sample of clinical records).

24. Daily, E. F., and Morehead, M. A.: A method of evaluating and improving the quality of medical care, Am. J. Public Health **46:**848-854, 1956.

25. Fitzpatrick, T. B., Riedel, D. C., and Payne, B. C.: Character and effectiveness of hospital use. In McNerney, W. J., et al.: Hospital and medical economics, Chicago, 1962, Hospital Research and Educational Trust, American Hospital Association, pp. 495-509.

26. Morehead, M. A., et al.: A study of the quality of hospital care secured by a sample of teamster family members in New York City, New York, 1964, Columbia University, School of Public Health and Administrative Medicine.

This study and its companion[28] perform an important social and administrative function by documenting how frequently the care received by members of a union through traditional sources proves to be inadequate. These studies also make a major contribution to understanding the relationships between hospital and physician characteristics and the quality of care they provide. Considered are physician classifications by ownership, medical school affiliation, approval for residency training, and accreditation status. The interactional effects of some of these variables are also explored. In addition this study pays considerable attention to questions of method, including representative versus judgmental sampling of hospital admissions and the reliability of record evaluations by different judges.

27. Morehead, M. A.: Personal communication.

28. Ehrlich, H., Morehead, M. A., and Trussel, R. E.: The quantity, quality, and costs of medical and hospital care secured by a sample of teamster families in the New York area, New York, 1962, Columbia University, School of Public Health and Administrative Medicine.

29. Maloney, M. C., Trussell, R. E., and Elinson, J.: Physicians choose medical care: a sociometric approach to quality appraisal, Am. J. Public Health **50:**1678-1686, 1960.

This study represents an ingenious approach to evaluation through the use of peer judgments in what is believed to be a particularly revealing situation: choice of care for the physician or members of his own family. Some of the characteristics of the physicians and surgeons selected included long-standing personal and professional relationships, recognized specialist status, and medical school affiliation. An incidental pearl of information is that although nine out of ten physicians said everyone should have a personal physician, four out of ten said they had someone whom they considered their personal physician, and only two out of ten had seen their personal physician in the past year!

30. Georgopoulos, B. S., and Mann, F. C.: The community general hospital, New York, 1962, The Macmillan Co.

The study of quality reported in several chapters of this book is based on the thesis that if one wishes to find out about the quality of care provided, all one might need to do is ask the persons directly or indirectly involved in the provision of such care. Although physicians may find this notion naive, the stability and internal consistency of the findings reported in this study indicate that this approach deserves further careful evaluation. A second study of a nationwide sample of general hospitals will attempt to confirm the validity of respondent opinions by comparing them to selected indices of professional activities in each hospital. The findings will be awaited with great interest.

31. Georgopoulos, B. S., and Tannenbaum, A. S.: A study of organizational effectiveness, Am. Sociol. Rev. **22:**534-540, 1957.

32. Evans, L. R., and Bybee, J. R.: Evaluation of student skills in physical diagnosis, J. Med. Educ. **40:**199-204, 1965.

33. Rimoldi, H. J. A., Haley, J. V., and Fogliatto, H.: The test of diagnostic skills, Chicago, 1962, Loyola University Press, Loyola Psychometric Laboratory Publ. no. 25.

    This study is of interest because it uses a controlled test situation to study the performance of medical students and physicians. Even more intriguing is the attempt to approach the question of the value or utility of diagnostic actions in a systematic and rigorous manner. While this particular study does not appear to contribute greatly to understanding the quality of care, this general approach appears to be worth pursuing.

34. Williamson, J. W.: Assessing clinical judgment, J. Med. Educ. **40:**180-187, 1965.

    This is another example of the assessment of clinical performance using an artificial test situation. The noteworthy aspect of the work is the attachment of certain values (helpful or harmful) to a set of diagnostic and therapeutic actions and the development of measures of efficiency, proficiency, and competence based on which actions are selected by the subject in managing the test case. Differences of performance between individual physicians were detected using this method. An unexpected finding was the absence of systematic differences by age, training, or type of practice in groups tested thus far.

35. Eislee, C. W., Slee, V. N., and Hoffmann, R. G.: Can the practice of internal medicine be evaluated? Ann. Intern. Med. **44:**144-161, 1956.

    The authors discuss the use of indices from which inferences might be drawn concerning the quality of surgical and medical management. The indices described include tissue pathology reports in appendectomies, diabetes patients without blood sugar determinations and without chest x-rays, and pneumonia without chest x-rays. A striking finding reported in this paper and others based on the same approach is the tremendous variation by physician and hospital in the occurrence of such indices of professional activity.

36. Furstenberg, F. F., Taback, M., Goldberg, H., and Davis, J. W.: Prescribing as an index to quality of medical care: a study of the Baltimore City medical care program, Am. J. Public Health **43:**1299-1309, 1953.

37. Peterson, O. L., and Barsamian, E. M.: An application of logic to a study of quality of surgical care. Paper read at the fifth IBM medical symposium, Endicott, N.Y., October 7-11, 1963.

    This paper and its companion[38] present a fairly complete description of the logic tree approach to the evaluation of quality. Examples are given to the logic systems for the Stein-Leventhal syndrome and uterine fibromyoma. No data are given on empirical findings using this method.

38. Peterson, O. L., and Barsamian, E. M.: Diagnostic performance. In Jacquez, J. A., editor: The diagnostic process, Ann Arbor, Mich., 1964, University of Michigan Press, pp. 347-362.

39. Lembcke, P. A., and Johnson, O. G.: A medical audit report, Los Angeles, 1963, University of California, School of Public Health (mimeographed).

    This is an extension of Lembcke's method of medical audit to medical diagnostic categories as well as a large number of surgical operations. Although this volume is a compendium of raw data, careful study can provide insights and limitations of the method used by the author.

40. Lembcke, P. A.: A scientific method for medical auditing, Hospitals **33:**65-71, June 16, 1959 and July 1, 1959, pp. 65-72.

41. Huntley, R. R., Steinhauser, R., White, K. L., Williams, T. F., Martin, D. A., and Pasternack, B. S.: The quality of medical care: techniques and investigation in the outpatient clinic, J. Chronic Dis. **4:**630-642, 1961.

    This study provides an example of the application of a routine chart review procedure as a check on the quality of management in the outpatient department of a teaching hospital. Routine procedures often were not carried out and abnormalities that were found were not followed up. A revised chart review procedure seemed to make a significant reduction in the percent of abnormalities not followed up.

42. Mainland, D.: Calibration of the human instrument, notes from a laboratory of medical statistics, No. 81, August 24, 1964 (mimeographed).

43. Joint Committee of the Royal College of Obstetricians and Gynecologists and the Population Investigation Committee: Maternity in Great Britain, London, 1948, Oxford University Press.

44. Yankauer, A., Goss, K. G., and Romeo, S. M.: An evaluation of prenatal care and its relationship to social class and social disorganization, Am. J. Public Health **43:**1001-1010, 1953.

45. Wylie, C. M.: Participation in a multiple screening clinic with five-year follow-up, Public Health Rep. **76:**596-602, 1961.

46. Commission on Professional and Hospital Activities: Medical audit study report 5: primary appendectomies, Ann Arbor, Mich., October 1957, The Commission.

47. Simon, A. H.: Social structure of clinics and patient improvement, Admin. **4:**197-206, 1959.

48. Lockward, H. J., Lundberg, G. A. F., and Odoroff, M. E.: Effect of intensive care on mortality rate of patients with myocardial infarcts, Public Health Rep. **78:**655-661, 1963.

49. Bakst, J. N., and Marra, E. F.: Experiences with home care for cardiac patients, Am. J. Public Health **45:**444-450, 1955.

50. Muller, J. N., Tobis, J. S., and Kelman, H. R.: The rehabilitation potential for nursing home residents, Am. J. Public Health **53:**243-247, 1963.

51. Getting, V. A., et al.: Research in evaluation in public health practices, Paper presented at the 92nd annual meeting, American Public Health Association, New York, October 5, 1964.

52. Ciocco, A., Hunt, H., and Altman, I.: Statistics on clinical services to new patients in medical groups, Public Health Rep. **65:**99-115, 1950.

    This is an early application to group practice of the analysis of professional activities now generally associated with the evaluation of hospital care. The indices used included the recording of diagnosis and treatment, the performance of rectal and vaginal examinations, the performance of certain laboratory examinations, and the use of sedatives, stimulants, and other medications subject to abuse. As is true of hospitals, the groups varied a great deal with respect to these indicators.

53. Myers, R. S.: Hospital statistics don't tell the truth, Mod. Hosp. **83:**53-54, 1954.

54. Cordero, A. L.: The determination of medical care needs in relation to a concept of minimal adequate care: an evaluation of the curative outpatient services in a rural health center, Med. Care **2:**95-103, 1964.

55. Butterworth, J. S., and Reppert, E. H.: Auscultatory acumen in the general medical population, J.A.M.A. **174:**32-34, 1960.

56. Evans, L. R., and Bybee, J. R.: Evaluation of student skills in physical diagnosis, J. Med. Educ. **40:**199-204, 1965.

57. Fattu, N. C.: Experimental studies of problem solving, J. Med. Educ. **39:**212-225, 1964.

58. John, E. R.: Contributions to the study of the problem-solving process, Psychol. Monogr. **71**(18):1-39, 1957.

59. Duncan, C. P.: Recent research in human problem solving, Psychol. Bull. **56:**397-429, 1959.

60. Fattu, N. A., Mech, E., and Kapos, E.: Some statistical relationships between selected response dimensions and problem-solving proficiency, Psychol. Monogr. **68**(6):1-23, 1954.

61. Stolurow, L. M., et al.: The efficient course of action in "trouble shooting" as a joint function of probability and cost, Educ. Psychol. Measurement **15:**462-477, 1955.

62. Ledley, R. S., and Lusted, L. B.: Reasoning foundations of medical diagnosis, *Science* **130:**9-21, 1959.

63. Lusted, L. B., and Stahl, W. R.: Conceptual models of diagnosis. In Jacquez, J. A., editor: The diagnostic process, Ann Arbor, Mich., 1964, University of Michigan Press, pp. 157-174.

64. Edwards, W., Lindman, H., and Phillips, L. D.: Emerging technologies for making decisions. In Newcomb, T. M., editor: New directions in psychology, New York, 1965, Holt, Rinehart and Winston, vol. 2, pp. 261-323.

Discussion

The feasibility of individual versus population level studies. Most of this discussion concentrates on the choice of the aspect of quality set forth in Dr. Donabedian's paper. While his focus on quality in the individual patient-physician relationship was acknowledged to be a traditional concern, a research approach from the standpoint of total target populations was advocated as a broader and more needed framework for studying quality in the future. In such a cast the assessment of quality should include such factors as the distribution, accessibility, and use of medical services relating, among other things, to the efficiency of providing and delivering services. Even though no new facilities become available, the quality of medical care received by particular population groups may change simply through a different pattern of use. While Dr. Donabedian provides examples of how the best quality of care for the individual may not be the best care for a community, unfortunately he does not develop this concept further but remains within the framework of the behavior of the individual patient and physician.

In reply Dr. Donabedian contends that if quality of care were defined to include the total medical care system and target populations, all research in health services involving values would become research into quality. The meaning of quality would lose the little precision it has and would be even more difficult to study than it is already. Introducing utilization and other socioeconomic variables would greatly multiply the factors to be integrated. Emphasis now should be placed on studies at the individual patient-physician level or on studies of the kinds of medical services offered to the public; the more complex variables could be introduced in subsequent investigations.

The most reputable findings in the social sciences appear to stem from studies of groups rather than of individuals. Likewise the natural sciences deal with the interactions of large populations. Similarly, while studies of the educationsl process at the individual pupil-teacher relationship have not been revealing, they have succeeded with remarkable precision in replicating relationships between settings, administrative structures, and outcomes. Since the whole patient care process cannot be brought into view and related even to a profile of outcomes, the study of process at the level of individual interactions would have to stop at immediate microcriteria and would not be fruitful. While complex variables do enter into the study of both the individual patient-physician relationship and populations at risk, the research problem is more within the investigator's grasp if populations rather than individuals are the object of study.

The importance of medical care outcomes. Also disputed is Dr. Donabedian's assumption that the more promising research strategy lies in studying process rather than outcome. The overall social circumstances in which medical care is provided today requires concentration on the issues and goals of the system and on outcomes rather than process. While the discussion brought out the difficulties of using the outcome approach, the obstacles are not considered insuperable. The difficulties cited by Dr. Donabedian reflected more on the ability of the investigators to define criteria relevant to the populations studied than on the power or desirability of the outcome approach. Divorced from the issue of context, any branch of study could be overwhelmed with methodologic problems. Acceptance of a margin of error is basic to all research, and the real methodologic issue for investigation concerns the degree of interference that bias can exert on conclusions concerning quality of care. Such determinations of the significant methodologic problems cannot be made in the abstract without discussion of the specific issues and goals of evaluating quality of care. Had Dr. Donabedian concentrated more on the issues and values of the medical care system he might have been led to a less pessimistic view of the importance of the outcome approach and to its more extensive treatment. In addition, he might have further clarified the gaps in methodology currently deterring research progress, the compromises that have to be accepted, and the priorities for sharpening existing research tools. While Dr. Donabedian agrees to the validity of introducing organizational changes, for example, and then observing the outcome in terms of care, he feels that such studies possess inherent limitations. The unknown variables involved prohibit generalizations about the ways such outcomes occur. The relationships between changes in settings and changes in outcomes can only be validated through studies of process. Also, outcomes may reflect the effects of two different processes; one that furthers, the other that detracts from good outcome. By themselves outcome studies cannot take account of such cancellation effects.

Since numerous variables other than medical care affect outcome, more research should be devoted to identifying the proportion of outcome that is related to medical care variables. The study of process at the individual level, aggregated to the population, is proposed as a way to define the contribution that medical care makes to outcome. Seen in this way the study of process at the population level would no longer be considered an inferior substitute for the study of outcome.

The need to separate values from the elements of the process. In Dr. Donabedian's opinion the issue is not one of process versus outcome but of choosing in any particular situation what is the most productive thing to do. While the ultimate concern in this field is indeed with outcomes, from certain vantage points he advocates concentrating on process and leaving the validation of the relationship between process and outcome to different kinds of investigators, clinicians in particular.

Furthermore he avoids reference to content issues and to the goals and values of medical care because he specifically argues for the need to separate value judgments from descriptions of the elements of the process. In Dr. Donabedian's opinion the approach to quality which maintains that, for example, continuity of care must constitute good care, is a naive approach. Research should transcend this limited stance and develop methods to define operationally what continuity means and to study its natural history, how and when it manifests itself. The study of the values and goals of the medical care process needs to be approached from a completely different and radically empirical point of view. Particularly important is the need to discover to what extent values in the medical care system agree or contradict each other. Whenever values conflict, medical care cannot be described as simply either good or bad. It can only be characterized as good in terms of certain specific dimensions and bad in terms of other dimensions. The elements of the process must therefore be dissected and understood more clearly before any value judgments can be attached to them in terms of their contribution to certain goals.

3

A matrix for assessing
health care quality

AVEDIS DONABEDIAN

To construct a frame of reference for reviewing the quality of health care let us first assume there are states of function or dysfunction that are the concern of the health professions (Fig. 3-1). Let us further assume that these can be classified as physical-physiologic, psychologic, and social. We could argue interminably about the way these states are classified, as well as about the nature, extent, and order of priority of our legitimate concern for each; and our judgments of quality would hang on the issue. But we shall not pursue this line further, since our current proposal is more illustrative than definitive, and we have yet a long way to go. So we move on to the second feature of our frame of reference, which is the level of aggregation of the patient, using that term to designate the entity for which we care and assume responsibility.

Traditionally this has been the individual patient who has come to us for help, but it could also be (1) the patient's family, (2) the caseload of a physician or institution, (3) a target population, varying in degree of formal definition from a clientele to an enrolled population, (4) a community, or (5) a society. This progression in the aggregation of the patient is the second aspect of the framework.

The third feature is a progression in the aggregation of the provider from (1) a single practitioner, to (2) a variety of professionals standing in various relationships to each other, from unorganized to highly organized, to (3) an institution, (4) a program, or (5) a system of health care. Thus these three features, aspects, or dimensions of our framework can be seen to subdivide the field of quality evaluation into various cells or aggregates of cells. But why the effort to do so? Because our definition of what is to be evaluated and what constitutes quality changes as we shift our attention from cell to cell and from sector to sector in this matrix. Nevertheless there also are threads that weave their way throughout, creating interdependence among the parts and an organic unity in the whole. Part of our purpose will be to show that this is indeed the case, but our major demand of this framework is not merely that it be logically persuasive or empirically valid but that it be useful in understanding the concept we call quality.

Given this frame of reference, let us move on to another organizing notion for which there is no fully appropriate name. We could call it the object or subject of evaluation. A simple trichotomy, structure, process, and outcome, has shown remarkable utility in ordering our thinking about

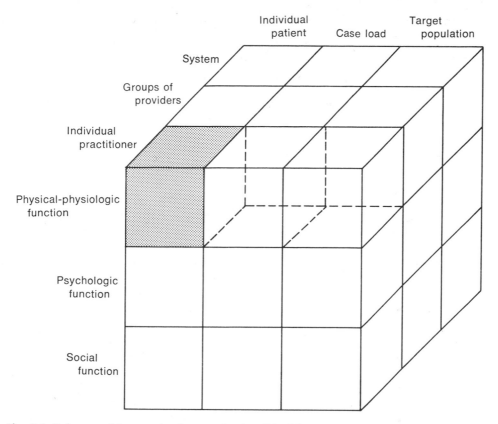

Fig. 3-1. Schema of frame of reference in simplified form. (From Donabedian, A.: Bull. N.Y. Acad. Med. **43:**52, 1967.)

the evaluation of health care quality. This formulation has also prompted important attempts at modification and extension, most notably that by De Geyndt, who has distinguished five approaches to assessing the quality of care: content, process, structure, outcome, and impact.[1] It seems to me that the two classifications are fully congruent and that the differences in detail, important though these are, have arisen from a shift in position within the frame of reference that we took some pains to construct. As one moves from concern with the care provided by one practitioner to that provided by aggregates or organized groupings of practitioners, the process of care appears to become readily differentiated into two components, one of which is what De Geyndt refers to as content. The other component, which would be called con-

figuration but which De Geyndt names process, includes properties such as continuity, coordination, sequencing, and even that yet undefined attribute or set of attributes that one might refer to as "teamhood." Similarly, as one moves from concern for individual patients to concern for a population, the logical category of outcome might bifurcate into end results, which describe states of individuals, and impacts, which describe states of populations taken in the whole. These relationships are schematically represented in Fig. 3-2.

In a more general sense one can postulate that there are different modalities of management and attributes of these modalities that correspond to each of the states of function-dysfunction at the several levels of aggregation. These include what is usually understood to constitute

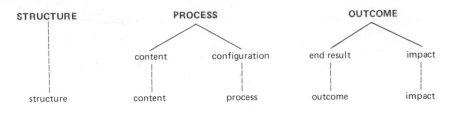

Fig. 3-2. Schematic relationships between concerns for the care of individuals and populations.

the technical management of illness and a variety of methods of managing the interpersonal and social aspects of care, which I can only dimly perceive and for which I have no names. Similarly the outcomes of care that are subject to evaluation would also vary according to dysfunctional state and level of aggregation of the patient. This is why there can be more than one way to view the quality of care. All are equally valid, provided the frame of reference has been properly defined.

Our purpose in all of this has not been to reassure ourselves that structure-process-outcome endures. On the contrary, we believe that the apparent usefulness and the seductive simplicity of this formulation can readily lead to its abuse so that it becomes an obstacle rather than an aid. This happens, for example, when there is insistence on assigning primacy to one of the elements over another. This has generally taken the form of a contest for preeminence between process and outcome; one or the other is held to be of primary importance. In fact, which of the triad is primary and which subsidiary arises from the context (or frame of reference) for evaluation rather than from the elements themselves. In the particular context of evaluating the performance of practitioners in caring for individual patients, I have felt it more appropriate to give primacy to the process of care and to consider structural attributes and outcomes as indirect measures or evidence of the quality of the process—on the assumption that certain attributes of structure are conducive to certain levels of

performance and these, in turn, conducive to the achievement of certain states of the patient. In another context outcome might be the primary object of analysis, and process or structure might be proxy measures of outcome. Few if any have championed the primacy of structure in evaluations of quality of medical care, but I can imagine situations in which the evaluation of structure might well be the primary focus of interest, and that process or outcome might serve as proxy measures of structure.

Besides the observation that each of structure, process, or outcome can serve as the primary focus of inquiry, depending on the context, one observes that aspects of structure, process, and outcome often flow into each other in a linear or branched chain of ends and means.[2,3] Hence we hear of intervening categories such as procedural end points,[4] proximate outcomes, intermediate outcomes, and remote or ultimate outcomes. Again, what segment of the chain is examined and what are the means and what the ends depend on the context. This formulation and the presence of intervening processes and states offer the prospect of reconciliation among formerly opposing positions.

There are problems of specification and measurement with each of the three approaches, or of any intermediate phenomenon. But the major problems in evaluation concern in one guise or another the causality of the relationships among the variables' measures—which itself is the justification for the choice of variables as tools for evaluation. Thus the major problem with the use of characteristics of process is their validity, which usually means their contribution to desired outcomes. Similarly the major problem with outcomes is that of attribution, which means the specification of the contribution to outcomes of the many intercurrent and intervening events that are additional to the care under evaluation. It follows that one of the most urgent needs in quality evaluation today is the development of a set of proximate, situation-specific outcomes that can be used with reasonable confidence for the monitoring of care. Since careful attention to clinically relevant states of the patient is a major characteristic of clinical management, it is difficult to understand why this approach to quality assurance has not received greater attention.

No system of monitoring can rest on attributes of structure, process, or outcome in isolation. Partly this is because we simply do not know enough to put all our eggs in only one of these three baskets. More fundamentally the object of evaluation is not simply measurement but an understanding of how desirable or undesirable results come about, so that action can be taken to encourage the former and prevent the latter. This means that structure, process, and outcome must be observed simultaneously, so that their interrelationships can be examined.

So much for the phenomenon or the category of phenomena, which is the object or subject of evaluation. Next we need to consider briefly what attributes are being evaluated. Under this heading one category is the power of the technology of health services: its ability under optimal conditions to bring about desired states in individuals or groups. There is no agreed-on name for this attribute. It might be called technologic efficacy or effectiveness. Elsewhere I have contended that this is not an object of study in the usual context of quality evaluation; that this is a matter for the clinical researcher

to pursue; that in our context health technology is a given. I suppose one could argue similarly concerning all the other modalities of care that pertain to the dysfunctional states we have identified, except that the technology of these modalities is often so poorly understood that the parallel may not be worth making.

If we have argued correctly, it follows that our particular concern is with the appropriateness of the application of the several modalities of care that correspond to the dysfunctional states for which we have a legitimate responsibility. This involves (1) the proper specification of the health situation, which is called diagnosis, (2) the decision whether to intervene, (3) the choice of the objectives of intervention, (4) the choice of the modalities, methods, and techniques meant to achieve these objectives, and (5) the properly skillful execution of these techniques. These are general categories that in theory apply to all the modalities of care. Almost always, however, attention has focused on the technical management of health states, which is generally regarded to constitute scientific medicine. It is fashionable to decry this restriction. We should remember, however, that this is the technology we understand best, the application of which is our most distinctive function, and which often makes the most difference in situations of acute peril to life and limb. We must be prepared to celebrate, therefore, those who practice "good medicine," even when so narrowly defined. But our best practitioners have always understood that health care is not merely the application of scientific technology but also an interpersonal exchange, which is itself a necessary vehicle for the application of the technology. But the interpersonal exchange has an additional and often deeper significance as a modality for the management of psychologic distress and social maladaptation. Consequently it is important to develop the necessary understanding of the proper role of health practitioners in the psychologic and social domains, of the uses and limitations of the methods available to modify psychologic and social states, and of the attributes that constitute goodness in these methods. This is an important area in the evaluation of the quality of care that has not received the serious and systematic attention it deserves, in spite of the lip service we have so easily offered. The result would be to enrich our concept of quality and almost certainly to bring it closer to the expectations of our clients. But there would be dangers as well. Chief among these is the conflict between our responsibility to the individual as compared to our responsibility to an aggregate of individuals. Whether a case of syphilis is to be reported, whether it is justifiable to engage in activities the chief purpose of which is learning or teaching, whether it is proper to curtail care to the individual to enhance access to greater numbers, whether it is justifiable to increase costs to the individual to reduce the financing program: all these are examples of the conflict between the responsibility of the practitioner to the patient as an individual and to society as a collectivity. Thus as we move from our concern with the evaluation of the technical management of health states at the individual level to the social management of these states at the collective level we are in danger of losing our initial innocence. Until then we thought quality could be built up from low levels to high by increments, each of which contributed positively to the total. Now we are no longer certain, and it looks as if to provide better care for all we may have to provide less good care to some. The concept of quality, no longer benignly seductive, looks us sternly in the face and offers a moral dilemma.

Faced with this dilemma and others of a similar nature, clinical medicine has resolutely looked the other way, seeking refuge in the less ambiguous ethical imperatives that govern the responsibility for the physical or psychologic health of individuals. But social medicine must face squarely the ethical and policy issues that arise out of the application of medical technology to achieve collective goals, for this is its proper and distinctive domain. To discharge its responsibility it must begin where clinical medicine appears to let go and develop a set of concepts and tools at least equal to those of clinical medicine in rigor. The evaluation of quality beyond the traditional management of disease at the individual level and in all its aspects at the collective level depends on this prior development in the conceptual and methodologic apparatus of social medicine. Which is not to say that the efforts to engage in evaluation will not themselves be the occasion and the incentive for the development of the basic science they require to succeed.

No matter what aspect of care is under evaluation, and at what level of aggregation, nothing can be done without criteria and standards of what constitutes degrees of goodness or badness. With respect to structure, our knowledge of such criteria and standards is rudimentary indeed; this is a prime area of research for social medicine to engage in. With respect to outcomes there appears to be a greater degree of agreement on what constitutes desirable states of physical, physiologic, psychologic, or social well-being at the individual and collective levels. However, as one moves within our framework from physical-physiologic to psychosocial, and from individual to collective, it becomes increasingly difficult to agree on what is desirable and therefore is the proper criterion of quality; and without such agreement, no socially legitimate statement concerning quality can be made. But even where there is agreement, so that our criteria enjoy the validity of social consensus, it may not be possible for clinical science to specify with a reasonable degree of certainty what outcomes are to be expected under optimal care.

The usual way of handling this problem is to engage in comparisons of alternative modalities of care under more or less controlled conditions. Another approach, developed by John Williamson, is to ask those who are responsible for care to specify the outcomes they expect at a given interval following the initiation of care for specified illness in the patients whom they have actually treated. The comparison between achievement and expectation, when disappointing, is often though not always a spur to critical self-examination, which should lead to better care.[5] There is the danger of course that by having lower aspirations to begin with, or by revising their expectations downwards after their first confrontation with reality, practitioners will continue in an unwarranted state of self-satisfaction. One antidote to smugness is to contend that the occurrence of any major adverse event that is significantly preventable, given present technology, represents a possible failure, which requires investigation, so that one may determine who or what must carry responsibility for its occurrence. This procedure, which some have called the "critical incident technique," uses each adverse event to evaluate prior care, seeking weaknesses subject to remedy. It is perhaps not overly fanciful to suggest that if a sufficiently broad range of adverse outcomes is identified, including psychologic and social states as well as physical or physiologic, one would have a "retroactive tracer" strategy of evaluation as a complement to the prospective "tracer methodology" formulated by Kessner.[6] One benefit of this would be a keener appreciation and a deeper understanding of all the risk factors that influence the outcomes of care and which must be taken into account in its evaluation.

With respect to the process of care, quality may be simply defined as normative behavior. The issue of course is where the norms come from and how valid they are. In the technical management of individual patients the norms arise ultimately from medical science, which is translated first into the opinions of the human embodiments of that science and then into their practice. We have said that the valid-

ity of medical science is primarily the concern of clinical medicine. But the degree of correspondence between practice and opinion and between opinion and science is central to our concern with evaluation— as is the degree of correspondence between the dictates of the science and our broader social objectives, particularly at the collective level. It is unfortunate that we have had little systematic exploration of this area, but a study reported by Hare and Barnoon offers a fascinating glimpse of what might be in store for the explorer.[7] The study is of the opinions and practice of self-selected members of the American Society of Internal Medicine (located in several regions of the United States) concerning the management of six clinical conditions. It was found that there was reasonable agreement among internists in the several locations concerning the importance of specified procedures in the management of each of the conditions. An analysis of records of office care that were kept specifically for this study showed there was also considerable agreement as to the frequency with which specified procedures were actually performed. All this is reassuring to those who would define quality as normative behavior. What comes as a disquieting surprise is that there is little agreement between the frequency with which procedures were actually performed and the prior estimate of their importance. This may be because freequency and importance are poorly related concepts. An alternative explanation is that physicians do not practice what they know to be good. Still another hypothesis is that actual practice represents an adaptation to a multiplicity of partially conflicting goals at least some of which are socially legitimate. If so, it would mean that the listings of all good procedures in the management of specified conditions represent the dictates of science essentially unmodified by considerations of relative priorities, patient acceptability, resource allocation, and benefits relative to costs. In contrast, the practice of good physicians in favorable settings would represent a more socially relevant standard of care. Having arrived at this hypothesis, it would be tragically dangerous to stop here and use it as a basis for accepting prevalent practice as the standard of care. This is emphatically not the intent. On the contrary, the intent is to stimulate conceptual development and empirical research to determine what styles and strategies of care are optimal in terms of multiple objectives at the individual and collective levels.

Styles and strategies are difficult to pin down. Styles may be defined as habitual ways of management of clinical situations in the behavior of individual practitioners. What is problematic is defining what properties of such behavior can be said to constitute categories of style, what constitutes goodness in style, and with what justification. With respect to problem solving one might suggest categories such as stereotypy or routinization versus flexibility, parsimony versus redundancy, degrees of tolerance of uncertainty, variations in the propensity to take risks, and a preference for type I errors versus type II.[8] With respect to the interpersonal relationship there are equally diverse styles including the hierarchical versus the egalitarian and the directive versus the participatory.[9] As to strategies, I do not know whether these can be clearly differentiated from styles. Possibly, strategies are more complicated game plans that represent a choice among alternatives because they are more likely to achieve a given objective or because they represent an optimal solution in the achievement of several partially competing objectives. Both styles and strategies are not simply aggregates of behavior but organizationally related configurations of behavior that require recognition and classification as organized wholes. Central to their evaluation is the recognition of the goals they pursue, monetary and nonmonetary, their success in achieving these goals, and their costs.

What makes the evaluation even more complex is that style, and possibly the choice of strategies as well, involves an adaptation to highly personalized aptitudes and needs. Hence we must be prepared to consider whether a set of behaviors that does not constitute the best modality of care, in general terms, may represent the best choice of care for a particular practitioner, a particular patient, or a conjunction of the two in some particular situation.

Some studies may indicate the direction of inquiry I have in mind. One is the study in 1963 of patients admitted to the Western Infirmary of Glasgow, Scotland, with possible appendicitis. The study was designed to determine which of the two approaches, one conservative and one radical, could be regarded the more successful.[10] The conservative approach demanded a greater degree of certainty to justify operative intervention and resulted in fewer operations and less frequent removal of normal appendices but a larger number of patients who came back with symptoms that required surgery within the following 2 years. The somewhat less conservative (but probably not radical) approach resulted in more operations, the removal of more abnormal as well as more normal appendices, and fewer recurrences during 2 subsequent years among those who were not operated on (Fig. 3-3). Under certain assumptions concerning the mortality from removing a normal appendix and that from not removing an abnormal appendix, the investigator demonstrates that the less conservative approach is associated with a lower avoidable mortality and therefore would represent higher quality. Table 3-1 is a computation of expected avoidable mortality for the conservative and radical approaches, based on estimates of risk, from the Glasgow study. I hold no brief for the accuracy of this study or for its conclusions. I use it here only as an illustration of an approach that examines more fully the consequence of alternative strategies of management—at

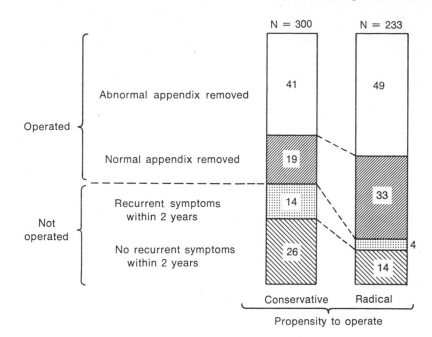

Fig. 3-3. Possible appendicitis by whether operated, nature of tissue removed and subsequent recurrence of symptoms, and by type of approach to surgery (Western Infirmary of Glasgow, Scotland, 1963). (Data from Howie.[10] From Medical care chart book, Ann Arbor, Mich., 1972, University of Michigan, School of Public Health.)

Table 3-1. Computation of expected avoidable mortality from the Glasgow study, based on estimates of risk*

State of appendix	Percent by state	Mortality risk	Expected mortality (%)†
Conservative approach			
Normal, removed	19	0.02	0.0038
Abnormal, not removed	8‡	0.04	0.0032
Both	—	—	0.0070
Radical approach			
Normal, removed	33	0.02	0.0066
Abnormal, not removed	0	0.04	—
Both	—	—	0.0066

*Adapted from Howie.[10] From Medical care chart book, Ann Arbor, Mich., 1972, The University of Michigan, School of Public Health.
†Product of preceding columns.
‡49% − 41% = 8%.

a conclusion that differs from what would have been concluded using, for example, the nonremoval of normal tissue as the sole criterion of quality. A more extensive and detailed consideration of costs and benefits, including monetary gains and losses, is to be found in a controlled comparison of treating varicose veins by surgery or by the injection of material that blocks the vein through causing a local inflammation.[11] An examination of the balance sheet is quite revealing, even though no measure is available that consolidates all categories of gains and losses into a single unit (Table 3-2).

In theory, cost is not a matter of con-

Table 3-2. Benefits and costs of treating varicose veins by each of two methods of treatment in a controlled trial, London, 1967-1968*

	Method of treatment	
	Injection-compression sclerotherapy	Surgery
Benefits		
At end of 3 years, no further treatment; considered to be improved†	86%	78%
Costs		
Did not attend‡	6%	15%
Mortality risk§	1 in 7000	1 in 4500
Immediate complications‖	28%	16%
Direct monetary costs per case:¶		
Capital costs	Not estimated	Not estimated
Current costs		
Actual	£9.77	£44.22
Hypothetical#		£16 or £12
Indirect costs		
Mean time for treatment and travel	30 hours	100 hours
Mean number of days taken off work	6.4 days	31.3 days
Average loss of earnings for those employed fulltime	£29	£118

*Data from Piachaud, D., and Weddell, J. M.: The economics of treating varicose veins, Int. J. Epidemiol. **1**:287-294, 1972.

†"There are at present no objective measures of the severity of either symptoms or signs, the limitations of the present methods of assessment are considerable and have to be recognized."

‡The injection-compression treatment was preferred by 14 of 18 patients questioned.

§Based on a review of the literature.

‖28% of those with sclerotherapy developed superficial phlebitis. Of those treated with surgery, 14% developed complications, mainly stitch abscesses and wound infection, and 3% developed neuritis and phlebitis.

¶Costs refer to 1967-1968 period.

#Under assumptions reducing hospital stay and providing treatment in smaller hospitals.

cern in formulating the criteria and standards of technical care for the individual. A state analogous to zero gravity appears to be assumed with respect to cost. In practice the issue of cost, in various guises, is implicit or explicit at all levels of evaluation, though to varying degrees. In the abstract the criterion applicable to cost is simple enough: the achievement of maximum benefits net of cost. In practice the application of this criterion is bedeviled by the absence of a common measure of costs and benefits and by variations in the various participants in the medical care transaction incur or enjoy various amounts of each under different strategies of care. Some examples may clarify the issue: in the technical management of individual patients the simplest decision rule is to say that procedures will be included as long as each additional procedure produces an increment of benefit. Procedures that produce no additional benefit in the information they yield or in their contribution to patient well-being are logically redundant and economically wasteful. Unfortunately it is difficult to apply the zero benefit rule, since one could argue interminably about benefits so minute they are almost beyond comprehension.

More fundamentally one must also look

at the costs. Medical procedures entail risks as well as benefits, and we must balance one against the other. Here the problem, in addition to defining and measuring the risks and benefits, is in finding a common unit of exchange between the two. Each medical procedure also entails monetary costs to the patient and to his family, which curtail their ability to purchase alternative goods and services. Should these considerations enter the calculus of costs and benefits and in what way? Perhaps of more immediate concern is the question of whether it is the responsibility of the practitioner to select that strategy of care which represents the least cost to the patient, to himself, to the institution of which the practitioner is a member, to the financing program, to the immediate community, or to the nation at large. The search for an answer leads to more aggregate levels of analysis. When we consider the entire case load of a practitioner, the limiting factor is most probably the practitioner's own time, which means that the optimal allocation of that time could well be an additional criterion of the quality of the total practice, quite distinct from the management of each individual episode. When one considers a target population rather than a case load, the issue of access to care looms large and one might well ask whether quality care for some is at the expense of less care or no care for others. Again the optimal allocation of resources is the central question. But the answer is by no means clear, since it depends in part on whether we must make the best use of the medical care resources we have or whether we must press for more resources in the medical care sector. When one considers the interests of the care-providing institution (for example, a hospital), the level of occupancy that represents efficient operation becomes an important issue. Even at the level of the financing program it is not completely clear what behaviors are optimal, since the answer depends, at least in the short run, on what happens to the

capacity released by the reduction in relatively redundant care to individual patients. If this is simply used up by other beneficiaries, the program is little advanced in its efforts at cost containment.

In more general terms the incidence of costs depends on the manner in which care is financed and paid for, what benefits are covered under prepayment (to what extent and under what terms), the availability of substitute modalities of care and their relative costs as well as their relative efficacy in assuring health and well-being, the presence of controls on the use and released capacity, the expansion of supplies in general, and the manner in which expansions in supplies are financed. Given these variables, it is easy to postulate circumstances under which it might be most advantageous to all local interests to admit patients to a hospital and keep them there until they are ready to go to work. The patient gets good care, the patient's family is relieved of expense and responsibility, the physician is able to see more patients at less cost to himself, the hospital is kept comfortably filled to a level of efficiency, there is a net flow of revenue to the local community through employment of residents and business for local tradesmen, and if the community plays its cards well, it could make a successful bid for an even larger hospital. It is only at the most aggregate level of social concern that this strategy begins to go sour. But even here one might well ask: What happens to the dollar that is saved through shorter hospital stays? Do I get to keep the money and spend it as I like? Do I get better schools? Or is the money spent on something else that is less valuable to me than an additional day in the hospital?

National policy has increasingly tended to use medical care institutions in general and physicians in particular as instruments of the social purpose—sometimes contrary to the more selfish interests of these providers but sometimes also contrary to their traditional role as advocates for the immediate and private interests of their patients. If so, we must be watchful to make certain that the benefits that accrue to the whole justify the assault on our more traditional roles and values and the diminution in our freedom to pursue more private ends for our patients as well as for ourselves.

REFERENCES

1. De Geyndt, W.: Five approaches to assessing the quality of care, Hosp. Admin. **15:**21-42, 1970.
2. Simon, H. A.: Administrative behavior, New York, 1961, The Macmillan Co., pp. 62-66.
3. Deniston, O. L., Rosenstock, I. M., and Getting, V. A.: Evaluation of program effectiveness, Public Health Rep. **83:**323-335, 1968.
4. Donabedian, A.: Evaluating the quality of medical care, Milbank Mem. Fund Q. **44**(part 2):166-206, 1966.
5. Williamson, J. W.: Evaluating quality of patient care: A strategy relating outcome and process assessment, J.A.M.A. **218:**564-569, 1971.
6. Kessner, D. M., Kalk, C. D., and Singer, J.: Assessing health quality—the case for tracers, N. Engl. J. Med. **288:**189-193, 1973.
7. Hare, R. L., and Barnoon, S.: Medical care appraisal and quality assurance in the office practice of internal medicine, San Francisco, July 1973, American Society of Internal Medicine. (A more complete report also is available.)
8. Scheff, T. J.: Preferred errors in diagnosis, Med. Care **2:**166-172, 1974.
9. Szasz, T. S., and Hollender, M. H.: A contribution to the philosophy of medicine: the basic models of the doctor-patient relationship, Arch. Intern. Med. **79:**585-592, 1956.
10. Howie, J. G. R.: The place of appendectomy in the treatment of young adult patients with possible appendicitis, Lancet **1:**1365-1367, 1968.
11. Piachaud, D., and Weddell, J. M.: The economics of treating varicose veins, Int. J. Epidemiol. **1:**287-294, 1972.

Critical issues of peer review

4

Functions of peer review

M. GENE ALDRIDGE

The vagueness concerning the role of peer review and the many reservations held about its more controversial aspects can probably best be understood when assumptions are made explicit. This chapter is written as an attempt at making explicit the functions of peer review that have been articulated in the literature.

A review of the literature since 1966 reveals well over 1500 different articles on either peer review, the quality of health care, or on PSRO. Investigations into this body of literature reveal several identifiable categories of functions for peer review that are currently being discussed. The following selected functions are not meant to be exhaustive but rather they were chosen because of their frequency of occurrence, their relevancy to Public Law 92-603 (and its current regulations), and because of their centrality to current national debate on peer review.

Serious unanswered questions exist about the role and relevance of peer review to the health care system. For example, to what extent is the cost of medical care affected by peer review? What variables can be systematically monitored by peer review that predict most accurately the quality of medical care and which variables reliably account for its cost? To what extent and in what way does the continuing education of health professionals affect the process or alter the outcomes

of medical care when conducted as a performance-based part of peer review? Does systematic peer review have a positive or negative effect on medical malpractice? Do the current PSRO organizations really encourage or practice systematic peer review? What is the minimum amount of data and information handling really necessary for systematic peer review? How does systematic peer review contribute to helpful public knowledge about medicine? What effect does the public disclosure of the results of peer review have on cost and quality of medical care delivery?

If there are to be answers to questions such as these they must come from an understanding of what functions apply to the peer review processes. Through this analysis it is hoped that groups who are interested in systematic peer review can have an understanding of what can and cannot reasonably be expected. A study of the functions of peer review is relevant for the following reasons:

1. Functional aspects explain the connections and relationships of the component parts of systematic peer review to each other and to the care delivery system.
2. Investigations into the functions of peer review can provide some sense of value comparison among the various components of peer review.

3. The study of functions should assist in developing adequate, appropriate, valid, and more reliable criteria for defining systematic peer review.
4. The order of parts (structure of peer review) requires the implementation of some notion of the order of functions (processes of peer review), which in the final analysis produces the order of results (the outcomes) of peer review.

The dictionary defines function as a "variable quantity or quantities."[1] The first important notion contained within this definition is that a function is a variable quantity; that is, it may vary depending on its relationship with other functions. Second, the dictionary definition suggests that there is a sensitive interdependent relationship between functions. That is, one function stands to be influenced by every other function. Finally, each function may be of more or less value (importance) depending on the goals and objectives established for the review system by the care institution in which the peer review system operates. Each of these concepts deserves some explanation and will be illustrated with an example based on the perception of color.

We could not understand the concept of "redness" in our universe if red was the only color to which our retina was sensitive. Without variability there would be no color contrasts and therefore no way to compare one color with another; that is, there would be no color values. Colors are thus interdependent and have value for the human enterprise because the existence of variety allows us to visualize various color values.[2] The traffic signal is a classic example of the purposeful exploitation of this idea as an instrument to fulfill a need or a useful objective. Similarly, if a peer review system is viewed as having as its only function an evaluation of the utilization of health services (via the cost function), then our vision would be limited, interdependent relationships would submerge, our approach to solving problems would be different, and our review objectives would be narrower than if we sought to develop a comprehensive peer review system to evaluate the health care services from multiple points of view.

Among the different objectives that could be addressed by a comprehensive review system are (1) accountability for the costs of care (for example, costing each service and comparing what one hospital charges in relation to various other services or in comparison with another hospital); (2) the educational aspects of upgrading care (to problem-solve in a learning situation that leads to the production of criteria sets for treatment and diagnosis and that encourages conformity of clinical performances with higher care standards); (3) the health research aspect to evaluate (retrospectively, concurrently, and prospectively) the efficacy and efficiency of clinical performances of physicians and other care providers in the hospital setting (to suggest new clinical research possibilities for patient care); (4) the advancement of any management strategy that might prove beneficial to patient care; (5) the opening of lines of communication (between the review system and all components of the care system); and (6) legal responsibilities to create an appeal system for health professionals (so that unfavorable decisions can be re-reviewed under due process in a system that protects the legitimate rights of the health professional and the institution from inappropriate malpractice problems).

Any particular hospital may have other goals or more specific objectives than these, but this listing encompasses those probably most shared by hospitals today.

By converting the foregoing issues into discrete functions of peer review, we come up with the following list:

1. Accountability function
2. Educational function
3. Research/evaluation function

4. Institutional and patient care management function
5. Communication function
6. Legal function
7. Innovation/change function

Too often these functions are discussed in isolation or in a way that suggests a lack of relationship between them. One of the main purposes of this chapter is to delineate the interdependence between the major functions of peer review. This chapter, then, is constructed to produce three outcomes. First, it is our hope to shed light on the relative importance of each function separately. Second, the relationship of all functions to each other is described. Finally, a matrix of functions for peer review will emerge that can be utilized by the reader to evaluate the extent to which current peer review systems manifest each or coordinate all of these functions.

Historically, single-purpose review systems dedicated mostly to the control of hospital utilization were among the first peer review programs to attain routine operational status. Most of these focused the review process on those service items that contribute to the costs of care and then established the control mechanisms to contain those costs. By contrast, a comprehensive or multiple-purpose system encompassing the functions described above becomes quickly complex and would require not only cost data but also a whole matrix of variables that must be analyzed to meet all the informational requirements for carrying out the additional education, research, management, communications, legal, and change functions. Establishing appropriate linkages between all these functions would also be essential before a comprehensive system of review can emerge in operational form (this is the subject of Chapter 10).

At this point in our discussion of the functions of peer review we would do well to recall the fundamental economic assumption cited by Victor Fuchs "that resources are scarce in terms of human wants."[3] Applied to peer review, some sense of priority for evaluating the medical care system must be made. But the priority health professionals might place on the various functions for systematic peer review may or may not fit the priority of society or government. This discussion will be conducted henceforth in cognizance of either possibility. What will be done first is to enumerate clearly the choices before us so as to make the options among evaluation mechanisms as respectable as resources will allow. In so doing, we will attempt to be equally mindful of the best interests of the public and of the profession.

Without an appreciation for the full range of review functions potentially available, however, no really clear choice of review methods and design strategies is possible. Forcing a choice among recognized review functions then provides a keener appreciation of the essential characteristics of peer review because this helps a group organization define its own goals, objectives, and desired outcomes relative to its own values and sense of commitment. From this perspective should emerge criteria by which a group (like a hospital) might weigh the alternatives just as it should help the reader define what an adequate systematic peer review approach might be for a given medical care setting. The functions of peer review will now be discussed in the order they were listed.

ACCOUNTABILITY FUNCTION

Public Law 92-603, Title XI, Part B, Section 1151, brings the accountability for health care clearly into focus when it states:

In order to promote the effective, efficient, and economical delivery of health services of proper quality for which payment may be made (in whole or part) under this Act and in recognition of the interests of patients, the public, practitioners and providers in improved health care services, it is the purpose of this part to assure, through the application of suitable procedures of professional standards review, that the services for which payment may be made under the Social Security Act will conform to appropriate professional standards for the provision of health care.[4]

An interesting debate raised by this legislation centers on three specific accountability functions in regard to health services. The most conspicuous of these is emphasized by the portion of the law that promotes accountability based on the economic aspect of delivering health care services. A second accountability function seems to focus on assessing the quality of health care delivery. The third accountability function is highlighted by the public disclosure issue associated with PSRO. Each of these issues is critical to this discussion of peer review, since any systematic approach to peer review, to be effective, should include all three accountability functions (economic, quality, and public disclosure) to comply with Public Law 93-641. For the purposes of discussion, economic accountability will be related to cost parameters involved in the provision of health services, quality accountability will relate to the effectiveness of the health care delivered, and public disclosure will relate to information-sharing issues associated with data from operating PSRO and peer review systems.

A society that does not take into account the enormous importance of the interdependence of these three accountability functions could end up with what Kenneth Boulding has described as a kind of profit-and-loss bookkeeping strategy for evaluating health services.[5] While Boulding's admonition was not point-specific to health care services, the principle behind his comment does relate in a general way to how, through shortsightedness, we occasionally limit our agenda when developing value functions and the indices for rational decision making. He further warns that "the quantification of value functions into value indices, whether this is money or whether it is more subtle and complicated measures of pay-off, intro-

duces elements of ethical danger into the decision-making process, simply because the clarity and apparent objectivity of quantitatively measurable subordinate goals can easily lead to a failure to bear in mind that they are subordinate."[5] Here Boulding argues for a wider perspective on issues associated with rational decision making.

His message for those of us in the health care field amounts to this question: how do we evaluate the health care system in respect to both accountability functions—economic accountability and quality accountability—while also disclosing the findings to the public without causing irreparable damage to the clinical care delivery process?

This general debate began a long time ago in the American political scene. As early as 1930 the book *Health Care for the American People*[6] cited issues on accountability that were already being publicly debated. Somehow the economic depression and the several wars that followed prevented the discussion from growing beyond its roots in legislative halls to open debate at the national level. This hiatus is somehow startling, since health legislation in America relating to accountability can be traced to the first public health law (1798). Even the direct linkage of the PSRO debate was spawned at least 40 years ago. The 1930s produced the social security legislation that introduced the doctrine of public obligations for personal financial security. The Hill-Burton legislation, which funded the physical development of medical facilities, came along in the 1940s. In the 1950s the national focus was on the National Institute of Health and its emphasis on health research. Finally, in the 1960s amendments to the social security legislation (Medicare and Medicaid) extended the concept of public obligations to medical security and unleashed resources into the health care system without an adequate means of accounting for the expended funds. And it was that which in 1972 sired the PSRO amendments to the original social security legislation.

During the decade since 1966 the accountability issue has progressively evinced broader concern not only from health officials at the federal level but also from virtually all segments of society, which now seem to agree that the taxpayer deserves some accounting for the health services supplied at public expense. What is not clear is what value functions will be used to determine which aspects of our health care system will be reported to the American people. What is clear is that public claims of fraud in these programs make more shrill the calls for an accounting.

The accountability function of peer review was certainly recognized among health professionals a long time ago, as it can be traced back to 1910 when Codman raised concern for evaluating the end results of medical care rendered to patients in surgery.[7] Brook (the author of Chapter 6) has clearly outlined the historical development of the accountability issue in another work,[7] so elaboration here is not necessary. What is important to point out is that peer review not only became a professional concern but also was being accomplished in some form long before the public became aware of it or the elected representatives of this nation got around to legislating accountability.

One could argue endlessly about the effectiveness of the form of peer review traditionally employed by physicians in the typical hospital setting, but the point is that until 1972 the accountability mechanism itself had been largely, if not exclusively, controlled by the health professional. But since 1972 the public has been injected into the accountability equation by legislative mandate. The accountability function in health care review thus contains two major identifiable threads: the thread that associates assumptions about public accountability with the rising cost of care and the thread that has arisen from the concern of health professions

and consumers for maintaining high quality of care.

Current review programs such as those advanced by the Joint Commission for the Accreditation of Hospitals and those described as medical care evaluation studies under PSRO largely represent or attempt to represent combinations of both parallel concerns. Clearly then any systematic approach to the assessments of health care services in our nation that purports to meet minimal requirements should consider carefully accountability for both the cost aspects and the quality aspects of medical care.

It is debatable whether peer review should treat both costs and quality as through they were of equal quantitative importance to medicine today or to its future. Indeed, maybe they should not be of equal importance, but what is important to note is that what is easily measured is also usually measured and therefore is emphasized over and above those functions that are not commonly measured[8] irrespective of the relative merits of each.

At the risk of oversimplification, let us illustrate with an example. Most utilization review systems in hospitals and nursing homes do measure the length of stay (LOS), which is regarded as an economic indicator for health services that have been provided. But to illustrate what is not usually measured, consider a patient who had a length of stay of 5 days for tonsillectomy. (Five days is well above the average in the nation.) Unquestionably the cost issue would be raised about this overstay, but as someone once said: "Who poses the question, did the patient stay for too short a time?" Other questions that might be addressed are, What was the quality factor associated with this tonsillectomy? What process was used to determine the need for surgical treatment in this particular case? Could other more appropriate alternatives of medical care be used? What clinical complications or patient behaviors may have intervened to prevent a shorter length of stay? In short, why must a longer than average stay be assumed to represent an excessive cost, and why couldn't other aspects of the care be more important—even from an economic point of view? Clearly then a peer review system that does not provide some functional relationship between economic indicators (cost) and quality indicators (care process and clinical outcomes) in evaluating health care could be called into question on the issues of validity, reliability, and full accountability. Further, some groups have asked, what is the central reason for existence of PSRO? Is it not to communicate the assessments of both cost and quality to the public? This aspect of accountability, if wisely done, can be an important positive evolutionary factor in the advancement of medicine as argued in Chapter 1. As so many researchers have found, it is not enough just to gather data and conduct studies; it is no less important to report those results to others. To fail in this is to lose an opportunity for stimulating further progress and support for health care efforts that otherwise could be forthcoming when full public disclosure results in increased credibility and public support.

The accountability issues raise questions of import for those who are in the process of constructing health care service evaluation programs at the local level whether associated with PSROs or not. There must be a clear vision of how to make accountability an effective instrument for change if it is to work for the good of the public and the profession. So often we are short-sighted in this regard, and like Mr. Magoo in the television version of Don Quixote, are left sitting on our ass, all the while thinking we are mounted on a magnificent steed performing great deeds.

One way that effectiveness can be assured is through the structure and content of the criteria sets professionals adopt. These can communicate not only to colleagues but also to society the functions of accountability that are held to be really important. But if professionals are then content to dispatch review personnel to hospitals armed only with utilization review criteria in a token effort to pacify the government, what will be communicated to the public is that cost alone is important. Should the standards of appropriate care be comprised of 80% cost criteria and 20% quality criteria, then the profession will have communicated that this is the proportion by which it favors cost over quality control. Similarly, if a hospital or regional peer review system is designed without a functional reporting mechanism for public disclosure, then it will have communicated that public disclosure is of little importance as a part of a peer review system. Intended or not, these will be the effects of disinterest or nearsightedness in understanding the total job that must be done. To the accountability functions of cost and quality one must add responsible and relevant public disclosure as a minimum accountability function for systematic peer review. The extent to which we design our accountability programs to evaluate each of these important aspects of health care and disclose meaningful results to the public will be the extent to which society can rely on the results that are produced from these systems. Whether expenditures of considerable resources (to produce a system of review that includes all conceivable functional parameters) can also be justified is another question open for debate. What is clear, though, is that choices among the options for developing mechanisms of accountability are being made whether knowingly or not. Why not add the functions and mechanisms systematically and explicitly?

EDUCATIONAL FUNCTION

In an article entitled "Education is PSRO Goal," Senator W. F. Bennett, the legislative author of PSRO, cited the educational function as an overriding concept for peer review as he saw it. He states: "The individual physician's sense of identification with and participation in the PSRO activities goes to the heart of what PSRO is all about—an educational process resulting from the broadest possible participation in the review experience by physicians in an area."[9] He further maintains that "the chief value and function of the review process becomes educational. It should never be punitive except in a case of blatant neglect or outright fraud."[9]

Senator Bennett's remarks find their historical roots in the attempts on the part of some educators to use the clinical data in hospital settings in such a way that practicing physicians could see an analysis of their own performance. Utilization review, medical audit functions, and special investigations, more recently termed "medical care evaluation studies," and instruction programs of a similar nature for practicing physicians have all been part of or outgrowths of the educational system in a larger sense. Like the accountability function, therefore, the educational function of peer review has interesting historical roots in the practice of medicine. The more recent history shows a string of educational contributions over the past decade by Dr. George Miller at the University of Illinois, Dr. John Williamson at Johns Hopkins University, and contributing author Dr. Clement Brown along with Dr. David Fleisher for their Bi-cycle concept of education to name but a few. These developments have contributed immensely to progress in the educational function of peer review as described here.

As pressure for accountability mounted, national groups like the American Hospital Association began building performance-based instructional programs like the Quality Assurance Program. Other educational mechanisms also appeared. The established precedent that preceded 1972 made it easier for Senator Bennett to include the educational function as an important component of Public Law 92-603. The educational function of peer review is based on several assumptions. First, that it is to be data based. This simply means that evaluating reliable information about diagnosis and treatment must be a part of the overall review process. The medical record of course is the prime source document for this data base, which means that it too takes on an important new function. Another assumption is that systematic peer review requires a performance base, that is, a prescribed basis for determining whether clinical performance was appropriate or inappropriate. This second assumption thus requires that explicit criteria be formed against which comparative judgments could be made about the appropriateness of diagnoses and treatment of specific problems and diseases. A third assumption, often implicit but nonetheless critical to the process, is that educational problem solving should be self-directed. This means several things. It means that physicians and not some other group should set the criteria for appropriate or inappropriate patient care. It also means that surgeons should not be setting criteria for family practitioners and urologists should not be setting criteria for orthopedic practitioners, and so on. However, it should be noted that wherever clinical problems with performance criteria overlap specialty areas, those problems should be resolved jointly by whatever specialties of disciplines are involved. Pretty much the same principle holds for the development of criteria for the care delivered by nonphysician clinical specialists.

Senator Bennett has referred to the intended purpose of criteria development in his written communication about PSRO when he stated, "These self-set parameters are not intended to be barriers to necessary medical care. They are simply local, professionally developed and accepted checkpoints that, to my mind, will be considered better than some of the arbitrary indexes we have used in the past."[9]

In an editorial written in 1973, Dr.

Ruttledge Howard of the American Medical Association's Department of Continuing Medical Education supported the self-directed aspects of the educational function of peer review when he stated, "Used in conjunction with self-evaluation techniques peer review can be of great value to the physician. . . . He need not fear this aspect of peer review, which in this role is fast becoming an educational necessity."[10]

During the early years of performance-based education efforts, computer analysis applied by CPHA in Ann Arbor, Michigan, became an invaluable source of descriptive data about physicians' use of hospital services. In 1971 Dr. Perlman and Dr. Slee of this group had written an article about how educational needs could be defined via PAS (Professional Audit Service) and MAP (Medical Audit Program)[11] for physicians in the hospitals that utilized their services. Dr. Slee and his team unquestionably have provided over the years a key component for the data-based approach that has now become a minimum requirement to fulfill the educational function associated with utilization review and medical audit.

It is now clear what the minimum requirements are for the educational function of systematic peer review:

1. The system should be data based.
2. The system should be performance based.
3. The system should be self-directed.

Future peer review systems will very likely require educational functions to be defined with even greater specificity to focus on the particular instructional needs of individual physicians. It is thus becoming clear that our concepts about medical education, and particularly about continuing medical education, are not going to be the same again.

To demonstrate this point, consider for a moment what we have recently learned from others about education or the learning process that can be applied to peer review. For example, Dr. Jerome Bruner, in a concise piece of research work, has demonstrated that there are two fundamentally differing styles of teaching: one of which is more productive toward behavior change than is the other.[12] He labels these styles or approaches as the expository model of teaching wherein the teacher lectures and exposes his knowledge base via his knowledge via his outline to the students. The other approach he labels the hypothetical model of teaching in which questions are generated usually on the part of both teacher and student. The way this works is that hypotheses are created with questions that usually begin with "what if . . ." In the expository method the student is passive. In the hypothetical method the student is active; that is, he participates actively in the learning process.

Physician education associated with most current systematic peer review approaches clearly calls for active participation on the part of the student (that is, the practicing physician). One of the important considerations that Bruner notes from his work is that contrary to prevailing opinion, this approach has the following benefits:

1. The shift from extrinsic to intrinsic rewards (rewards now come from within the individual, not just from the teacher)
2. The pleasure to discover
3. The aid of conserving memory
4. An increase in intellectual potency (the increased ability of a person to seek out patterns and relationships on his own)[12]

The implications of these findings with regard to systematic peer review cannot be overlooked without paying a price for doing so. Review systems that bypass local clinicians in the criteria-setting phase cannot fulfill one of the basic intensions of current peer review strategies. If, for example, 14 to 20 physicians set the criteria for the clinical management of a hip fracture for an entire region, then valuable and unique educational opportunity will be experienced by those 14 to 20 physicians but not by any of the other physicians who treat that condition in the region. A basic educational function will have been bypassed for all those physicians who were just handed the criteria and asked to comment on them because that is not a situation which supports active learning. It has been suggested that the justification for "a proposed gathering together of all the criteria that have already been devised" (for the purpose of assembling and distributing a national criteria set) was that there was not enough time to produce them any other way, that is, from the bottom up. All that we remember about that kind of an explanation is that "schools and prisons are the only place where time takes precedent over the job to be done."[13]

Other research into education and learning also contributes directly to the educational function of peer review. For example, Guilford published some interesting research on *The Nature of Human Intelligence* well over a decade ago. In that work he identified "convergent" and "divergent" types of thinking in people. Divergent thinkers tend not to seek quick solutions to problems. Convergent thinkers, on the other hand, do and converge immediately on the answer.[14]

The familiar clinical-pathologic conference and the radiology conference are typically convergent; that is, they are conducted by the expert who has information the conferees do not have and who figuratively says to the group, "I have an answer in my head to this most difficult radiologic or pathologic problem." The learner or problem solver is then forced to converge on the "right" answer or predetermined categorical responses to the questions that are raised. It should be quickly noted that this in itself is not really such a bad thing provided that opportunities for divergent thinking are also provided in the learning process. What we are doing when we confine our educational process to only answer seeking is

destructive of building options and alternatives into the problem-solving process and to seeking new solutions to problems.

Recent experiences would suggest that more convergent than divergent thinking pervades the generation of criteria for peer review. That is, a few physicians usually wind up setting the criteria for those conditions commonly encountered in an entire region. Feedback on predeveloped criteria sets from local practitioners is sought only after an initial model set has been generated. Those who do respond to criteria that are already prepared have not had an opportunity to contribute their divergent thinking during the critical formulation stage and thereby potentially worthy options are lost to the final product, but an educational opportunity has surely been lost to the nonparticipants. Passing already established criteria sets to practicing physicians for review and comment should not suffice for active learning either.

A critical point in this discussion is that the educational functions of peer review are probably as important to practicing clinicians in the early stages of developing criteria sets as they are in the later full operation of the review system when educational intervention may be required to correct their inappropriate performances. In other words two critical points of educational intervention exist in a systematic peer review process. It would seem important to enlist the participation of all those care providers in the original development of criteria whose performance will later be evaluated by them. It is recognized that involving all clinicians in criteria development is such a sizable undertaking that it may be challenged on the grounds that its benefit may not be worth the effort, and for that reason this topic deserves discussion.

Some basic research conducted in 1964 in a totally unrelated field has some interesting implications for criteria development. Fattu's work had to do with problem solving in relation to troubleshooting equipment malfunctions.[15] Most problem solving typically focuses on end results, but Fattu examined how the process of problem solving produces an outcome or solution. He was primarily interested in being able to formulate a generalization as to what were the thinking processes in a typical problem-solving setting so that he might predict which are the more useful in finding solutions.

Fattu's work utilized a concept called *réflexion parlée.* It simply means spoken reflections. To tap the problem-solving process of his subjects, Fattu used a method that required persons to talk about the process of problem solving while they were actively engaged in seeking solutions. The educational value of this technique for peer review can be found in this intriguing methodology itself.

It is hypothesized that when people explicitly speak their mind out loud in the process of solving problems, they are most often communicating their beliefs to themselves. That is, the value of saying something out loud to myself (with others present) gives me a chance to speak about my reflections. Thus when physician groups go about the business of setting criteria for *x* diagnosis or treatment, it may be just as important that they articulate to the group how (and why) they arrive at a given criterion as it is to articulate the criterion itself. The very thought processes that lend validity to the criterion become more evident and are shared. Brook and Ertel (see Chapters 6 and 10) will describe the applications of this concept for assessing the extent to which quality can be measured in systematic peer review.

An example of the rewarding payoffs of the *réflexion parlée* methodology was typified in the experience of a working interdisciplinary criteria development panel. An internal medicine group (cardiologists) and a group of family practitioners were engaged in setting criteria for diagnosing heart problems in their hospital. The cardiologists had been concerned for some time about the quality of care given to heart patients by family practitioners as frequently evidenced by an apparent failure to diagnose serious cardiac disease in their parents. Cardiologists had observed that many patients admitted by family practitioners carried diagnoses at both admission and discharge of chest pain, respiratory problems, and other nonspecific symptoms. Yet it was clinically apparent that they suffered from cardiac problems that warranted attention in coronary care units. In other words heart patients admitted to the hospital by family practitioners were being distributed to other hospital services when they should have been in coronary care units. Yet family practitioners readily revealed in the criteria development session that they had for the most part more than adequate knowledge to diagnose those same cardiac conditions properly. When confronted by this issue in the problem-solving environment of a criteria-setting session, the family practitioners revealed why these medical labels were used by them to describe their patients. This behavior had become their response to the rule the cardiologists had approved as hospital policy. The rule held that any serious cardiac diagnosis (like myocardial infarction) would automatically require a cardiology consultation if the patient was sent to the coronary care unit. Finally, the question was posed by the frustrated cardiology group: "How does that explain why you don't follow your own criteria for diagnosing myocardial infarction in the first place—and why, then, do you send your patients all over the hospital diagnosed as 'chest pain' when in fact, their cardiac problems are evident?" One family practitioner responded, "Because we lose control of our patients to you when we diagnose them properly and send them to the coronary care unit." If the discussion had not focused on the process by which the family practitioners arrived at their solution for the setting of diagnostic criteria, there would have been little hope for understanding this most usual dichotomy between knowledge and behavior.

Réflexion parlée it is hypothesized, can become an extremely important educational function of peer review. That is why it is not enough just to obtain criteria sets from some external source no matter how good (valid) they are. What is also important is the problem-solving process that encourages individuals and groups to weigh each possible criterion as being of more, less, or equal importance to all the other candidate criteria. Consensus opinion in this way illicits behavioral commitment (or the last opportunity for behavioral commitment) through the democratic process.

This opens up a new alternative to the didactive teaching session for continuing education (for example, a speaker from the medical school lecturing on the use of antibiotics in colon surgery). The continuing education committee may be better advised to sponsor a problem-solving session to establish criteria for antibiotic usage in colon surgery. In this way all the practitioners benefit from learning not only which antibiotics are chosen by their colleagues, and with what priority for x condition, but they benefit also from actively sharing with colleagues the reasons why a specific antibiotic is thought more or less efficacious under clinical conditions that exist in their own institutional practice (which may be quite unlike conditions in the big medical centers).

More will be said in later chapters about how the continuing education subcommittee might function as an integrated component of operating peer review systems (see Chapters 9 and 10) with an active role in correcting care deficiencies. Suffice it to say here that specific educational needs identified for individual physicians can seldom be met by shuffling them off to some educational session that is didactic and expository in method (and that also happens to be located next to a golf course).

What then is the role of the expert in educating physicians with regard to new knowledge? Basically the educational function of the expert should likewise be incorporated into more problem-solving experiences whenever possible. The expert could, for example, better assist criteria development groups by reserving his own considered opinion until others have exhausted their supply of explicit judgments in a give-and-take criteria-setting experience. When the learner group has first established a set of its own criteria, then they should have the opportunity to compare their approach and reasoning with that of the expert. A final common set of criteria can by synthesized from both inputs. Subsequent behavior change on the part of the practitioners to keep up with information communicated by the expert has a better chance for occurring under this method than under didactic and expository modes of education.[12] We cannot leave this point, however, without sharing one other notion about this process, which is that the "expert" often learns some medical facts from the community practitioners in the exchange.

One last note on the all-important educational function of peer review. We have discussed a number of rapidly developing areas, but one unresolved task is associated with unequivocally demonstrating how the educational process improves the outcomes of care. As others have pointed out (see Chapter 6), we will not have completed our educational feedback to practitioners if we remain unable to communicate what effect all of the assessment strategies of peer review actually have had on the health status of the population served. This not only is essential to convince practitioners of the value of their continued support of peer review but it also gets directly at the very reason for their professional existence. Thus all the goals of the evaluation methodologies we have discussed are really subordinate goals to the educational process. Evaluation technologies can only lead in setting the direction in which the educational function should move.

RESEARCH AND EVALUATION FUNCTION
External research/evaluation

An unequivocal external demonstration of the effectiveness of systematic peer review will require answers to questions like, In what ways and to what extent are the utilization of resources and costs of health services affected by peer review? How does systematic peer review affect the quality of medical care services? How does peer review, working through local health facilities, affect the health status of a given community?

Most of these research questions will not be resolved immediately, but any peer review system that does not explicitly take into account the need to research these questions can expect long-range if not short-range problems from fiscal agents (including government) who pick up the bills for the current health system.

Internal research/evaluation

Besides the above external research/evaluation questions, there are also internal research questions that must be addressed by health facilities for their own needs and benefit. Examples of those questions are as follows:

1. How many and what kind of medical care evaluation studies are most appropriate to conduct within our own institutional setting?
2. Were our medical audits conducted in a way that related to educational needs of staff members (as evidenced by performance of physicians or other health professionals)?
3. In what ways has medical audit in conjunction with continuing education programs changed the practice behavior of health professionals?
4. What specific utilization review strategies have led to either a cost reduction or cost increment in our health facility?

There are four generally recognized kinds of research, and all are applicable in some way to examining some aspect of peer review. Table 4-1 describes which kinds of research are useful in addressing the kinds of questions often encountered.

Probably the type of research most employed in peer review studies is descriptive in form and function. Descriptive research is the kind reflected in ongoing surveillance activities that produce the utilization patterns, physician or patient profile analyses, and the typical retrospective statistical summaries derived from abstracted hospital records.

The second form of research most applicable to peer review relates to determining which topics and study methods would be most useful to special medical care evaluation studies (MCEs) that examine diagnosis and treatment modalities in depth. Beyond descriptive data like length of stay, cross-infection rates, and mortality indices, these types of studies can be expected to take on characteristics of experimental research to measure, for example, the extent to which one drug or treatment strategy may prove more appropriate than another. It can also be expected that research plans such as these will be linked to cost analysis, since in the final analysis a selection between two treatment strategies that produce the same outcomes, for example, may well lead to the question of which one should be advocated on the basis of cost parameters.

Formulative or exploratory research is particularly useful for developing instruments to assess the human impact of peer review. If, for example, it was important to assess patient satisfaction encountered in the management of a specific condition, an instrument for measuring patient attitudes and perceptions of their care experience would first have to be developed (formulated). Gilson et al. appear to have been successful in the development of an outcome measure using the patient's own assessments of illness level.[16] This approach combines an instrument development approach and an outcome approach in the formulation of a research strategy. With an increased emphasis on consumer

Table 4-1. Types of research applicable to peer review

Kinds of research	Application to peer review	Sample peer review questions
Historical	Prime use in demonstrating historical trends that have occurred on specific methods, concepts, and issues	How did concern about medical outcomes enter peer review processes? How successful and why?
Formulative/ exploratory	Prime use in generating adequate hypotheses about structure of criteria sets or development of instruments for evaluating process and outcomes of medical care	What kind of instrument will best assess the clinical outcomes of medical care rendered for a given diagnosis?
Experimental	Prime use in identifying variables that predict the most appropriate strategies for assessing diagnosis and treatment; employed especially in validating review procedures or choice of one diagnosis or treatment strategy over another	Which antibiotic should be cited as the drug of choice for use in a given infection under what clinical circumstances?
Descriptive	Prime use in describing patient populations, utilization patterns, physician treatment profiles; also in establishing norms for screening and in linking important relationships between costs, use patterns, and outcomes	What is the frequency (by diagnosis) of x disease for y population at this health institution, how well do they respond to z treatment, and how much does it cost per case?

input into the evaluation of the health system, the formulative approach will likely be considered more often in the developmental stages for criteria sets in peer review systems.

The research method least employed for peer review to date is probably historical research. However, this is not to say that this strategy has nothing to offer peer review. Certainly in planning implementation of particular review programs it can be helpful to know both the historical development and the level of acceptance for similar review concepts that may have been attempted previously. For example, in developing outcome studies it may prove useful to know that Codman attempted end-results studies way back in 1914 and encountered great resistance from his colleagues. Awareness of what has gone on before—especially in this field—may be of material assistance in alerting the developers of peer review systems to where the conceptual obstacles

and operational difficulties are likely to lie. Hopefully it may also provide clues in how to deal successfully with them.

More complete discussions of data requirements and information management systems necessary to support these research approaches can be found elsewhere in this text (see Chapters 6 and 7). For the present it is relevant to observe that most existing external and internal peer review exploratory research activities appear to focus on three specific areas. Those areas are

1. Institutional management research
2. Medical (patient) care research
3. Professional continuing education research

It can be seen from Fig. 4-1 that overlapping informational requirements to support such research can be best met by organizing the research functions in such a way that they are integrated with care activities through a common data base. To achieve this, research functions must be

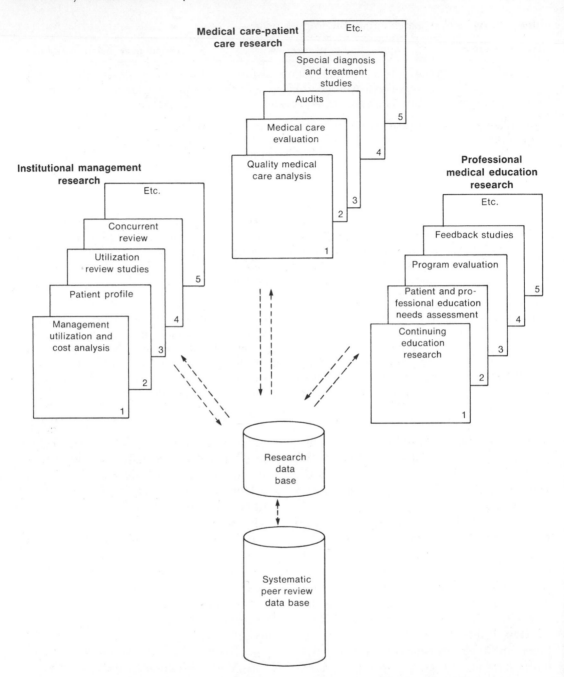

Fig. 4-1. Research function of systematic peer review.

well defined and not buried within the organizational structure if they are to contribute much to solving the management problems inevitably associated with both care delivery and the evaluation of it.

It now begins to appear that existing review programs have established the first operational data base on which broader research strategies are becoming possible. Farrell, in 1963, cited several desirable populations for future systematic study that are now included under a variety of operating peer review programs.[17] His list included hospital inpatients, emergency patients, outpatients in clinics, long-term care patients, and patients in psychiatric hospitals. But compatible data bases, research methods, and strategies will be essential if cooperative research activities of this nature among local hospitals or across regions are to become a practical reality.

One last note on the research function concerns the role that medical records personnel might play not only in respect to data collection but also in coordinating data-handling policies. There are ample opportunities for records personnel to establish close liaison with the hospital administrative structure internally and with the PSRO externally to maximize the coordination of research in all three areas of major interest (institutional management, patient care, and continuing education). Some of the organizational issues associated with developing these relationships are included in the discussion of operational peer review systems in Chapter 10.

INSTITUTIONAL MANAGEMENT/ PATIENT CARE MANAGEMENT FUNCTION

Modern management strategies encourage the creation of an environment conducive to assisting work groups in developing initiative, creativity, and self-directed approaches to solving management problems.[18] Management of this sort requires a system that brings forth good questions for group problem solving and not those like the sign on the wall of one health institution that read: "Just about the time I learned all the answers to life's questions, they changed the questions!" If the management data base is utilized in a way that generates good management questions (in addition to good research questions), then there is hope for progress in a particular health institution.

Peer review that is conducted in a systematic way and that generates meaning-

ful data can be an immeasurable aid to both institutional (hospital) management and patient care aspects of medical management. In fact, both may be well served by the managerial functions of peer review.

For purposes of discussion, institutional management will refer to the management of the health institutions, that is, hospital administration, budgeting, productivity, overhead, and so on. Medical or patient management will refer to the care of individual patients within the institution, for example, diagnosis and treatment with associated studies and evaluative reports including medical care evaluation studies, physician profiles, and patient care studies.

In many ways these two aspects of management overlap as discussions associated with reimbursement rates have established. For example, it is pointless to talk about costs of medical care without also talking about the utilization of medical care. It may be possible to reduce acute inpatient hospital days by denying the coverage of inpatient services, thereby reducing costs of care associated with hospitalization. However, those same patients denied inpatient services may begin using outpatient services in even greater numbers, thereby increasing the overall utilization. In addition the medical management of those patients can be subject to other influences on the cost and utilization of medical care. The fear of malpractice actions, for example, has caused many physicians to practice "defensive medicine." This means that more ancillary services are ordered than may be strictly indicated so that the physician can feel comfortable in the fact that he has ordered everything possible for a patient to cover contingencies no matter how unlikely, thereby driving costs up again on both the inpatient and outpatient side.

Without detailing all the existing possibilities, an examination of how overlapping institutional and patient management functions are related seems to be in

Table 4-2. Institutional and patient care management functions of systematic peer review

Management issues	Peer review considerations
Reimbursement/ budgeting in the hospital setting	Accurate, prompt documentation of patient care services required for prompt reimbursement. Utilization of peer review data on on utilization, cost, and quality of care can assist in predicting next year's staffing needs and costs and in preparing a budget.
Productivity measures in the hospital setting	Process (and eventually outcome) data can assist in defining units of service consumed in direct patient care. A well-developed data base, using systematic data acquisition techniques, can provide more clearly defined patient care, cost, and utilization data by service department; in essence, this distinction will separate direct care costs from other departments in the hospital, e.g., medical records, comptroller, and administration.
Patient and physician profiles for hospital planning	Adequate and accurate planning begins with the ability to reliably recognize problems. The patient profiles and physician profiles of systematic peer review can contribute to hospital care program development and planning through enhanced problem recognition. Projected case loads can also predict staffing and resource needs.
Institutional accountability to the public	Identification of specific relationships between the cost and the quality of care rendered advances public understanding and provides a rational basis for establishing social priorities for resource allocations.

order. Table 4-2 suggests some of the possible relationships that might be established between hospitals' (or patient care) management objectives and those of the systematic approach to peer review.

A more specific example of the utility and impact of peer review data in the management of both the institution and the care of patients can be cited from experience. The experience of one health institution is particularly instructive in regard to an unexpected impact from a reduction of length of stay via their utilization review–education program. At the same time medical professionals were documenting success in their efforts to reduce the length of stay of their patients, the hospital administrative team was faced with a disproportionately increasing debt (by over $8 million). This apparent paradox prompted further investigations, which found that increases in per diem costs for patients were responsible for the indebtedness and not professional ser-

vices. It was the comparison of peer review data with financial data that demonstrated the rising hospital costs could not be attributed to professionals but were clearly the result of administrative actions, many of which were under institutional control and therefore manageable.

Many other potentially helpful peer review management functions are just beginning to be recognized by hospitals as having a positive value to its administrative staff in much the same way that the educational function of peer review has a positive value to its clinical staff. Still other potential benefits from the change and communication attributes of peer review are discussed under the next two functions of peer review.

COMMUNICATION FUNCTION

In a way the communication function is one of the most intriguing functions of peer review. The fact that the peer review process intrinsically places professionals (and especially specialties) in an open and meaningful discourse one with the other is so conspicuous that it is often overlooked as a functional property for examination. When professionals of any kind insulate themselves from the world of knowledge or experience of other professionals, they become locked into their own peculiar form of circular reasoning.[19] At least some of this is inevitable in modern medical specialization. In the kind of cycle that results, men and organizations are forced to repeat the same way of doing things, the same set of basic assumptions, and the same mistakes. Men and women in this condition become at least to some degree blind to the limits of their own knowledge and to the potential benefits from doing things differently.

Communication, on the other hand, enables men and women to share their inner worlds with one another, thereby opening the possibility for exchanging their knowledge, skills, and perhaps most importantly, enhancing the will to change. There is an interesting parallel between the communication aspect of peer review and that of the problem-oriented medical record. Both provide a mechanism whereby "students" and "teachers" share (communicate) information through a common data base and can also share their thinking about clinical problems to establish a more open dialogue in working for quality patient care.

In much the same way the establishment of measures for clinical effectiveness via the development of explicit criteria and standards of comparison constitutes both an invitation and a vehicle for open communication. It is interesting, for example, to observe the discourse of physicians who share the same specialty as they attempt to set criteria for a specific diagnosis. Often what is communicated within the group is an appraisal of the state of the art in the process of defining what constitutes a professionally acceptable diagnostic approach or treatment for the conditions their specialty manages. Communication of this kind among professional equals can evolve into a kind of collective consciousness for recognizing better ways of doing things within the limits of current medical capabilities. This collective consciousness can be shared not only within specialties but also between specialties and across professional disciplines as well.

For example, it was most instructive to us to observe how general surgeons, family practitioners, and pediatricians worked cooperatively with otolaryngologists to develop a single criteria set on the indications of tonsillectomy. Agreement was not often previously found among the individual practitioners of these specialties on specific indicators for surgical intervention. Nonetheless, over time, one professional group was able to communicate (via research data on their own patient population) to the others why the therapeutic criterion or approach favored by them should be sanctioned as an acceptable alternative to the criteria already proposed by others. An essential step was conveying the fact that clinical outcomes in differing populations served by these various disciplines can differ and thus explain the need for one treatment rationale over another treatment rationale.

Besides the value of this type of communication between groups of physicians, there is also the intergroup communication of study results between physicians, other professionals, and the hospital administration, and between the hospital and the community. All of these links can be stimulated to varying degrees by systematic peer review that clearly defines its role and function as an instrument of change.

Both intraorganizational and interorganizational communication are important to the process of peer review. One illustration of such an intraorganizational program for communication was established for developing care criteria in a hospital setting. It went something like this:

1. Each criteria development session

was assigned a physician leader for each specific diagnosis. The goal of the physician leader was to have the panel arrive at consensus criteria for both the diagnosis and treatment of the given problem.

2. Prior to calling the panel into session, each physician leader first met with the director of medical education to decide by frequency, severity, and correctability which clinical entity should be chosen for examination at each meeting.

3. Once the entity was chosen, preliminary criteria for establishing the diagnosis and managing the therapy were developed by the physician leader in concert with the director of medical education. Data from a retrospective analysis of records were then reviewed to ascertain the extent to which these particular criteria were currently being met by fellow professionals.

4. At the actual meeting of the full criteria development panel the physician leader refrained from revealing either his own criteria or his data from the review of records until the specialty representatives independently went through the entire criteria-setting process.

5. A comparison was then made of the two criteria sets for diagnosis and treatment. A consensus method was subsequently used to get agreement on a single common criteria set. An analysis of conformity to these criteria was performed on retrospective data following that. The group then agreed to mount a similar analysis of prospective data to determine the degree of compliance with the consensus criteria. This latter analysis provided feedback data to the group to see whether a performance change (via the new criteria set) did or did not occur as a result of this mutual agreement to recognize a single standard of care.

This process produced some interesting communication events. First, it allowed each physician to take a position of leadership within his own specialty group. Second, it provided an opportunity for all members to share their knowledge. Third, it provided an open communication climate wherein feedback on results could be communicated via objective data to the entire group.

The educational value of criteria-setting activities using these theoretical constructs of communication becomes invaluable in itself as a mechanism for changing behaviors among professional groups. This effectiveness, through communication, may pose some possibilities for the dilemma Confucius wrote about when he said: "The way out is through the door. Why is it that no one will use this exit?"[2]

LEGAL FUNCTION

While a number of important legal matters associated with peer review and Public Law 92-603 (PSRO) are not sufficiently clear to warrant much discussion yet, there are nevertheless some interesting concepts that deserve attention because certain legal functions clearly are provided by most peer review systems whether intentionally so or not, and a few of these will be briefly reviewed here.

In a short article in 1974 Welch wrote some thoughts about the question of whether PSROs would reduce malpractice actions. According to Welch, an analysis by David Willett revealed the answer to be both yes and no.[20] The explanation offered can be summarized as follows: (1) If a physician were to provide patient care along the lines of PSRO-specified criteria, then cause for malpractice actions should be diminished. (2) If the physician's care did deviate from the criteria but a review of his records by the PSRO found the care to be innovative yet proper and effective, this community endorsement for the physician's methods would protect him. (3) If the physician did not stay within the criteria and his actions did not receive endorsement by the local PSRO, then the physician's position would be less secure in a liability context.

On the balance the legal function of PSRO, it is hypothesized, should have an overall effect of reducing malpractice considerably under the above gradient conditions. It should also be noted, however, that individual states can enact their own regulations thereby creating local and independent evaluative standards for medical care irrespective of PSRO standards.[21] In any event a well-established and systematic approach to peer review in local hospitals with medical society support probably has the best chance for providing reductions in malpractice actions in the years to come.

It is increasingly apparent that regardless of the form future third-party expenditures will provide for medical and health care (national health insurance, private catastrophic illness insurance, and so on) the monitoring of the medical care process and its clinical outcomes will likely be critical elements in reimbursements and resource allocations. If PSROs become the evaluative mechanism for such monitoring of medical care reimbursement, then the delegated review status concept for local hospitals could also extend to cost control measures and add critical new importance to peer review. Delegated status in this context would probably require a demonstration that the peer review system of the local hospital monitors care with sufficient effectiveness, reliability, and fiscal integrity to be trusted by the payor and that the review mechanism will not become self-service to the hospital. The delegated status for payment determinations would then also have specific legal ramifications for the local peer review group.

As reported by Curran and Moseley,[21] payment for treatment of a patient can be denied by a PSRO. This means that if a patient still wants the given care, he will have to pay for it himself. Under the condition of a PSRO denial of specific care

services, practitioners and other providers appear to be expressly protected from liability. The immunity clause has some qualifications, though, as cited by Curran and Moseley: "This immunity, however, is conditioned upon the physician having exercised due care in all professional conduct taken or directed by him and reasonably related to, and resulting from, the actions taken in compliance with, or in reliance upon, such professionally accepted norms of care and treatment."[21]

It should be noted, moreover, that there are several definable conditions under which an attending physician may not be legally secure.

1. The immunity clause seems least challengable if a physician seeks approval for a specific treatment that is denied.
2. The physician is still obligated to provide other modes of treatment even if a PSRO has rejected that one option.
3. If norms do not exist for specific treatments, the immunity clause apparently does not apply.
4. If a physician applies the norm of the local PSRO, but believes it to be incorrect, it is unclear whether the immunity will apply.[21]

If the above considerations exist in relations between the PSRO and the attending physician, these same questions can also be raised regarding immunity contingencies for a hospital's own peer review program (under the delegated status), since the same or similar professional norms and standards may apply.

The definitive legal functions of peer review will likely be clarified and developed over time, so it can only be said now that the direction and outcomes of the current direction are as yet unclear. However, what does seem to be abundantly clear about the legal functions associated with peer review is that the norms, standards, and criteria used are going to be taken seriously by the courts.

Peer review, which is a system for applying these professionally derived norms, standards, and criteria, could play an accelerated role in reducing the malpractice epidemic by becoming the stabilizing intervening variable. The extent and impact of that function and role is yet to be determined. As Carl Sandburg reflected: "Time is a great teacher. Who can live without hope?"

INNOVATION/CHANGE FUNCTION

In a 1973 monograph on quality assurance there was a thought-provoking article entitled "Diffusion of Innovation and Change in Health Systems" by Samuel Betty and Everett Rogers.[22] In that article they outline some important variables that seem to characterize innovation. The variables, which have implications for our functional discussion of peer review, are as follows:

1. Relative advantage: this concept suggests some advantage to adopting any one idea over another, which might also affect the rate of adoption of new techniques on the part of the individual being asked to change.
2. Compatibility: this has to do with whether the specific innovation is compatible with the values of the individual.
3. Complexity: this relates to the level of difficulty in understanding the proposed change. The less understood, the more slowly will be the acceptance of any proposed change.
4. Trialability or experimentation: if the suggested change is introduced as an experiment to be tried and tested, adoption of the change has less risk associated with it.
5. Observability: if the suggested change is observable and somewhat tangible, the chance for acceptance will be greater.

What is most interesting about these variables is that they are generalizations distilled from the results of some 2000 different studies on change and innovation.[22] Further, when these same variables are applied to the theoretical suggestions concerning peer review functions discussed in this chapter, some compatibility seems to emerge.

Simply stated, any systematic peer review approach that does not take cognizance of the function of change may lose some of the inherent potential value of the peer review process. In fact, when the above variables are utilized as criteria for evaluating the function of changes considered appropriate to operational peer review systems, some interesting hypotheses emerge.

First, peer review places the capability to implement change strategies with the physicians who participate in the review process itself. This places in their hands the basic tools to guide the process of evolutionary change. The extent to which peer review systems monitor such changes, using the aforementioned variables, is the extent to which the function of change can become explicitly operative within a peer review system.

Second, the more involved the local physicians are in setting criteria for and monitoring patient care, the more internalized becomes the adoption of new standards and the greater practice conformity can be expected from the peer review system. If any discrepancies associated with the physician's stated criteria for excellence and his actual behavior (as performed in clinical practice) are to be successfully dealt with, it will be necessary to measure these changes via systematic peer review.

Third, the more open, adaptive, and flexible the system of peer review, the greater the chance for survival of new values, norms, standards, and criteria for patient care. The benefit of an open system concept is that new clinical values, skills, and practices (as derived from new medical research) have a better chance for implementation into the medical practices, if the criteria, norms, and standards are flexible and not written into concrete.

While these particular variables basically

apply to the development of a system of peer review, they also apply internally to the operation of a peer review program, which is the guide to its optimization as a system. It can be said then that one function of peer review we cannot afford to forego is the innovation-change function of peer review.

CONCLUSION

While this chapter has by no means exhausted all the possible functions of peer review, we can say that the functions discussed are the ones we found to be the most frequently cited in the literature. From this composite of expressed interest emerges a matrix on which peer review systems can be evaluated. If it is agreed that the functions itemized in Fig. 4-2 are the critical ones, then we will be that much closer to defining the entity we have been calling peer review. In addition it would be possible to cross-compare various peer review systems using this matrix

to gauge the extent to which these functions are in fact made operational. If, on the other hand, a given peer review system only developed one function well (say accountability), then its usefulness to the local hospital would depend on the priority the hospital has for this function over all others. In like manner this matrix could be applied to evaluate the completeness of a comprehensive model of the review process in terms of serving all seven functions and the various levels of implementation for peer review (see Chapter 10). Finally, the above functions matrix could also be used as a guide in gauging the need for further development and implementation of operational peer review systems or their components.

REFERENCES

1. Webster's New World Dictionary of the American Language, college ed., New York, 1960, The World Publishing Co., page 586.
2. Watzlawick, P., Weakland, C. E., and Risch,

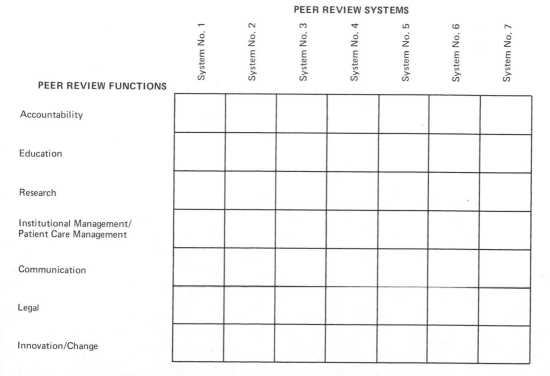

Fig. 4-2. Matrix assessment for systematic peer review.

R.: Change, New York, 1974, W. W. Norton & Co., pp. 4, 77.

3. Fuchs, V.: Who shall live: health economics and social choice, New York, 1974, Basic Books, Inc., Publishers, p. 4.

4. Public Law 92-603, Designation of Professional Standards Review Organization, The Social Security Act (as amended through January 4, 1975) and related laws, Committee on Finance, United States Senate, Section 1152 (a), pp. 322-341.

5. Boulding, K.: The ethics of rational decision-making, Science, February 1966, pp. 161-169.

6. Lee, R. I., and Jones, L. W.: The fundamentals of good medical care, Chicago, 1933, University of Chicago Press.

7. Brook, R. H.: Quality of care assessment: policy relevant issues, Policy Sciences **5:**318-320, 1974.

8. Galbraith, J. K.: Economics, peace, and laughter, New York, 1972, Signet Classics, pp. 17-18.

9. Bennett, W. F.: Education is PSRO goal, Hospitals, J. Am. Hosp. Assoc. **48:**53-58, 1974.

10. Howard, R.: Peer review—an educational necessity, J.A.M.A., **225**(7):731-732, 1973.

11. Perlman, J. M., and Slee, V. N.: Defining educational needs, PAS and MAP, N. Engl. J. Med. **284**(20) (suppl):74-81, 1971.

12. Bruner, J. S.: On knowing, New York, 1962, Atheneum Press.

13. Glasser, W.: Quotation from a film: Glasser on schools, 1970.

14. Guilford, J. P.: The nature of human intelligence, New York, 1967, McGraw-Hill Book Co.

15. Fattu, N. A.: Experimental studies of problem-solving, J. Med. Educ. **39:**212-225, 1964.

16. Gilson, B. S., Gilson, J. S., Bergner, M. et al.: The sickness impact profile, Am. J. Public Health **65**(12):1304-1310, 1975.

17. Farrell, J. R.: PSROs and internal hospital review, **2**(11):1-7, 1973.

18. McGregor, D.: The human side of enterprise, New York, 1960, McGraw-Hill Book Co., p. 132.

19. Barnland, D. C.: Communication: the context of change. In Larson, C. E., and Dance, F. E., editors: Perspectives on communication, Milwaukee, 1968, University of Wisconsin, Speech Communication Center, p. 34.

20. Welch, C. E.: PSROs—pros and cons, N. Engl. J. Med. **290**(23):1319-1323, 1974.

21. Curran, W. J., and Moseley, G. B.: The malpractice experience of health maintenance organizations, Northwestern Univ. Law Rev. **70**(1): 78-79, 1975. Arizona has required hospitals via physician groups to review the medical practice.

22. Betty, S. A., and Rogers, E. M.: The diffusion of innovations and change in health systems (monograph on quality assurance of medical care), Washington, D.C., February 1973, Regional Medical Programs Service, Health Services and Mental Health Administration, U.S. Dept. of Health, Education, and Welfare, pp. 403-424.

5

Quality assessment: issues of definition and measurement

ROBERT H. BROOK
ALLYSON DAVIES-AVERY

Quality of medical care is a concept in search of measurement. As with any other concept, it must first be defined in order to be validly and reliably measured. Furthermore the validity and reliability of the measurement process itself must be considered before it is used in an operational context to alter the manner in which medical care is provided. Unfortunately concepts encountered in the health field are often both poorly defined and measured, and methods problems are frequently ignored. Despite this, concepts are measured and conclusions reached. This sequence must be carefully avoided when dealing with quality of medical care, since inadequate definition and invalid or unreliable measures may produce considerable harm in the name of doing good.

This chapter discusses six major issues in the conceptualization and measurement of the quality of medical care. These issues include

1. How quality should be defined

2. How medical care problems should be selected for quality assessment activities
3. What type of data should be used to measure quality
4. What data source should be used to measure quality
5. How criteria to determine whether quality is good or bad should be set
6. What values should be applied to these criteria

The history of quality assessment activities, current political controversies over approaches to quality assessment and assurance, and the ways in which measurement data can be used to improve quality of care are not specifically considered here. For discussion of these broader issues (to put those considered here in perspective) the reader is referred to references 1 through 6.

DEFINITION OF QUALITY OF CARE

To measure quality and have some confidence that the concept has been truly measured, one must first try to define it. The definition of quality of medical care can be approached from several different vantage points. Two in particular are worth discussing. The first is how to define the quality of the physician-patient inter-

The research reported herein was performed pursuant to a grant from the U.S. Department of Health, Education, and Welfare, Washington, D.C. The opinions and conclusions expressed herein are solely those of the authors and should not be construed as representing the opinions or policy of any agency of the United States government.

action itself, and the second is how to define the quality of the medical care system as a whole.

Quality of physician-patient interaction

Regarding the physician-patient interaction, the following variables have been considered important: (1) the adequacy of the technical management of the symptoms or signs with which the patient presents to the physician, (2) the adequacy of the art of care, and (3) the adequacy of the efficiency of care. Technical medical care here is taken to represent the adequacy of the performance of preventive, diagnostic, and therapeutic procedures vis-à-vis the patient's needs or conditions. Art of care refers to the manner of physician care relative to the patient as an individual, as measured by its sensitivity, openness, and non-authoritarian nature. Efficiency refers to the ability of the physician to arrive at a favorable solution to the patient's problem while consuming the minimum amount of resources necessary.

Most work in quality assessment has concentrated on measuring the quality of the physician-patient relationship. In particular it has involved measuring the technical aspects of the physician-patient relationship. Little attention has been paid to measuring the art of care aspect of medical practice. Similarly, efficiency has rarely been measured, and many people still argue that this concept should not be considered as part of the quality of the physician-patient relationship. Examination of the work in this field indicates that to many people quality of medical care, at least as presently measured, is synonymous with the technical management of health and disease. That in itself is not harmful as long as the reader is aware that investigators have chosen to limit their definition of quality and thus measure only some part of it.

Quality of medical care system

Many experts, especially operations researchers and health services researchers,

when formulating their concept of quality of care, are implicitly considering the quality of the entire medical care system. In taking this viewpoint they further broaden the definition of quality by including at least two additional concepts: (1) accessibility of medical services and (2) availability of medical services. They also broaden the definition of quality by considering health professionals other than physicians and by considering an entire episode of illness as opposed to an isolated visit. Virtually all measures of the physician-patient relationship are physician centered; virtually all measures of the quality of the medical care system are patient centered. For example, the input of nurses, physical therapists, pharmacists, and all other health professionals who make independent decisions would be considered in a statement about the quality of the medical care system. Although measurement of all components is rarely possible in a single study, it is important to keep in mind, at least at a conceptual level, that quality concerns more than just physician actions and includes variables other than the technical management of health and illness.

This broad definition of the quality of medical care—the one we prefer—provides much guidance to the developer of a quality assessment or assurance program. Since quality is seen as a multidimensional concept, it is readily apparent that construction of a single index of quality will be difficult if not impossible. Instead, multiple indicators will be necessary to describe the functioning and impact of a quality assurance program on quality of care. Furthermore, in particular situations some variables under the quality rubric might be more critical to improvements in health status than others; a multidimensional construct can be adapted to reflect this fact.

Purpose of improving quality

Clearly the purpose of improving quality of care is to improve the health status of the patient. In this case health status should be defined broadly to include physiologic, physical, social, and mental health concepts and to take account of both the positive and negative dimensions of these concepts. Improvement in health status is thereby the criterion by which quality can be validated, and the value of any program that attempts to improve quality of care can be assessed by whether it improves a patient's health status.

A person presents to the medical care system for one of three reasons: (1) he is seeking preventive medical services or health maintenance; (2) he is seeking services for acute problems; or (3) he is seeking services for care of problems that have existed for a long time. In each case considerations of accessibility, availability, efficiency, the technical management of care, and the art of care combine to determine whether the interaction of the patient with the system will improve his health status, maintain it, or at least prevent it from deteriorating as fast as it might if there were no interaction with the system. The quality of the services rendered will at least in part determine that patient's outcome. However, different components of those services will be more or less critical in producing a good outcome, depending on the patient's needs. A patient presenting with chronic nonspecific joint pain due to osteoarthritis, for which definitive medical care is not available, will be very dependent on the quality of the art of care for a good outcome. A patient presenting with a fractured femur will be most dependent on the quality of the technical care in achieving a good outcome. Finally, a patient presenting for health maintenance or preventive services may be most dependent on the accessibility and availability of these services if a good outcome is to be achieved. Clearly when quality assessment is being done, a model that links these variables together in some a priori manner should be built so that the points at which the quality of care given is critical can be identified.

An example of how this can be done is given for hypertension. To maximize the health status of a patient with hypertension to reduce the incidence of strokes, the following steps must be accomplished: (1) hypertension must be identified through some type of screening program; (2) the type of hypertension that the patient has must be identified; (3) the severity of the hypertension must be determined; (4) therapy must be instituted; and (5) a recursive cycle must be set up so the ability to control the hypertension can be determined. To carry out these tasks many providers other than physicians must be involved in the care of the patient, variables other than the technical management of the disease are important, and considerations of quality extend beyond a single visit to consider at least an episode of illness or multiple visits for this chronic disease. A study done by Brook at a large city hospital indicated two major problems in the quality of care given to hypertensive patients: (1) since the blood pressure taken by the nurse was recorded at the top of the chart, it was not noted by the physician, and thus medication was not altered to lower the blood pressure in the considerable number of patients who remained hypertensive; and (2) a large proportion of patients were noncompliant and did not return for appointments or did not take medication. This was at least in part due to the fact that the art of care was not emphasized in this institution; written instructions were not given to patients regarding how they should take their medication, and follow-up of missed appointments was minimal. On the other hand, the diagnostic investigations done on these patients were superb and met the highest standards of quality. Overall, if only the adequacy of the diagnostic investigations had been measured (and this is usually as far as measures of quality go, especially those focused on the technical aspects of the physician-patient relationship), then the quality of the care would have been judged as very adequate. Of course this would have been a misleading conclusion, since problems in the art of care and follow-up prevented adequate control of these patients' blood pressure. As a result, about half of the patients showed no improvement in health status, remaining hypertensive at the end of the study.[1]

Summary

This rather lengthy, albeit oversimplified, discussion of how quality of medical care should be conceptualized is necessary because most studies of quality in the literature rely heavily on only one, or at the most two, components of the quality matrix. In many studies only a single visit or a single hospitalization is considered. Criteria established for quality assessment often relate only to the physician. Furthermore, most criteria are heavily weighted toward diagnosis, with therapy and management being distant cousins. Finally, concepts such as efficiency, accessibility, availability, and the art of care are hardly ever studied. Nevertheless the authors of such studies conclude, often without qualification, that quality of care is either good, bad, or indifferent. The reader of such studies should be aware that such conclusions may be erroneous, especially when only diagnostic interventions were measured and care was judged good on the basis of the results of such measures.

For patients who present to the medical care system with acute problems, a narrow definition of quality of care may be adequate. However, for the majority of patients who present to the medical care system for health maintenance or preventive services or who have chronic problems demanding long-term care, a physician-oriented, diagnosis-specific quality of care assessment is inadequate. In the future operational quality assurance programs will begin to pay attention to broader considerations and to measure multiple variables during a single quality assessment study; this level of sophistication, however, is at least 5 to 10 years away. At present, as long as one has a model for how these multiple variables relate to health status for a given set of patients in a given set of institutions, measurement of one component of quality may suffice for most operational programs. This observation is based on the fact that hundreds of studies of the quality of care using a narrow conceptualization have been performed, and most have shown remarkable deficiencies in the level of care given, no matter what variable was measured for what group of patients in what set of institutions. What has not been shown is that improvement in the quality of that particular service will improve the health status of the patient. This is probably due to the fact that the link between health status and quality was not conceptualized at the beginning of the study. For instance, in the earlier example recognition of the high blood pressure by the physician and change in medication would not have significantly improved health status in the absence of attempts to improve the art of care given and thus the compliance of patients. If the latter variable had not been measured, people could have assumed that increased recognition of hypertension by the physician would automatically have led to improvements in health status. Thus measurement of one or two components of quality may be appropriate in a quality assessment study; in a quality assurance program, however, unless one is virtually positive that the improvements made will affect health status, changes in health status per se must be assessed to determine whether the quality assurance program actually worked.

SELECTION OF STUDY POPULATION

The first major methodologic question to be addressed in a quality assessment study is: which patients with what medical problems should be studied? Quality assessment is expensive. This usually means that only a small proportion of patients can be studied or, if large numbers of patients are studied, that superficial measures must be used. Although the issue of systematic sampling is critical, the major problem in the selection procedure is the content of the sample, that is, the sampling frame. Almost all quality of care studies start from a list of diagnoses. In the hospital this might be a diagnosis-specific list of conditions completed at the time of discharge from the hospital. Such lists are generally easy to compile and readily available. Development of a comparable list in ambulatory care requires examination of medical records from which diagnoses are abstracted. This is extremely difficult to do, since ambulatory records are sketchy at best; often too the ambulatory visit does not result in a definitive diagnosis. Lists of diagnoses for ambulatory problems can also be obtained in some instances from fiscal intermediaries or from laboratories that maintain duplicate copies of results. In any event, however, lists of problems or symptoms (as opposed to diagnoses) for which ambulatory care is sought do not now generally exist.

For many conditions the critical question in assessing quality may be the accuracy or reliability of the diagnosis itself. Identifying a patient sample via a diagnostic list does not permit the quality assessment study to address the issue of the probability that the diagnosis is correct or that false-negative and false-positive errors in diagnosis are at a minimum. It is preferable therefore to begin a quality assessment study from a defined symptom, sign, or problem. In most cases, however, the basic clinical research that would relate signs and symptoms to prognosis and outcome has not yet been completed, which makes the use of signs and symptoms as a sampling frame somewhat premature. In addition, such data are not recorded for either ambulatory or hospital patients in an easily retrievable form. In the future a symptom-oriented coding system such as that now being developed by the National Center for Health Statistics for the National Ambulatory Medical Care Survey might be incorporated routinely into both ambulatory and hospital records.[7] Such a system might also stimulate necessary basic clinical research so that signs and symptoms can be used as the sampling frame for a quality assessment system.

One other possible type of sampling frame involves health status indices, which are now in the process of development; over the next 5 to 10 years their reliability and validity will undoubtedly increase.[8,9] Most are being developed in a manner that permits self-administration by patients and thus decreases their operational cost when used in a real-life situation. In the future it may be possible to send such questionnaires to a sample of patients discharged from a hospital, enrolled in a health maintenance organization, or in the care of a solo practitioner or group of physicians. The results of such questionnaires could be analyzed to indicate which patients have relatively good or poor health. For the latter a detailed investigation could be undertaken to determine whether changes in the level of quality of care could have resulted in better current health status or would result in improvement of future health status.

At the moment the sampling frame must be derived from diagnoses, not signs and symptoms or health status indices. Given the limitations inherent in this approach the next question to be addressed is: how should the diagnoses be chosen? Five basic approaches have been suggested: (1) choose the most frequent diagnosis; (2) choose the diagnosis for which the product of the frequency times the ability of medical care to make a difference is maximal; (3) choose the diagnosis for which we know problems exist in the care rendered; (4) choose a rare diagnosis, since we may learn something more about the pathophysiology of that disease; and (5) choose the diagnosis that will make us look good. These five approaches are not mutually exclusive; they all possess some positive characteristics. For instance, choosing a disease for which the results of quality assessment are expected to be good may increase the acceptance of the quality assessment program by a group of physicians. Similarly, studying a rare disease in a university medical center may facilitate the acceptance of a quality assessment program in that setting. We believe that neither of these two approaches is warranted because each consumes scarce resources and very likely does not actually improve the health status of patients. The first criterion (frequency alone) as a variant of the second criterion (frequency times ability of medical care to alter the natural history of the disease) is overly simplistic and will be discarded for that reason. This leaves two criteria: either choose a problem area in which you know deficiencies exist or attempt to determine which conditions in your population have a maximum score on a product between frequency and the ability of medical care to make a difference. At the beginning of a quality assessment program the data to develop the latter criterion will be unavailable and literature reviews and educated guesswork will be required. For this reason it is probably legitimate to begin any quality assessment program by studying those problems for which physicians as a peer group believe care to be deficient.

The New Mexico Experimental Medical Care Review Organization (EMCRO) began in this manner. The physicians involved believed that injections were being given with great frequency in their state, and they undertook a scientific study of the problem. They found that injections were being given at a rate of about 0.4 per ambulatory visit and that some physicians administered more inappropriate injections than others. EMCRO established criteria for the proper use of injectables, mounted an educational program, and then implemented a sanction system based on denial of payment for claims for medically unnecessary injections. This peer review quality assessment program dramatically curtailed the use of unnecessary injectables. Since over half of the improper injectables were antibiotics, reduction in their use would be associated with reduction in adverse reactions such as rashes, drug fevers, and even an occasional anaphylactic reaction or death.[10]

The principle to be kept in mind when selecting diagnoses or problems for study is that generalization from study results to other diagnoses and problems is fraught with error. There are no convincing data to indicate that physicians manage all their patients, even those with similar diseases, at the same level of quality. Payne and Lyons assessed the quality of care given to people hospitalized for some 20 different conditions in all nonfederal acute short-stay hospitals in Hawaii; they did a similar study on problems seen in office-based practice.[11,12] They observed that for some conditions physicians in group practice provided better care than did solo practitioners; for other conditions the statistics were reversed. Furthermore, for similar conditions such as acute urinary tract infection or diabetes mellitus or hypertension, physician performance varied widely from what was expected and varied from condition to condition, so that generalizations about overall quality of care from the few conditions studied would be inappropriate.

A study done by Brook examined the quality of care given by interns and residents to patients presenting to a large teaching hospital with urinary tract infections, duodenal or gastric ulcers, or hypertension, and found similar results. Even though the same interns and residents were treating patients with three common chronic medical conditions, the quality of care given to patients varied as a function of the condition.[1] Thus generalization of the quality of care given by an internist to patients with diabetes mellitus is impossible if only patients with hypertension are studied. Clearly generalization of the quality of hospital care given is impossible when, for instance, only one or two surgical conditions are studied and no obstetric, gynecologic, or medical conditions are studied.

This problem of generalization is unavoidable at present. In the future it may be partially overcome by sampling on some health status measure, as discussed above. At present, readers of quality assessment studies must be cognizant of the manner in which problems are identified. An organization or group of physicians can determine the image of quality of care they present to the community by controlling the selection process. If only problems or diagnoses that are known to be managed adequately are selected, then the level of quality reported will be high. Similarly, in those institutions that attempt to maximize the impact of a quality assessment program on health status and thus select areas for study in which they know they are deficient, a low level of quality will be reported. Thus quality assessment activities must be put in context; otherwise reported results will inhibit the development of programs that really aim to improve the health status of patients.

TYPE OF DATA
Structure

Donabedian, in what is now a classic article, identified three different variables by which quality of care can be measured: structure, process, and outcome.[13] Structural measurements are concerned with descriptive characteristics of facilities or providers or both such as the number of hospital beds, the ratio of physicians per population, the number of nurses per physician, or whether the physician is board certified or has attended postgraduate education courses. Quality assessment in its infancy was concerned chiefly with measuring structural factors; without testing the validity of the assertion, people argued that better scores on these structural variables would automatically indicate, for example, which physicians actually delivered better care or which nurses cared most about their patients.

When these variables were studied, variation in performance of physicians and hospitals was found to be a function of structural variables. The study of the use of the anesthetic halothane in various hospitals showed that mortality rates for common operations varied tenfold as a function of the individual hospital in which the operation was performed.[14] The recent Institutional Differences Study, refining the methodology of the halothane study, has shown a two and one-half to threefold difference in mortality rates for common operations, again as a function of the individual hospital in which they are performed.[15]

For those structural variables that have been validated against the actual care delivered, however, inconsistent and unexpected correlations have been found. Studies done in both Vermont and Kansas showed that operative rates for common conditions varied two to fivefold by regions within each state as a function of the number of surgeons in that region. Areas with the greatest ratios of surgeons per population (a structural measure of better quality) had the highest operative rates; however, the studies suggested that many of the operations done appeared to be unnecessary and that better care was probably not associated with a greater number of surgeons.[16,17] Another study found that even if a patient goes to a physician who is board certified, graduated from a good medical school, graduated high in the medical school class, or reads a large number of medical journals, he has no guarantee of high quality of care on the basis of those physician characteristics. The only two structural variables that seem to relate consistently to better quality of care are the age of the physician (as the physician ages, the technical care delivered becomes worse) and whether the physician is a modal specialist (a modal specialist is a physician who is trained to treat the condition for which the patient presents; a urologist would be the modal specialist for a child with a kidney stone, rather than a pediatrician).[11]

Process

Because of these problems in the validity of structural measures, that is, their relationship to changes in health status of patients, recent attempts to assess quality of care have turned to process and outcome measures. Process measures are those that evaluate how a person is moved into and

Table 5-1. Process criteria for pneumonia: Hawaii Medical Association*

Services recommended†	Weights
History: specific reference to:	
Character of sputum	2.0
Pain in chest	2.0
Duration and degree of fever	2.0
Onset of illness	1.0
Previous episodes and social history	1.0
Contact history	1.0
Physical examination: specific reference to:	
Breath sounds, character, presence or absence of	2.0
Friction rub	1.0
Rales	1.0
Chest movements	1.0
Percussion	1.0
Cyanosis	2.0
Vital signs—temperature, pulse, respiration, blood pressure	2.0
Character of respiration	2.0
Laboratory:	
CBC	2.0
Blood culture in seriously ill patient (temperature equal to or greater than 104°, cyanotic, needs oxygen)	3.0
Sputum or throat culture with sensitivities	3.0
Roentgenology:	
PA and lateral of chest on admission	3.0
Follow-up chest X-ray in seven days or before discharge	2.0
Therapy: appropriate antibiotics (not sulfa drug or chloramphenicol)	3.0

*Adapted from Payne, B. C., and study staff: Methods of evaluating and improving personal medical care quality: episode of illness study, Chicago, 1976, Hospital Research and Educational Trust, appendix C, p. 38.
†Indications for admission: presence of proven or suspected pneumonia.

out of the medical care system, that is, what is done to or for the patient with respect to his particular disease or complaint and how well it is done. Outcome measures describe what happened to the patient's health status in terms of palliation, cure, rehabilitation, or whatever other descriptors are applicable.

Considering process measures first, Table 5-1 illustrates a set of process criteria that were developed by the Hawaii Medical Society to measure the quality of care given to patients who present with pneumonia, from which some generalizations about process criteria can be made. First, process measures are usually disease- or diagnosis-specific, and the limitations of such an approach were discussed previously. Second, most process measures are

applicable only to the types of care rendered in inpatient settings; very few have been developed to assess care in outpatient settings. Third, process measures usually are confined to the following procedures: history, physical, laboratory tests, and occasionally therapy; the tender-loving-care aspect of medical care is not measured. The reason for this is that the data source from which most process information is obtained is the medical record, which rarely contains information about the art of care provided. Fourth, although process measures are usually weighted, the weighting scheme is simplistic and by no means reflects the decision-making process of a physician. For instance, a doctor could receive a near-perfect score (97) if he performed every task listed in Table 5-1 except the one that requires giving the pneumonia patient an antibiotic, yet the patient probably would suffer a great deal of unnecessary morbidity and might even die. Fifth, process measures are usually limited to the services a physician provides and do not include services provided by other personnel such as nurses who make independent decisions. Process criteria are thus provider centered and not patient centered, resulting in the probability that multiple audits may be done on a single patient, none of which will give a true picture of the care received. Finally, development of these lists of process measures depends largely on clinical judgment. This last point needs emphasis and underscores the problem of validity of the use of process measures in quality assessment, since it raises the issue of the validity of clinical judgment. Can physicians distinguish those components of the process of care that relate to improved health from those that do not? Corollary questions are: what do we know about the efficacy of certain procedures that are judged medically necessary? Do they actually promote better health?

A problem in relying on clinical judgment in the setting of process criteria lies in the fact that medical students and physicians in training programs are taught to minimize type I errors at the expense of type II errors. A story that paraphrases a real event illustrates this problem. A nephrologist was called to see a seriously ill patient at 2 AM. The patient had had a renal transplant and was now suffering the symptoms of an acute abdominal attack. The decision to be made was whether an immediate operation was necessary. The nephrologist asked the following questions of the surgeon: What was the probability that the patient really had an acute abdomen? The answer was 25%. What was the probability that the patient would die if indeed he had an acute abdomen and was not operated on? The answer was 100%. What was the probability that the patient would die if he had the operation,

regardless of whether an acute abdomen was present? The answer was 50%. What was the probability that this patient would die if not operated on, if he did not have an acute abdomen? The answer was zero percent. Both physicians agreed that these were the best possible estimates of the Bayesian probabilities. Given this, the patient was clearly better off if treated medically. However, the surgeon (a senior member of a prestigious medical faculty) refused to accept this conclusion, probably for two reasons. First, he had never used this simple type of decision logic to arrive at a solution to a clinical problem. Second, he had been taught implicitly that death produced in a heroic effort to save a life is less criticized than a death produced by not making the same effort. Thus errors of judgment involving the overuse of aggressive therapy are criticized far less than errors associated with not doing enough.

Similar problems in clinical judgment have been more formally documented for a broader physician population in research done by Leaper and associates. They initially collected uniform data on patients who presented with acute abdominal symptoms.[19,20] Using these data and a Bayesian approach, they programmed a computer to predict both the diagnosis and the probability that the patient needed an operation. The probability decision is the crucial decision in treating these patients. In a prospective study, Leaper and associates then matched the computer against the senior consultant surgeon. As can be seen in Table 5-2, the computer's error rate was 8.2%, as compared to 20.4% for some of the best surgeons in the area; this difference was significant at <0.0001. (The surgeon's error rate is considered by United States standards to be very good.) Following the physicians' clinical judgments would have resulted in six patients with appendicitis having their operations delayed over 8 hours (clinical false-negatives) and in 27 patients having an unnecessary operation (clinical false-positives) because their nonspecific pain was

Table 5-2. Comparison of diagnosis made by senior clinician and computer prediction with final diagnosis—304 patients with acute abdominal pain*

Condition	Final diagnosis (number of patients)							
	Appen.	Divert.	Perf. D.U.	N.S. pain	Chole-cyst.	S.B. obst.	Pan-creat.	Other
Appendicitis								
Clinician	75	—	1	27	—	—	—	3
Computer	84	—	—	6	—	—	—	3
Diverticulitis								
Clinician	1	2	—	—	—	—	1	1
Computer	1	4	—	—	—	—	1	3
Perforated duodenal ulcer								
Clinician	—	—	5	1	—	—	1	—
Computer	—	—	7	1	—	—	1	—
Nonspecific pain								
Clinician	6	1	—	117	—	—	—	1
Computer	—	—	—	136	—	—	—	1
Cholecystitis								
Clinician	—	—	—	2	10	—	1	—
Computer	—	—	—	1	26	—	—	1
Small bowel obstruction								
Clinician	—	—	—	—	1	17	—	1
Computer	—	—	—	—	—	16	—	—
Pancreatitis								
Clinician	—	—	—	1	3	—	5	—
Computer	—	—	—	3	—	1	6	—
Other								
Clinician	3	1	1	1	2	—	—	2
Computer	—	—	—	—	—	—	—	—

*Adapted from de Dombal, F. T., Leaper, D. J., Staniland, J. R., et al.: Computer-aided diagnosis of acute abdominal pain, Br. Med. J. **2:**9-13, 1972.

misdiagnosed. If the computer predictions had been followed, the numbers of patients mistreated would have been zero and six, respectively. Both numbers are far superior to the two generated by the clinicians. Following computer predictions would have resulted in significantly lower false-negative and false-positive rates than following physicians' clinical judgments.

Subsequently the investigators attempted to determine the reason for these differences. They asked each surgeon to complete a table relating the probability of making a diagnosis, such as appendicitis or diverticulitis, to a process element, such as the age of the patient or the results of a white blood cell count. They compared the surgeon's responses to computer-generated probabilities based on experience with 2000 patients and found major differences (see Table 5-3). In the absence of published information that related the probability of a particular diagnosis given a set of multiple symptoms, the surgeons were working from sets of personal probabilities that were inherently wrong. In addition, when the correct computer-generated tables were released to the surgeons and their comments solicited about the correctness of the results, virtually all results were changed by the surgeons back to their original (incorrect) probabilities. Not only were the surgeons wrong, they were adamantly wrong. If good process criteria

Table 5-3. Comparison of frequency of actual diagnosis estimated by senior clinician and by computer as a function of patient age in cases of acute abdominal pain*

Condition	Frequency in patient age group (%)							
	0-9	**10-19**	**20-29**	**30-39**	**40-49**	**50-59**	**60-69**	**70+**
Appendicitis								
Clinician	30	20	20	10	5	2	1	2
Computer	22	33	22	8	5	5	4	1
Diverticulitis								
Clinician	0	0	0	5	20	30	20	25
Computer	0	0	2	2	10	10	28	48
Perforated duodenal ulcer								
Clinician	0	0	10	20	30	20	15	5
Computer	0	4	7	9	26	22	20	12
Nonspecific pain								
Clinician	30	30	20	10	5	2	1	2
Computer	14	41	19	7	5	3	7	4
Cholecystitis								
Clinician	0	0	10	30	40	10	5	5
Computer	0	1	8	4	9	19	26	33
Small bowel obstruction								
Clinician	0	5	10	20	25	20	10	10
Computer	2	6	24	6	14	14	18	16
Pancreatitis								
Clinician	0	0	5	15	30	30	15	5
Computer	0	2	8	6	14	16	30	24

*Adapted from Leaper, D. J., Horrocks, J. C., Staniland, J. R., and de Dombal, F. T.: Computer-assisted diagnosis of abdominal pain using estimates provided by clinicians, Br. Med. J. **4:**350-354, 1972.

are to be developed for quality care assessment, this misuse of information must be corrected.

These two problems, lack of knowledge about decision making and the ready acceptance of aggressive therapy, have led and will continue to lead to serious problems in the use of process measures in the assessment of quality of care. A typical table from a standard medical textbook (Table 5-4) lists the symptoms associated with a given diagnosis, giving the impression that the symptoms occur independently. This independence does not accurately reflect the true situation—if it did, there could be no classic case of this or any condition—but the student of medicine is not taught this. Eventually the student, probably through luck, develops a diagnostic method that takes into account the interrelationship of presenting symptoms; with such a diagnostic approach he may practice medicine as a physician at a reasonable level. In setting process criteria, however, the physician probably reverts to old habits and develops tabular lists again (see Table 5-1). It is only very recently that any principles of decision making or clustering of symptoms have been applied to the development of any criteria by which the process of care could be judged.

Given these problems in clinical decision making and in setting criteria that reflect the decision-making process, it is evident that process criteria require careful analysis in terms of implied or potential impact on delivery of care and health status. This requirement applies even to those criteria that seem to be relatively simple to implement and that may have received widespread approval. One seemingly simple and widely accepted process criterion is

Table 5-4. Typical table of symptoms: frequency of manifestations of acromegaly*

Manifestation	Percent
Parasellar manifestations	
Enlarged sella turcica	95
Headache	85
Visual impairment	54
Uncinate fits	7
Rhinorrhea	15
Pituitary apoplexy	3
Papilledema	3
Growth hormone excess	
Weight gain	64
Hypermetabolism	52
Hyperhidrosis	73
Impaired glucose tolerance	36
Clinical diabetes mellitus	17
Acral growth	96
Enlarged hands	82
Prognathism	88
Arthritic complaints	64
Osteoporosis	80 (estimated)
Soft tissue growth	100
Hirsutism	60
Pigmentation	40
Fibroma molluscum	27
Visceromegaly	80 (estimated)
Serum PO_4 over 4.5 mg/100 ml	50
Fatiguability	60
Insulin sensitivity (does not include patients with clinical diabetes mellitus)	71
Disturbance of other hormones	
Lactorrhea (LTH excess?)	4
Hyperadrenocorticism	Rare
Hyperthyroidism	Rare
Increased libido	38
Decreased libido, male	23
Menstrual disturbances	89
Goiter	25

*Adapted from Hume, D. M., and Harrison, T. S.: Pituitary and adrenal. In Schwartz, S. I.: Principles of surgery, ed. 2, New York, 1974, McGraw-Hill Book Co.

that all children should have a cardiac examination during the first year of life. The purpose of this examination is to identify those children with congenital heart disease and to correct the lesions before harm is done. The prevalence of congenital heart disease is low (less than 1%), but the prevalence of innocent heart murmurs in children may approach 50%. There is plenty of room for diagnostic error, even by the most skilled cardiologist. Indeed, in a follow-up study at the junior high school level of all children previously labeled as having cardiac disease, Bergman[21] concluded that the morbidity from cardiac nondisease was greater than the morbidity from cardiac disease. Thus the health of the community was adversely affected by this screening process. This situation is similar to countless others in which the prevalence of a condition is extremely low. For virtually all these situations false-positive rates on screening or diagnosis might be unacceptably high and could result in the creation of more morbidity than was cured.

In the therapeutic area insistence on an aggressive therapeutic approach in the absence of information can lead to similar problems. Consider the following process criteria that were accepted by most physicians a few years ago and would still be accepted by many physicians today:

1. Most patients with varicose veins should be treated by surgical therapy rather than injection-compression therapy.
2. Most adult-onset diabetics should be treated with oral hypoglycemic agents if diet alone does not control the disease.
3. All patients who suffer an acute heart attack should be hospitalized in a coronary care unit.
4. All women who develop breast cancer should have a radical mastectomy.

All of these widely agreed-to criteria support aggressive medical or surgical intervention. Yet each has been shown in randomized, controlled clinical trials to have questionable or no validity. Patients with varicose veins pay five times more for care when treated by surgery, are exposed to all the morbid events of an operation, and have a cosmetic result no better than the patients treated by the simpler outpatient therapy.[22,23] Diabetics treated with oral hypoglycemic agents die sooner of cardiovascular disease, and the late complications of diabetes are not prevented.[24] The survival rate for at least one third of patients with an acute heart attack (the low-risk group) is no higher in a coronary care unit than at home. Indeed, for people over age 65 who suffer a heart attack, home care yields higher survival rates than does hospital care.[25] Finally, there is no evidence that a radical mastectomy for some groups of women who develop breast cancer increases their chances for survival

over the use of a simple mastectomy, but the former group suffers a great deal more morbidity.[26]

Development of process criteria may result in the legitimization of aggressive therapies that are both costly and produce more harm than good. This must be avoided by questioning the judgments concerning both efficacy and effectiveness that are implicit in each criterion. The actions implied by all the above criteria are not efficacious and, by extension, not effective, but many efficacious criteria may still be ineffective. For instance, the replacement of an aortic valve in a university hospital that does many such operations annually may be extremely efficacious, but the same operation performed in a hospital that does four a year may produce more harm than good and be ineffective.

This problem of process criteria based on implicit judgments of effective and efficacious medical care is critical. The percent of the gross national product spent on health care is rising. If the use of invalid process criteria accelerates this process by promoting the use of nonefficacious and inefficient medical therapies, large problems in resource allocation will develop. It has been estimated that if existing lists of process criteria were implemented, ambulatory services would increase by 150% and inpatient services by about 50%.[27] Many of these criteria are probably invalid, and it is imperative that better quantitative techniques be brought to bear to separate valid from invalid process criteria.

Outcome

After reviewing these drawbacks in the use of structural and process measures to assess the quality of medical care, the use of outcome measures would appear to be the only answer. This conclusion is not warranted, however; outcomes of care are largely determined by the natural history of the disease and other factors outside the personal medical care system such as patient behavior. Unless the more important extrinsic circumstances influencing outcomes are clearly understood and controlled, valid assessment of the quality of care will be impossible. Unfortunately, since clinical research generally concerns itself with length of life rather than quality of life, we know little about the natural history of many diseases, especially in terms of outcomes other than death. For instance, if we wanted to assess the care given to patients with leukemia in terms of outcomes such as number of days the patient was in pain, able to perform his usual activities, or able to function as a member of a family, we would not be doing quality assessment but basic clinical research. The total lack of this type of information is one reason why clinicians often hide behind the mantle of clinical judgment when making therapeutic decisions.

Despite the lack of information about the natural history of disease, outcome measures are very useful in assessing the quality of medical care. First, they represent the measure of most interest, since their focus is on the patient's health status following the intervention of medical care. A quality assurance system that can state only that it increased the number of ECGs taken per heart attack patient is less impressive than one that says it halved the death rate or doubled the percentage of heart attack patients who returned to work.

Second, outcome is a multidimensional concept, as are health status and quality of care. Therefore one cannot measure all outcomes of care by just examining mortality, morbidity, or disability; all appropriate or possible outcomes must be conceptualized and either included in the measurement effort or excluded for explicit reasons. One conceptual framework for outcome assessment recently developed by Starfield[28] includes the following variables and categories:

Resilience	Resilient versus vulnerable
Achievement	Achieving versus not achieving
Disease	Not detectable, asymptomatic, temporary, permanent
Satisfaction	Satisfied versus dissatisfied
Comfort	Comfortable versus uncomfortable
Activity	Functional versus disabled
Longevity	Normal life expectancy versus death

Third, outcome measures implicitly take into account the quality of the art of care provided. Virtually all process measures are related to technical aspects of care. An outcome such as the return to work rate or longevity following a heart attack measures both the physician's technical ability to manage this complex entity and the physician's ability to relate to the patient and convince him to change his personal habits to maximize his life expectancy.

Finally, outcome measures bridge the gap between efficacy and effectiveness. An ideal pattern of care as measured by the process of care in one hospital may not be ideal in another hospital, and dissimilar outcomes may be obtained. Surgeons operating in two different hospitals may have the same process scores but different postoperative death rates. Outcome measures could identify these differences in quality of care while process criteria would not; explanations for the differences, such as the quality of the knots tied at surgery or the care with which the surgeon washed his hands preoperatively, could then be sought.

Summary

In choosing the type of measure by which to assess quality of care one must pick valid measures, whether they be structural, process, or outcome. Failure to do this will result in the expenditure of billions of dollars to fulfill invalid criteria that produce no change in health status.

One study that demonstrates this point vividly was performed by Fessel and Van Brunt, who abstracted the medical records of patients who presented to one of three hospitals with the symptoms of acute appendicitis.[29] First, they compared this information to a list of process criteria indicative of good care; on this assessment hospital A did best. Second, they measured the outcome of care by examining the appendix removed at operation to determine if it was removed for appropriate pathologic reasons. As judged by this technique hospital C, not hospital A, was the better hospital. Most patients certainly would prefer to have their abdominal pain treated at hospital C rather than hospital A.

DATA SOURCE

The fourth major methodologic issue involved in measuring quality of care is: what data source does one use when assessing quality of care? Fig. 5-1 summarizes the numerous options available. As one proceeds down the list the expense of collecting the given data generally increases; however, the face validity of the information obtained also increases. The more expensive methods of data collection need to be employed if outcome measures are to be tested. Unfortunately no single study has yet been done that compares the assessment of quality of care based on data obtained from a medical record with information obtained from an insurance claims form or from direct observation of the provider. Thus critics of Fessel and Van Brunt's study argue that they did not compare process measures with outcome measures in assessing quality of care but instead compared process data obtained from the medical record with outcome measures. The argument continues that if they had compared data on process measures obtained by directly observing the patient-doctor encounter with outcome measures, the results of the study would have been more congruent.

This debate over whether one has measured the recorded process of care or what was actually done is not a trivial one. Virtually every large quality of care study has used recorded information to judge the process of care. All these studies discovered major deficiencies in the level of care provided; most concluded that this finding must be due to the recording of information and not to the actual level of care provided. An example is the recently completed study by the Joint Commission on Quality Assurance for Children and Youth on the quality of care given to chil-

METHOD OF COLLECTION	TYPE OF DATA			
	Structure	Process	Outcome	Combination
Routinely reported data	X			
Hospital discharge abstract		X	X	X
Claims form		X		
Encounter form		X	X	X
Source-oriented medical record		X	X	X
Problem-oriented medical record		X	X	X
Direct observation of physicians		X		
Simulation techniques	X	X		
Patient interview		X	X	X
Tracer disease strategy		X	X	X
Population survey		X	X	X
Combination of above	X	X	X	X

Fig. 5-1. Method of collecting data for quality of care assessment.

dren.[30] They studied six conditions and disease entities (for example, health supervision, asthma). Although major deficiencies in the recorded process of care as judged by explicit criteria were found, the conclusion was that these deficiencies were most likely due to the recording of information and not to the care given.

Obviously not much progress can be made until this circular logic, which is most prevalent in the field today, is disproved or substantiated. A series of well-designed, well-performed studies that test judgment of quality of care as a function of the method used to gather the data is clearly needed, although this will not be very helpful to people who are beginning quality assessment activities today. What rule regarding data source should they use when undertaking such assessment activities?

Certain general rules seem applicable in this situation. First, outcome data are generally not available from many recorded documents. Most outcome data must be collected directly from the patient, especially when outcomes other than mortality are used. For instance, if one wants to assess the quality of care given to a patient with urinary tract infection by examining work-loss days, pain, disability, or social-psychologic outcomes, a questionnaire must be administered to the patient, since such data are not routinely recorded in the medical record. Second, the amount of information available from the medical record or insurance claims forms on the process of care is drastically limited to the technical management of illness. Very little is reported on patient education or art of care. Furthermore, in the technical area one is likely to find only that information the physician thinks is needed for subsequent management of the patient. Thus a child with a fever and otitis media presenting to a physician may have nothing more in his record than the statement of the fever, the diagnosis of otitis media, and the type of drug prescribed. Descriptive data concerning the history of this episode or the appearance of the ear and other organs assessed by physical examination may be totally absent from the medical record. Therefore if the medical record or claims data are to be used to assess the quality of the process of care, the criteria used in such assessment must be based on a limited set of information. For instance, regarding otitis media, it certainly would be possible to answer the question whether the correct antibiotic was chosen. Clearly it is not possible to answer the question of whether otitis media was really present, whether the physician really examined the child's ear, or whether the physician took a history of previous episodes of otitis media. Yet the absence of such examinations would be considered evidence of poor care.

Thus the source from which the data are to be gathered severally constrains the criteria that can be established. We believe it is better to confine criteria to elements of care that when done are virtually always recorded than to include elements of care that are often done but never recorded. Stimulation of additional recording is not necessarily the purpose of a quality assessment system. The physician should be expected to record only information necessary for future management of the patient; he should not be expected to record information for the sole use of a quality assessment system. It is probably cheaper for the quality assessment system to gather that information directly from the patient than to require uniform recording of such data.

Although this section concludes on a pessimistic note, one study of the validity of recorded data provides a more optimistic view. Payne and Lyons in their Hawaii study found marked differences in the level of the process of care provided by physicians[11,12] (see Table 5-1). In a subsequent analysis they examined the correlation between items performed by the physician and recorded by another professional (for example, laboratory tests) and items performed and recorded by the physician (for example, certain physical and historical findings). The correlations were weak but positive, suggesting that those physicians who do more of the appropriate laboratory tests also do and record more of the basic history and physical findings appropriate to a given patient. The correlation, however, was not high enough to make use of this information in an operational quality assurance program.[31]

SETTING CRITERIA

Many issues are involved in setting criteria for judging quality of care. This paper will discuss one of them: should explicit or implicit criteria be used to judge care? An example of explicit process criteria was previously given (see Table 5-1). Explicit criteria are predetermined criteria generated through a process of physician consensus. They should be specific enough to allow a nonphysician data abstractor to generate a score without consulting the physician. Implicit criteria are really criteria that exist in the mind of the physician and generate a gestalt view of the care given. In general a physician is given a medical record and asked to judge from it the level of care given the patient. It is a time-consuming and expensive method, since each chart must be read by one or more physicians.

A methodologic study by Brook compared the use of outcome and process data and implicit and explicit criteria in judging quality of care.[1] Each method was applied independently to about 300 patients with either hypertension, urinary tract infection, or an ulcerated lesion in the stomach or duodenum. Five methods were tested: (1) implicit process, (2) implicit outcome, (3) implicit process plus outcome, (4) explicit process, and (5) explicit outcome. The proportion of patients judged to have received adequate care varied from 2% with the explicit process method to about 63% with the implicit outcome method, a considerable variation.

The most valid assessment method, that

is, the one most likely to maximize health, is the implicit outcome method. Yet the method likely to be implemented for quality assessment is the explicit process method, which produced the worst score in Brook's study. If this latter method is implemented carelessly, the number of procedures performed might double or triple, yet the health level of the population might be improved only minimally. One major reason that a list of explicit process criteria produces this effect is inherent in a way explicit process criteria are formulated. Initially, lists of criteria are developed for a given diagnosis. Thus a patient with pneumonia would need x, y, and z. These criteria would be weighted, and the final score would be calculated according to criteria fulfilled. Medicine is simply not practiced this way, however. Physicians make clinical decisions such that the performance of one aspect of the process of care is conditional on previous results. Criteria lists have traditionally not been established in a conditional probability framework. Furthermore, medicine is both an art and a scientific discipline. This implies that multiple paths can be used to arrive at a single solution. In many cases the value of each pathway may be virtually identical. Thus explicit process criteria developed in the next few years must incorporate both concepts: conditionality and multiple pathways. An approach such as that recently published by the UCLA Experimental Medical Care Review Organization[32] is now feasible in an operational quality assessment program; in its simplest form it should be attempted when the process of care is to be reviewed against explicit process criteria using data from a medical record or claims form. In implementing this approach only those processes known to be related to outcome should be measured. For some diseases development of such lists of explicit process criteria may be impossible; in those instances an implicit approach to measurement should be used. Difficulty in developing a list of explicit process criteria is no justification for ignoring quality assessment in certain areas such as mental health.

VALUES APPLIED TO THE CRITERIA

No matter what criteria are selected to assess quality of care, some value judgment must eventually be placed on the results. Consider, for instance, a cancer screening test recommended as part of good quality of care for health maintenance and, specifically, the frequency with which it should be done to indicate good quality of care. Assume that the prevalence of cancer in the population is 1 per 100; the sensitivity of the test (the ability of a test to detect a disease if present) is 0.99; and the specificity of the test (the ability of the test to determine that a person does not have the disease, given the disease is absent) is also 0.99. These three statistics represent a very favorable screening situation, since virtually all tests are neither that specific nor that sensitive and disease prevalence is usually far lower.

Table 5-5 indicates what would happen if the screening test were applied to 10,000 people.

Thus for every person identified on screening who truly has the disease (cell a), an additional person would be identified who did not have the disease (cell b); that is, one true-positive would be identified for each false-positive. In addition, one person who truly had the disease would be missed (cell c). If it were desirable to identify every person who has the disease, then the 9802 people in whom the disease was declared absent must be rescreened. The prevalence of the disease in this smaller population is 1/9802 or 0.001; the results of the rescreening are shown in Table 5-6. Applying the test to this population twice results in identification of 100 true-positives, 0 false-negatives, and 197 false-positives. To decide whether applying the test twice is worth the cost, society must place a value on the desirability of detecting every patient with the disease; the harm done to patients falsely labeled as

Table 5-5. Example of cancer screening test results

| Test result | True result | | Total |
	Disease present	Disease absent	
Disease present	a	b	a + b
Disease absent	c	d	c + d
Total	100 = a + c	9900 = b + d	10,000

Sensitivity = a/(a + c) = 99/100 = 0.99
a = 99; c = 1
Specificity = d/(b + d) = 9801/9900 = 0.99
b = 99; d = 9801

Table 5-6. Rescreening test results

| Test result | True result | | Total |
	Disease present	Disease absent	
Disease present	a	b	a + b
Disease absent	c	d	c + d
Total	1	9801	9802

Sensitivity = a/(a + c) = ≃ 1/1 = 0.99
a ≃ 1; c = 0
Specificity = d/(b + d) = 9703/9801 = 0.99
b = 98; d = 9703

positive must be compared to the good done to those appropriately labeled as positive.

The actual situation is even more complex than that illustrated by the no-risk cancer screening test. Modern therapeutics involve potent medications and technologies that may at great monetary cost extend the life of a few while producing suffering for many. Questions to be resolved are: how should these therapies be applied? Is their application evidence, in general, of good or poor medical care? How much is society willing to spend for an additional year of life? How much value does society attach to improvements in care that increase quality at the margin?

Acton has outlined several different

ways in which values can be applied in this area.[33] The traditional approach used by economists to estimate the cost of illness or the benefit of additional medical care is the human capital approach, in which the worth of an individual is approximated by the present discounted value of lifetime productivity. Major conceptual problems (for example, how to value the life of non-productive members of society such as retirees or housewives) have cast serious doubt on the validity of this approach. Newer ways of assigning values include the use of explicit criteria generated by individuals themselves or their representatives in Washington; this has been termed the "willingness-to-pay" approach. In this approach people are asked about their willingness to pay for a given improvement in medical services (for example, a mobil coronary care unit) or for the availability of additional tests to rule out unlikely events (for example, an EMI scan for a patient with a headache or skull x-rays for a child with a bump on the head). Willingness to pay is equated with the benefits of these services and procedures. Thus a person might be willing to spend two tax dollars a year to increase his chances of surviving a heart attack by 10%, given a 0.1% probability of its occurrence in the next year. Similar although perhaps less accurate results could be arrived at through the use of implicit criteria or a gestalt feeling.

To complicate the situation even further, many therapies incur costs in the present but produce benefits only in the future. For example, a screening test to measure cholesterol levels could be applied to 10 year olds, and those in the upper 10% of the distribution could be treated with low cholesterol diets. Some 20 to 30 years later a difference in the incidence of symptomatic coronary artery disease might be detected; a few deaths might have been prevented, life expectancy for some might be extended, and the amount of symptoms due to coronary artery disease might be less. The value society places on such a treatment will be reflected in the way future benefits are discounted against present costs. A high discount rate implies a low social value on future benefits; a low rate, by contrast, implies a higher social value on the longer-term project. Choice of a high or low discount rate will result in vastly different costs for a year of life saved. Creton found that with a high discount rate (for example, 10%) a year of life saved would cost $94,000 by initiating a cholesterol screening program and $5000 by upgrading coronary care units; by comparison, at a low discount rate (for example, zero), the costs per year of life saved would be $2355 and $1780, respectively, for the cholesterol and coronary care unit programs.[34]

For the future the willingness-to-pay approach may offer the best approach to the evaluation of how much quality of care society really wants, although severe methodologic problems remain to be solved. At present few data exist in this area, and directors of operational quality assessment programs must use their own values in setting standards for the quality of medical care. The authors recommend that personal values be used cautiously, although explicit definition of such values helps to minimize the risks involved. As argued above, most assessments of the quality of medical care will show major deficiencies, especially when such studies concern themselves with the links between ambulatory and hospital care. In addition, many deficiencies will be so major that assigning values to their correction is moot. Clearly priority lies on the side of correcting the major deficiencies in quality of medical care wherever they may lie; determining the value of correcting minor deficiencies is of secondary importance.

SUMMARY

Six issues in assessment of the quality of medical care have been raised. This chapter also demonstrates the rationale for defining quality in a broad sense and for examining all of the critical components of quality that affect the health status of patients with a given problem at that moment in time. For different problems, certain variables in the conceptual outline of quality will be more pertinent and need to be emphasized. In terms of data used in quality assessment, the state of the art is such that a combination of structural, process, and outcome data is necessary if a truly valid assessment of quality of care is to be obtained. Particular attention needs to be paid to measuring the art of care and to measuring a broad spectrum of outcomes. The data source from which to gather pertinent information should be carefully studied. Quality assessment should not be overextended in a manner that places unreliable data in a complex analytic framework that itself masks the unreliability of the data. These problems are compounded when one attempts to establish criteria for judging these data. Criteria should be established in accordance with the sequential procedures available in decision analysis; they should, where appropriate, permit multiple paths to the same goal. Most criteria should be conditional, that is, dependent on successful completion of previous criteria. Finally, in placing some value on these results the analyst must be careful to exclude values that are not widely held by society. For instance, an individual may not be willing to pay hard-earned tax dollars for the amount of quality a professional wishes to deliver.

It is perhaps fitting to close this discussion on a more optimistic note. At least another 5 to 10 years of hard research will be needed before many of these methodologic and conceptual problems are adequately resolved. In the meantime quality assessment activities should be continued. Most physicians know what the major problems are in the delivery of optimal quality of care. Reasonable criteria and standards can be developed using that as a cue to address these problems. Through a quality assurance mechanism these problems can be detected and corrected. By the time most of the major deficiencies are dealt with, refinements in methods of assessing quality of care will have been made. These will allow a second generation of quality assessment activities in which questions of efficiency versus effectiveness and society's value of health and quality can be considered.

REFERENCES

1. Brook, R. H.: Quality of care assessment: a comparison of five methods of peer review, publ. no. HRA-74-3100, Rockville, Md., 1974, U.S. Dept. of Health, Education, and Welfare.
2. Brook, R. H.: Policy issues in quality assurance, publ. no. P-5517, Santa Monica, Calif., October 1975, The Rand Corporation.
3. Brook, R. H., and Davies-Avery, A.: Mechanisms for assuring quality of U.S. medical care services: past, present, and future, publ. no. R-1939, Santa Monica, Calif., 1977, The Rand Corporation.
4. Brook, R. H., Williams, K. N., and Davies-Avery, A.: Quality assurance today and tomorrow: forecast for the future, Ann. Intern. Med. **85:**809-817, 1976.
5. Brook, R. H., Brutoco, R. L., and Williams, K. N.: The relationship between medical malpractice and quality of care, publ. no. P-5526, Santa Monica, Calif., October 1975, The Rand Corporation.
6. Williams, K. N., and Brook, R. H.: Foreign medical graduates and their effects on the medical care in the United States, publ. no. R-1698-HEW, Santa Monica, Calif., January 1976, The Rand Corporation. An earlier version of this paper was published as Williams, K. N., and Brook, R. H.: Foreign medical graduates and their impact on the quality of medical care in the United States, Milbank Mem. Fund Q. **53:**549-581, 1975.
7. National Center for Health Statistics: The national ambulatory medical care survey: 1973 summary, publ. no. HRA-76-1772, Rockville, Md., October 1975, U.S. Dept. of Health, Education, and Welfare.
8. Bergner, M., Bobbitt, R. A., Pollard, W. E., et al.: The sickness impact profile: validation of a health status measure, Med. Care **14:**57-67, 1976.
9. Fanshel, S., and Bush, J. W.: A health index and its application to health services outcomes, Operations Res. **19:**1021-1066, 1970.
10. Brook, R. H., and Williams, K. N.: Evaluation of the New Mexico peer review system, 1971 to 1973, Med. Care **14** (suppl.), December 1976.
11. Payne, B. C., and study staff: Methods of evaluating and improving personal medical care quality: episode of illness study, Chicago, 1976, Hospital Research and Educational Trust.

12. Payne, B. C., and study staff: Methods of evaluating and improving personal medical care quality: office care study, Chicago, 1976, Hospital Research and Educational Trust.

13. Donabedian, A.: Promoting quality through evaluating the process of patient care, Med. Care **6:**181-202, 1968.

14. Bunker, J. P., Forrest, W. H., Jr., Mosteller, F., and Vandam, L. D.: The national halothane study, Washington, D.C., 1969, National Institute of Health, p. 193.

15. Staff of the Stanford Center for Health Care Research: Comparison of hospitals with regard to outcomes of surgery, Health Serv. Res. **11:**112-127, 1976.

16. Wennberg, J., and Gittelsohn, A.: Small area variations in health care delivery, Science, **183:**1102-1108, 1973.

17. Lewis, C. E.: Variations in the incidence of surgery, N. Engl. J. Med. **281:**880-884, 1969.

18. Peterson, O. L., Andrews, L. P., Spain, R. S., et al.: An analytical study of North Carolina general practice—1953-1954, J. Med. Educ. **31**(p. 2):1-165, 1956.

19. de Dombal, F. T., Leaper, D. J., Staniland, J. R., et al.: Computer-aided diagnosis of acute abdominal pain, Br. Med. J. **2:**9-13, 1972.

20. Leaper, D. J., Horrocks, J. C., Staniland, J. R., and de Dombal, F. T.: Computer-assisted diagnosis of abdominal pain using estimates provided by clinicians, Br. Med. J. **4:**350-354, 1972.

21. Bergman, A. B., and Stamm, S. J.: The morbidity of cardiac nondisease in school children, N. Engl. J. Med. **276:**1008-1113, 1967.

22. Chant, A. D. B., Jones, H. O., and Weddell, J. M.: Varicose veins: a comparison of surgery and injection/compression, Lancet **2:**1188-1191, 1972.

23. Piachaud, D., and Weddell, J. M.: Cost of treating varicose veins, Lancet **2:**1191-1192, 1972.

24. University Group Diabetes Program: A study of the effects of hypoglycemic agents on vascular complications in patients with adult-onset diabetes, J.A.M.A. **19**(suppl. 2), 1970.

25. Mather, N. G., Pearson, H. G., Reed, K. L. R., et al.: Acute myocardial infarction: home and hospital treatment, Br. Med. J. **3:**334-338, 1971.

26. Meier, P.: Statistics and medical experimentation, Biometrics **31:**511-529, 1975.

27. Brook, R. H.: Quality assurance: the state of the art, Hosp. Med. Staff **3:**15-26, 1974.

28. Starfield, B.: Measurement of outcomes: a proposed scheme, Milbank Mem. Fund Q. **52:**39-50, 1974.

29. Fessell, W. J., and Van Brunt, E. E.: Assessing quality of care from the medical record, N. Engl. J. Med. **286:**134-138, 1972.

30. Osborne, C. E.: Criteria for evaluation of ambulatory child health care by chart audit: development and testing of a methodology, final report on contract no. HSM 110-71-184, Evanston, Ill., 1975, American Academy of Pediatrics.

31. Lyons, T. F., and Payne, B. C.: The relationship of physicians' medical recording performance to their medical care performance, Med. Care **12:**463, 1974.

32. Greenfield, S., Lewis, C. E., Kaplan, S. H., and Davidson, M.: Peer review by "criteria mapping": criteria for diabetes mellitus, Ann. Intern. Med. **83:**761-770, 1975.

33. Acton, J. P.: Evaluating public programs to save lives: the case of heart attacks, publ. no. R-950-RD, Santa Monica, Calif., January 1973, The Rand Corporation.

34. Creton, S.: Comparing strategies for the treatment and prevention of myocardial infarction, Health Serv. Res., summer 1977.

6

Measurement of outcomes: primary health care evaluation in the United Kingdom

CARLOS J. M. MARTINI
IAN McDOWELL

Commentators on the development of health care evaluation have concentrated on two fundamental points of choice: what aspects of care should be measured in making evaluative judgments, and by whom should such judgments be made? Possible answers to the first question have been reviewed by several authors, generally following Donabedian's basic structure-process-outcome framework.[1] The decision on who is to make the evaluative assessments has commonly been answered in favor of peer review. The Professional Standards Review Organization (PSRO), for example, which "is an organization of physicians and should not be considered an entity separate from the physician community,"[2] has as its role to define norms and criteria "against which aspects of the quality of a medical service may be compared."[2]

As the demand for medical evaluation spreads from hospital systems into primary and community care, it is an opportune moment to comment on the assumptions that have commonly been followed in making these basic choices and to assess how adequate they may be within the expanded scope of evaluation. Criticisms that have already been made cover three basic points

and are reviewed in other chapters. These criticisms concern the emphasis on measuring process to the exclusion of outcome and the narrow orientation of the measurements used, which commonly reflect only the major decisions taken in caring for a patient, and this in isolated parts of the whole spectrum of care, such as the hospital episode. Such measurements do not indicate the consequences of these decisions for the patient, nor do they assess the long term care he receives.

It is the purpose of this chapter to review some alternatives to the established evaluative methods and to suggest how these may be applied in evaluating primary medical care. The study in which the ideas outlined are being applied is being undertaken in England, although it is estimated that the principles involved may be more broadly applicable. The first section summarizes the reasons for the orientation towards primary care and indicates some of the bases for claiming that it represents a special case in terms of evaluative methods. The following three sections discuss the basic choices of methods in primary medical care evaluation, while the final section of the chapter presents examples of applications of the ideas outlined.

THE EMPHASIS ON PRIMARY MEDICAL CARE

Primary medical care may be defined as the point in a chain of referrals of an individual with a health problem where he or she leaves the lay referral system and contacts a professional health practitioner. As the work of the same practitioners includes the care of chronic patients, the elderly, and even terminal patients at home, the term primary care will also be used to cover these aspects of care.

There are many examples of the growing attention paid to such care; for instance, a recent policy document published by the Department of Health and Social Security in England formulates a national strategy for expanding family practitioner services, noting: "The degree of priority given to primary medical care and its associated expenditure is thus higher than for any other group of services of comparable size, and it can be achieved only by restraining growth in other services."[3]

In the United Kingdom the primary care doctor provides the only method of access to hospital treatment with the exception of emergency services. In determining initial contact with primary care, the doctor refers the patient into the hospital system, where the patient becomes dependent on the proposals of a number of doctors. The responsibility of the primary care doctor is therefore not only economic in terms of intensity of services but also directly concerned with protecting the patient's freedom. These two aspects of the centrality of this type of health practitioner in the health care system underline the importance of monitoring this work.

Furthermore, to judge by the numbers of patients seen, primary care is the most important part of the health care system; in England the average individual makes about three visits to his health practitioner each year, and the practitioner will see annually at least 70% of the population registered with him.[4]

With modern medicine accepting a growing responsibility for high risk groups in the community, the question of when to intervene and how to do it is becoming one of the crucial problems in medical care. Two recent areas of study in epidemiology have contributed to answering this question: first, the growing understanding of the multifactorial etiology of disease, and second, the concept of increased vulnerability of certain groups in the population. Both have relevance for primary care.

The implication of multifactorial etiology is that treatment should cover more than just the medical aspects of disease. The second development, the concept of vulnerability, linked with outgrowing ability to predict disease, forms the basis for all the new developments in high-risk strategies. The population for which the primary care doctor in England is responsible makes an ideal target for the application of high-risk strategies based on registration systems and continued surveillance. Because of limited resources, intervention must clearly be carried out on the basis of those at highest risk of disease. The primary care doctor's responsibility in these choices again indicates his strategic position in the total system of care. This is appreciated by some new medical schools (for example, at Nottingham and Leicester Universities in the United Kingdom) where the teaching of primary medical care and social medicine form part of the medical curriculum in an integrated manner.

These cumulative indications of the importance of the primary medical care sector make the need for appropriate health indicators one of the most pressing requirements in medical care evaluation. Our ability to measure the effectiveness of the services we provide is only just beginning, and the traditional health indicators such as mortality and morbidity rates are still the only outcome indices widely used in the health services. These measures are, however, especially inappropriate in the area of primary medical care.

Primary care is only marginally concerned with mortality, as life-threatening conditions are generally referred to other sources of care (with the possible exception of some terminal care). Morbidity indices also present a related limitation, deriving in part from the lack of appropriate systems of classification. It has been estimated that up to one-half of patients[5,6] attending primary care either cannot be labeled by the conventional medical classifications or the doctor is unable to reach a diagnosis, which in any case reduces the applicability of such indices.

Even more important, these indices do not reflect the full impact of a good primary medical care team, which is concerned with the total presenting problem, and where the diagnosis, like the treatments, should be expressed in emotional and social terms, and not merely physical.

The relevance of such dimensions is illustrated in some recent information systems where description of the broader social context of the patient's illness is included (as would be done in problem-oriented medical records).

These difficulties associated with selecting adequate outcome indices and the knowledge of their poor sensitivity to medical care, as discussed below, may explain the greater emphasis put on process indicators in most peer review systems. Although understandable, this situation by our criteria does a disservice to the area of primary medical care where the use of suitable outcome measures such as sociomedical or subjective indices presents a number of advantages we would like to discuss further.

RELEVANT ISSUES IN EVALUATION

Three aspects of evaluative methodology can be selected for further investigation: the stage of care at which the measurement is made, the scope of the indices used, and the issue over who makes the judgment.

Stage of measurement

Donabedian's basic triad of structure, process, and outcome (see Chapter 2) forms the basis for a number of studies in the evaluation of medical care and is discussed more fully in other chapters. Most of the interrelationships between these stages (for example, between process and the outcome of care) have not yet been fully explored.

Comments on the limitations of indices of process are made by Brook and Avery in Chapter 5. While process measures can be undoubtedly useful in monitoring the quality of care given, the ultimate judgment must be made in terms of outcome if we are to accept responsibility for the patient's welfare (as in primary care) rather than for a limited range of interventions on his behalf, and especially if we want to avoid judgments of the type that goes something like this: "the operation was a success but the patient died." These two stages of measurement (outcome and process) may not be highly correlated.

Outcome in the present context refers to the possible impact, in terms of quality of life, that a certain process of care may produce. It is usually measured at the end of the interaction of the individual with an organized system of care (examples being survival or residual disability rates), but in the sense of intermediate results outcomes may also be accounted at any stage in this process after the initial consultation. The validity of many commonly used outcome indices for evaluating changes produced by medical care is, however, low, as they are affected more than process indicators by nonmedical factors in the environment such as crowding, housing, and social class. Certain outcomes such as infant mortality or specific death rates for pneumonia[7] are predominantly influenced by socioeconomic factors and should be used with great care in the comparison of different medical systems. There exists, however, another group of outcome indicators designed to reflect not only the medical aspects of morbidity but also the patient's social functioning; the term "sociomedical" has been used to describe indices of this type.[8]

Type of measurement

Sociomedical indicators would appear especially relevant in evaluating primary care, particularly where a patient is still able to perform many of his normal activities of daily life. These measurements frequently assess the patient's level of functional abilities, considering his total experience of disease and its termination, and may thereby reflect the whole spectrum of care provided, thus adding new dimensions to laboratory and clinical information. Their appropriateness when the subject of inquiry is the health of an entire population (as in profile analysis) makes them potentially useful as screening measures applied through normal survey techniques.

The implications for evaluative methodology of this approach are crucial. The whole concept of peer review implies that the main responsibility for evaluation is in the hands of professionals who are assumed to be better judges of what is proper in terms of "norms, criteria, and standards that are non-professional." However, the PSRO review system also accepts within this organization of physicians the care provided by nonphysician health care practitioners and even invites the involvement of such practitioners.[2] Sociomedical indices may be a vehicle to move even several steps further and make consumer participation a real and live issue, since the patient is able to express his subjective reactions to disease and treatment. He then will be able to participate actively, first in the evaluation of his own case, enabling a consideration of the patient's personal experience by the evaluator, and then in the longer term in the establishment of priorities for medical care. By consideration of social as well as medical outcomes we may avoid anomalies such as the misjudgment of poor medical care by counting deaths of terminal patients instead of looking at the alleviation of pain and discomfort on the same patients as criteria for good medical care. (This last aspect of care to our knowledge is not yet included in any outcome or process indicators in use).

Approach to measurement

There are two main approaches to applying sociomedical measurements: the choice between using a trained assessor to judge the quality of the patient's functioning or relying on the patient's own assessment, his subjective report of his condition. It is the second approach we suggest provides benefits in evaluating health care outcomes for several reasons. The basic motivation for a person to seek care relies more closely on his subjective perception of his condition than on objective medical criteria, and similarly his satisfaction with the treatment received is not only a reflection of the objective aspects of his condition. Much of primary care is concerned with treating nonorganic disease, and ultimately the diagnosis of such conditions relies on the patient's own description of his problem: to formalize this and render it more reliable would benefit the process of communication between doctor and patient. Finally, as the basic aim of providing health care is to make people feel better, the most direct as well as the simplest way of judging its success is to ask the patient how he feels.

At the same time, subjective measurements have been criticized as being too soft or unreliable, and if asked, most physicians will probably favor harder information on the health of an individual, such as biochemical profiles or the measurement of physiologic variables like blood pressure or weight. There is evidence, however, that the objectivity and reliability of medical diagnosis and many such tests do not stand up to careful examination.

For example, the accuracy of medical diagnoses has long been doubted by epidemiologists. A survey of deaths carried out by the Registrar General in England[9] in 1955 and repeated by Heasman[10] in 1966, showed that in only 51% and 45.3% of the cases, respectively, was there agreement between clinical and pathologic diagnoses. Of the disagreements, one-half were on questions of fact, where the clinician's underlying cause of death was not mentioned in the pathologist's report or vice versa.

The issue of definition of a case for many medical diagnoses is also a matter of debate. Many studies attest to the arbitrary ways in which the definition of abnormal values is established.[11-21] This is in part due to the fact that values for many physiologic and biochemical variables are not normally distributed. Criterion values should be adjusted by age and sex at least, and in some cases (as with serum cholesterol concentration) significant changes can occur even from month to month. It is claimed that in some cases these seasonal variations might be large enough to obscure interpretation of values.[22]

The medical literature on screening gives many examples of the so-called "borderline problem." If the distribution of values for a physiologic variable is bimodal, as might be expected in some genetically transmitted characteristic such as phenylketonuria,[19] the borderline group of individuals (between health and disease) will include some with the disease and others without, but all with values within the same range. This problem originated the need to classify medical tests according to their sensitivity and specificity (false-positive and false-negative rates). If, instead, the distribution is unimodal, we still must determine a cutoff point, and on this will depend the identification of an individual as normal or sick. Conditions in which this is a problem are diabetes, hypertension, obesity, glaucoma, and so on.[23]

The objectivity of medical tests also has been questioned before. The finding of unexpected abnormal results has been studied by Bradwell et al.[11] and Whitehead.[16] The first investigators made a follow-up study of 200 patients with unexplained abnormal results in a biochemical profile on admission to the hospital. They found that after 5 years 3.5% of the patients still showed persistent abnormal

results that could not be explained on clinical grounds. Thirty-seven percent initially had anomalous results that were later explained by gains in knowledge relating to reference values and the biochemical changes occurring in disease, while a further 35% had results that were normal on repeat.

Laboratory errors may also be common, as most doctors would accept. These may be classified as random errors (for example, incorrect labeling, accidental switching of specimens, clerical error) and systematic errors like the case of measurement of potassium in urea being affected by the shorter length of time that blood was centrifuged on Saturdays, reported by Whitehead.[16] Many other authors have mentioned other examples of observer and instrument errors.[13,15,18,22-23]

Considered in this light, sociomedical indices may not be any less valid than many traditional medical tests, and in some cases high correlations have been shown between both types of measurements. For example, it is well established that there is a close association between subjective ratings of energy expenditure and physiologic parameters. This has been demonstrated by several investigators who found that there is a linear relation between heart rate and ratings of perceived exertion during submaximal exercise[24] and that perceived effort is an indicator of metabolic strain, work intensity, and muscular and articular stress.[25]

POSSIBLE DIRECTIONS IN THE EVALUATION OF PRIMARY CARE

The idea of recording standard information on the social aspects of a case is not new and forms part of any good case notes. It was formalized 25 years ago in the Cornell medical index.[26-27] The approach outlined below extends this by concentrating not only on the patient's symptoms but also on the implications they hold for his style and standard of living.

The fact that such measurements would rely on self-assessment has made them the object of the type of criticism leveled at all subjective indices as representing value judgments. Bush and Fanshel,[28] in commenting on this point, note that the whole concept of health and the actions made to promote it are so heavily value laden that it is probably no longer desirable to develop value-free operational definitions of it. This, it is argued, need not be a disadvantage as long as it is recognized, and as subjective reactions already represent a major component in social and political judgments of care, a standard method of assessing them as objectively as possible should be formalized.

A review of the main trends in current research on sociomedical indices will indicate which type is potentially most suitable for application in primary care. The criteria for selecting a suitable index demand[29] that it should reflect social and psychologic states before and after care,[30] that it be judged by the individual himself rather than by the physician,[31] and that it be applicable to as wide a spectrum of conditions as possible.

Because of the diversity of existing definitions of health there has been no consensus over an appropriate measure of it, and this, modified by diverging demands placed on health indices, has led to a diversity of types of sociomedical indices. Within this diversity three general approaches may be identified. First, there has been an attempt to provide an aggregated single index of health based on the weighted sum of various individual indicators, which commonly include a social dimension. Second, for use where only a limited view of health is required, its concept and measurement have been limited to a single dimension such as disability.[32-33] The third major approach has aimed at creating a broad spectrum type of measure, differing, however, from the first in not attempting to aggregate the component indices.[34]

Work on indices that summarize health status in a single value has met with a variety of problems.[35] The problems of aggregating the various component indices have been discussed in several sources.[36-37] Fundamentally, as health represents a multifaceted concept, it is difficult to conceive of a single or even several simple indices capable of summarizing the possible range of health levels in a heterogeneous population. At the same time summary indices of health can be extremely useful to compare geographical areas in planning. In evaluation of primary care (and not using a purely descriptive research model) the problems are different. For example, to make it possible for any evaluation to make sense, a matrix (multifactorial) approach becomes essential. Since health is also multifactorial, a single aggregated index to measure specific components on the input of primary physicians is not entirely satisfactory, but rather it seems more appropriate to report a patient's status on each of several dimensions of health, social and behavioral as well as physical.

Within the second approach, the measurement of a single dimension of health, a number of relatively specific disability indices have been developed, which are commonly used in assessing the impact of a particular type of handicap or disease on selected aspects of a patient's functioning.[28,33,38] One of the best known and most broadly applicable indices in this category is the Activities of Daily Living scale of Katz et al.[39] For use in primary care evaluation, however, their specialist nature makes many of these indices too narrow, although the general dysfunction approach is suitable.

The third approach has so far received less attention but may prove to have most relevance in evaluating primary care. Measures of this type consider many aspects of a patient's welfare and may include morbidity, activity levels, pain, and satisfaction with care so that their broad scope reflects many of the features associated with primary care. Such measures have been suggested by May,[34] who emphasizes a need to "devise some basic measures of generic

ITEM STATEMENTS

2   I go out less to visit people.

5   I often act irritably towards people.

8   I worry about my state of health.

11   I get upset more easily.

19   I am cutting down on physical activities.

24   I do not finish work that I start.

32   I act irritably towards my family.

38   I express worries about the future.

42   I tend to cook simpler meals.

68   I eat less than usual.

mothers with young children

pregnant women

0 10 20 30 40 50 60 70 80 90 100

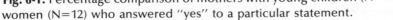

Fig. 6-1. Percentage comparison of mothers with young children (N = 15) and pregnant women (N=12) who answered "yes" to a particular statement.

health which would apply to each whole person, and beyond that, to each whole family," and have also been the subject of intensive studies by Bergner et al. in Seattle, who have concentrated on the development of the Sickness Impact Profile.[40-42] This provides an extremely flexible index that may be self-administered, enabling the assessment of the effects of almost any type of illness on a wide range of behavioral functioning. As well as providing a description of the impact of illness, the statements may be scaled for severity to provide a numerical indication of the degree of impairment. The scope and flexibility of this approach make it it most promising for assessing the outcomes of primary care.

To illustrate the scope of this type of index the following results are taken from our studies[43] done as part of an investigation into the area of primary medical care in Britain.

The interview schedule was adapted from Bergner's original, modified by the addition of 20 locally collected statements (provided by patients) by preliminary pilot studies. It covers 13 aspects of everyday living, ranging through social relationships, sleeping, eating, doing housework, the respondent's job, going out and walking, speech, recreation, body movements, mental activity levels, family relationships, feelings of health, and dressing and toileting. Within each of these areas the level of impairment of what the respondent judges to be his normal functioning is assessed by referring to a list of 85 statements, which other sick people had stated described their disabilities. Relating to behavior rather than purely to feelings and emotions, each statement describes a change in a common daily activity that can result from current illness, for example, "I no longer go out to visit my friend," or "I sit down to rest more often during the day." The respondent is asked to indicate whenever he hears a statement that aptly describes his present condition, where the impairment is associated with sickness (de-

scribed to the respondent as not feeling completely well). From his responses a descriptive profile of the effect of any illness on the individual is built up. Both interview and self-administered applications (each containing identical items) have been tried.

Figs. 6-1 and 6-2 and Table 6-1 illustrate some of the uses of this type of sociomedical index in the types of setting described in discussions of peer review systems. The first application is in giving a profile measurement (a broad description of the health status of a group of people) and the second is in terms of longitudinal health measurements that may be used in evaluating the care given to individual patients. The reason for applying sociomedical indices in this context is to extend the range of the normally applied indices rather than to replace them and to offer an evaluative approach based on assessments by both doctors and patients.

In making a cross-sectional type of health profile, two sets of data have been selected. These are intended for illustration only and do not in any way represent fully validated descriptions of the groups involved. The first example shows how individual items in a questionnaire of the type described above can be used to highlight contrasts between different groups. These need not necessarily be ill patients. The method is flexible and broadly applicable. To indicate this Fig. 6-1 presents results of interviews with a group of pregnant women (on or above the twenty-eighth week of pregnancy) compared with a group of women who had recently given birth to their first child. The items were all worded so that a positive response indicated illness or disability, and the results show the proportion of positive responses for each group for a selection of items.

In terms of psychologic concomitants of sickness (for example, concern over their health status, anxiety about the future), the pregnant women realistically show a higher positive response rate. But in terms of the indications of disruption of their

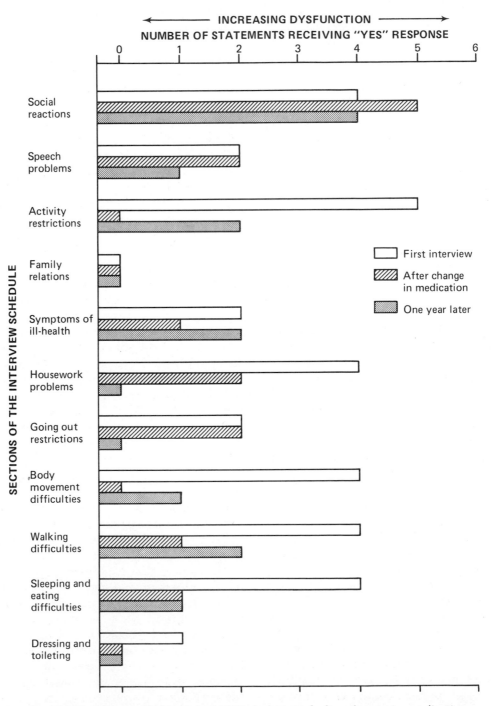

Fig. 6-2. Single case of regional enteritis before and after change in medication.

Table 6-1. Comparison of ratios of affirmative responses of patients and students

	All patients (N = 85)	Patients under age 23 (N = 35)
Social reactions	5.36	5.76
Speech problems	5.34	6.38
Activity restrictions	4.12	5.03
Family relations	8.36	8.98
Symptoms of ill health	2.76	2.83
Housework problems	4.40	3.33
Going out restrictions	7.85	8.84
Body movement difficulties	6.41	6.38
Walking difficulties	7.05	3.55
Sleeping problems	3.54	3.49
Eating problems	8.69	8.24
Working patterns	3.37	6.10
Dressing and toileting	2.42	2.35

normal routine, the women with a small baby are clearly badly affected. This is not to say that they are ill, but simply they are suffering difficulties in their normal lives similar to that found in many people who are unwell in medical terms, and which of course frequently does lead to various manifestations of ill health. The strength of this method in drawing attention to this type of problem may make it suitable to reflect the input of care from paramedical workers or of preventive medical inputs designed to help the new mother with the strains of motherhood.

Table 6-1 illustrates the use of material from the same interview schedule presented not in terms of individual items but by aggregating the items in each section to give more general and reliable indications of levels of disability of dysfunction in each aspect of daily living. The groups were chosen deliberately to illustrate the general level of difference to be expected between a supposedly healthy population (for which a group of active young students was selected) and a typical group of patients attending their family practitioner's surgery.

The scores for each group, aggregated from a mean of 6.5 statements per section in the schedule, are presented as the ratio of positive response rates for the patients to that of the students. Thus a figure of 5.0 would indicate that the patients' replies were five times as serious as the students'. The results consistently indicate a contrast between the two groups, falling in the expected direction. In case this difference might have been an artifact of the contrasting ages of the patients and students, the same information has also been presented for the 17 youngest patients whose mean age compares closely with that of the students, the differences remaining clearly marked.

For the second general type of application of such material, that of describing longitudinal changes over time (for example, before and after treatment), Fig. 6-2 indicates some results based on a single chronic case. The woman concerned was suffering from regional enteritis (which ranks as number 560 in the World Health Organization classification of diseases, injuries, and causes of death), and the patient's condition was adequately stable to make traditional medical indices insensitive to the minor changes she experiences in her daily life. However, her family practitioner believed that a change in her medication would improve her general well-being, even without affecting her medical condition.

At the first interview (before the introduction of the new medication) she was shown to suffer from severe restrictions in many aspects of her life. Three months later, after she was put onto steroid therapy, a second interview indicated many improvements in her subjective condition, although it also showed one area of slight regression. A third administration made one year later indicated that the improvement (confirming the physician's impression) had been in general maintained. Again, this type of index is of use in drawing attention to some of the desirable components of care that are not expressible in purely medical terms.

The results outlined above give nothing more than the most preliminary indication of the types of material to be collected by indices of this type; it is to be stressed that this does not supplant conventional medical information, but it is our belief that information of this type is the only method of providing a basis for evaluative judgments that can reflect the diverse aspects of the work not only of the primary medical care doctor but also of his whole team.

REFERENCES

1. Donabedian, A.: Promoting quality through evaluating the process of patient care, Med. Care **6:**3, 1968.
2. Goran, M. J., Roberts, J. S., Kellogg, M. A., et al.: The PSRO hospital review system, Med. Care **13**(suppl.):4, 1975.
3. Department of Health and Social Security: Priorities for health and personal social services in England: a consultative document, London, 1976, Her Majesty's Stationery Office.
4. Royal College of General Practitioners: Present state and future needs of general practice, report from general practice no. 16, London, 1973, The Royal College.
5. Cassell, J. C.: Information for epidemiology and health services research, Med. Care **11**(suppl. 2):76-80, 1973.
6. Research Committee of College of General Practitioners: Records and statistical unit; perspective studies: disease labels, J. R. Coll. Gen. Pract. **6:**197-204, 1963.
7. Martini, C. J. M., Allan, B., Davidson, J., and Backett, E. M.: The impact of medical care in health outcome indices, occasional publ. no. 10, Nottingham, England, 1975, University of Nottingham, Department of Community Health.
8. Elinson, J.: Toward sociomedical health indicators, Paper presented at the International Conference of Medical Sociology, Warsaw, Poland, August 1973.
9. Registrar General's statistical review, part III, London, 1956, Her Majesty's Stationery Office.
10. Heasman, M. A., and Lipworth, L.: Accuracy of certification of cause of death, studies on medical and population subjects, no. 20, London, 1966, General Registry Office, Her Majesty's Stationery Office.
11. Bradwell, A. R., Carmalt, M. H. B., and Whitehead, T. P.: Explaining the unexpected abnormal results of biochemical profile investigations, Lancet **2:**1071-1074, 1974.
12. Doyle, J. T., Kinch, S. H., and Brown, D. F.: Seasonal variation in serum cholesterol concentration, J. Chron. Dis. **18:**657-664, 1965.
13. Grasbeck, R., and Saris, N. E.: Establishment and use of normal values, Scand. J. Clin. Lab. Invest., suppl. **110:**62-63, 1969.
14. Pryce, J. D.: Level of haemoglobin in whole blood and red blood cells and proposed convention for defining normality, Lancet **2:**333, 1960.
15. Pincharle, G., and Shanks, J.: Value of the erythrocyte sedimentation rate as a screening test, Br. J. Prev. Soc. Med. **21:**133-136, 1976.
16. Whitehead, T. P., and Wootton, L. D. P.: Biochemical profiles for hospital patients, Lancet **2:**1439, 1974.
17. Holland, W. W.: Taking stock, Lancet **2:**1494, 1974.
18. Levin, G. E., McPherson, C. K., Fraser, P. M., et al.: Long-term variation in plasma activities of aspartate transaminase and alkaline phosphatase in health, Clin. Sci. Mol. Med. **44:**185-196, 1973.
19. Wilson, J. M. G., and Jungner, G.: Principles and practice of screening for disease, public health paper no. 34, Geneva, 1968, World Health Organization.
20. Oliver, M. F.: The early diagnosis of ischaemic heart disease, London, 1967, Office of Health Economics.
21. Graham, P. A.: The early diagnosis of visual defects, London, 1968, Office of Health Economics.
22. Browne, R. C., Ellis, R. W., and Weightman, D.: Inter-laboratory variation in measurement of blood-lead levels, Lancet **2:**1112, 1974.
23. Cochrane, A. L., and Holland, W. W.: Validation of screening procedures, Br. Med. Bull. **27:**308, 1971.
24. Borg, G.: Physical performance and perceived exertion, Lund, Sweden, 1962, C. W. K. Gleerup.
25. Pandolf, K. B., and Noble, B. S.: The effect of pedalling speed and resistance changes on perceived exertion for equivalent power outputs on the bicycle ergonometer, Med. Sci. Sports **5**(2):132-136, 1973.

26. Brodman, K., Erdman, A. H., Lorge, I., Wolff, H. G., and Broadbent, T. H.: The Cornell medical index, J.A.M.A. **145:**152-157, 1951.

27. Brodman, K., Erdman, A. J., Lorge, I., Wolff, H. G., and Broadbent, T. H.: The Cornell medical index, J.A.M.A. **140:**530-534, 1949.

28. Bush, J. W., and Fanshel, S.: Basic concepts for quantifying health status and program outcomes, San Diego, Calif., 1970, University of California (mimeographed).

29. Henderson, M. M., and Meinert, C. L.: A plea for discipline of health and medical evaluation, Int. J. Epidemiol. **4**(1):11-23, 1975.

30. Doll, R.: Surveillance and monitoring, Int. J. Epidemiol. **3**(4):305-314, 1974.

31. Goldberg, G. A., Needleman, J., and Weinstein, S. L.: Medical care evaluation studies, a utilization review requirement, J.A.M.A. **220**(3):383-287, 1972.

32. Sullivan, D. F.: Conceptual problems in developing an index of health, publ. no. 1000, series 2, no. 17, Washington, D.C., 1971, National Center for Health Statistics, **2**(42):1-35.

33. Sullivan, D. F.: Disability components for an index of health, Vital Health Stat. **2**(42):1-35, 1971.

34. May, J.: Indicators and predictors of health status and health action, Paper presented at the 1973 Engineering Foundation Conference on evaluation in health services delivery, Berwick Academy, Berwick, Me., 1973 (mimeographed).

35. Patrick, D., and Bush, J. W.: Toward an operational definition of health, Paper presented at 99th annual meeting of the American Public Health Association, Minneapolis, Minn., October 1971 (mimeographed).

36. Cazes, B.: The development of social indicators: a survey. In Schonfield, A., and Shaw, S., editors: Social indicators and social policy, London, 1972, Heinemann Educational Books, pp. 9-22.

37. Balinsky, W., and Berger, R.: A review of the research on general health status indexes, Med. Care **13**(4):283-293, 1975.

38. Ekwall, B.: Method for evaluating indications for rehabilitation in chronic hemiplegia, Acta Med. Scand. **180**(suppl.):450, 1966.

39. Katz, F., Ford, A. B., Moskowitz, R. W., Jackson, B. A., and Jaffe, M. W.: Studies of illness in the aged, the index of ADL: a standardized measure of biological and psychosocial function, J.A.M.A. **185:**914-919, 1963.

40. Gilson, B., Gilson, J., Bergner, M., Vesselago, M., Kressel, S., Bobbit, R., and Pollard, W.: Development and application of the sickness impact profile, Seattle, 1973, University of Washington, School of Public Health and Community Medicine.

41. Pollard, W. E., Bobbitt, R. A., Bergner, M., et al.: The sickness impact profile, reliability of a health status measure, Med. Care **14:**2, 1976.

42. Gilson, B., Gilson, J. S., Bergner, M., et al.: The sickness impact profile: development of an outcome measure of health care, Am. J. Public Health **65**(12):1304-1310, 1975.

43. McDowell, I., and Martini, C.: Problems and new directions in the evaluation of primary care, Int. J. Epidemiol. **5**(3):247-250, 1976.

Organizational issues of peer review

7

Organizational issues in systematic peer review

GORDON C. BLACK
PAUL Y. ERTEL

The boundaries of peer review are wide, the content massive, the tools unproven, and the health care system it monitors is constantly undergoing change. In the past, peer review methods and procedures understandably reflected considerable variability in organization, scope, and practice from hospital to hospital. But such variability can be expected to gravitate toward greater uniformity as the informational demands of governmental agencies and third party payors come closer together and the conceptual basis for professional obligations of public accountability become better appreciated.

The major task of this chapter is neither to applaud the inevitable nor campaign for an alternative but to sensitize the reader to the organizational aspects of peer review independent of the specific content or hospital in which it is found. We will attempt to present an overview of those organizational and management variables that are essential to designing and implementing within a hospital a comprehensive type of medical peer review system as defined in the Glossary.

Accounting is said to be the language of business, yet the act of determining if medical care meets professionally recognized standards amounts to an accounting system in that it requires an organizational structure for monitoring performance and a data capturing system for recording the results. But there the resemblance ends as peer review involves so much more. What is therefore germane is to review the important organizational concepts that make the highly complex task of launching a peer review system manageable. This discussion will focus on (1) stages and phases of project development, (2) project organization and management, (3) design considerations, and (4) a discussion of specific items dealing with alternatives and problems that should be considered before settling on a final configuration of the review system. Although operating and optimizing a review system normally are considered part of the overall organizational task, the sheer volume and complexity prohibits discussion in this chapter. The operational aspects of peer review are presented in Chapter 8. It should be clearly recognized that the systematic approach to the entire development project has interactive feedback within and between all phases and that the entire process is a continuum rather than a linear stepwise sequence. In discussing this systematic approach the organization imposed for descriptive clarity should not be interpreted as hard boundaries in the development or operation of peer review systems.

From an organizational standpoint the care evaluation function is (for convenience only) considered independent of the care delivery function. Accepting this premise, it follows that an organizational entity that is external to existing administrative structures should be charged to perform this function regardless of whether the hospital received the delegated status from its professional standards review organization (PSRO) or not.

A systematic approach to any planning activity starts with a "conceptual base." This is described as a definition of the job to be done, and it requires that the objectives of the project must be clearly defined. To do this the decision makers within the hospital hierarchy must recognize operative values for the institution and also develop a familiarity with the technical aspects of what systematic peer review really entails. This orientation aspect is normally achieved through a "systems survey" or an evaluation of existing review systems and a comparative analysis of modern peer review concepts, methodologies, and techniques. The objective is to weigh the advantages against the drawbacks of all possible variables for incorporation into the local functioning system. The design objectives that are simply too important to overlook in the planning phase are as follows: optimization of the care system in a way that enhances the medical care delivery, conformity to mandated external standards and guidelines established for utilization review under PSRO, and considerations for an efficient review process and flow of information between reviewers, functioning hospital components, and external review bodies.

Prior to discussing the optimal approach to a systems design of a comprehensive hospital-based review mechanism, it is necessary to first focus on certain organizational issues that can have a far-ranging impact on the design of any peer review mechanism. Among the major discussion topics to be addressed here are the following: planning, designing, methods development, implementation, and finally, the evaluation of peer review.

CRITICAL VARIABLES ASSOCIATED WITH ORGANIZATIONAL ISSUES IN PEER REVIEW
Planning

Appropriate and effective planning of systematic peer review is an essential ingredient to the success of both the short-range and long-range goals of the medical organization. Planning is a critical stage because a successful review system implies that it will introduce second-order change in the care system. In other words, there is an underlying assumption that systematic peer review will effect some change in the care system and that change had better be in the right direction for everyone concerned. The kind of change suggested in this chapter involves strategies that call not only for institutional policy realignments but also for behavioral realignments of the health professional's attitudes, beliefs, and assumptions. Planned change affects individuals at several different levels. Health professionals who work with peer review systems can be expected to be involved in planned change at the "people technology" level.[1] Deliberate change of this type calls for planning that will affect cognitive behavior, emotional behavior, and skill behavior. Systematic peer review, more than most health technologies, is a people technology that involves planning for behavior, both individual and social. Good planning can prevent behavioral difficulties and organizational problems in operationalizing systematic peer review and in dealing with the changes invoked by peer review.

Designing and developing

While planning requires the creation of an explicit set of assumptions on which systematic peer review can be built, design and development strategies require a commitment to define the boundaries of the system. This means to delineate the specific review elements such as criteria, monitoring strategies, review programs and subprograms, peer judgments, corrective actions, management information system, education component, and so on. These are all part of system design.

Designing becomes the next critical stage, since it entails a crystallization of relationships within the review organization that can then be seen with the greatest clarity. The design stage is in essence the architectural rendering that produces sufficient specificity for the review approach (or methodology) to become testable. In being specific about information flow, data systems requirements, and database requirements, for example, the organizational staff can predict error sources in the review process before the system is actually operating. It is this prediction capability through manipulating the system in model form that many valuable dollars can be saved prior to full implementation. This is what development is really all about.

Implementation

With the planning, designing, and development of systematic peer review well underway, the actual implementation of the program can be made much smoother and easier. Preparation for implementation, however, can be as critical as actually carrying out review activities. This chapter explores the critical theoretic implementation processes and sequences with "make or break" capabilities for launching the actual successful operation of systematic peer review (which is described in the next chapter).

Evaluation

It has been suggested that research is that discipline which develops or generates criteria, while evaluation measures the extent to which the criteria have been met (see Chapter 4). Evaluation as presented in this chapter will explore two specific considerations: first, that evalua-tion is essential in determining the extent to which previously set planning and design criteria for the management of the peer review systems have been met; and second, that evaluation is critical in determining the extent to which systematic peer review has been effective in impacting on patient care processes and their clinical outcomes. It is theoretically possible to have a well-developed and well-managed peer review system that has virtually no impact on patient care at all. The converse of this hypothesis is also theoretically possible: namely, that a review system can become blind and deaf to its impact on the care system. Neither should be tolerated, as the first is a waste of time and resources better spent on care delivery, and the latter can be downright dangerous to life and limb for the patients. Evaluation of peer review systems is therefore explored in earnest, since it represents perhaps the most critical single variable of a comprehensive peer review system.

PLANNING AND MANAGING THE PEER REVIEW DEVELOPMENT PROJECT
Conceptual base

From an organizational standpoint the project to develop (or redesign) a peer review system requires (1) dedication: establishing clear project objectives and obtaining authoritative commitments to proceed; (2) planning: determining what is to be done and how to do it (for example, select review strategies); (3) organizing: obtaining necessary personnel, facilities, equipment, methods, process, and operational decision making; (4) directing: setting up a time and cost framework for what and when intermediate objectives are to be achieved; and (5) controlling: measuring performance of the developmental process against the project plan and initiating all actions necessary to assure that the review system fulfills institutional goals.

The sequential steps in the overall review system development project might be summarized as follows: (1) study existing review systems, (2) design an inhouse system, (3) implement it, (4) test it, (5) operate it, and (6) evaluate how well it meets institutional needs. Presumably the ideal inhouse review system would also meet the requirements for delegation of review authority by the local PSRO. This delegation can be given only when it can be documented that an efficiently and effectively functioning review system is in place in a given institution. Such documentation will require the development of explicit criteria and review methodologies for certification of hospital admission, concurrent review of patients at specific points in time, and for the retrospective review of provider and disease profiles. If the external (PSRO) requirements also represent institutional objectives, then the process of creating such a system can begin. It is described as a series of logically discrete stages as modeled below, but the reader is reminded that in the real world these stages should blend and interact with each other.

Stages of project development

There are three stages in the life cycle of a system. Each stage has certain phases that form the framework for the orderly accomplishment of specific tasks required for developing, installing, testing, implementing, operating, and evaluating a new system.

Each of the three major developmental stages is comprised of a series of discrete organizational subsets of phases (Table 7-1). Approximate completion times are given below in parentheses.

Stage I: Study and design of candidate review systems

Phase 1: The study phase. Stage I begins with a detailed analysis of current peer review systems including their scope, organization, staff, procedures, methods, forms (input and output), and so on. (Time requirement for completion: 1 to 2 months.)

Phase 2: Determine systems requirements. Phase 2 consists of a study of new methods in response to projected future conditions. It is based on the analysis of each major review activity in terms of process inputs, operations, outputs, and resources required for each review function included in the total system (1 to 2 months).

Phase 3: Design the new system. The design phase is concerned with the development, evaluation, and description of the new or redesigned institutional system. Various design approaches must be considered in the process of arriving at the final one (2 to 4 months).

Stage II: Implementation and testing of the selected system (6 to 12 months)

Phase 1: Preparation, demonstration, and implementation. The first phase of stage II consists of the following functions and processes: issue directives, organize

Table 7-1. Suggested stages and phases of developing, testing, implementing, operating, and evaluating a peer review system

Stage	Phase				
	1	2	3	4	5
I. Study and design	Study/survey	Determine systems requirements	Design new system	—	—
II. System implementation and testing	Preparation	Installation	Silent running	Pilot test	Implementation
III. System operation and maintenance	Observation	Evaluation	Maintenance (optimization)	Impact	—

review teams and committees, train and select personnel and staff, and order equipment and supplies.

Phase 2: Installation of review system. Equipment and personnel are placed into operational status while the system is being tested in pilot operation within selected wards or facilities.

Phase 3: Silent running. The system is operated in all its functions but for the rendering of peer judgments while the evaluation process proceeds (shakedown and debut phase).

Phase 4: Pilot testing phase. The whole system is tested, including the judgmental (accountability) function, in selected hospital service areas for the identification of problems and elicitation of suggested corrections to meet program objective.

Phase 5: Implementation. The revised and debugged program is made fully operational in the total facility.

Stage III: Operation and maintenance of peer review system

Phase 1: Observation. Data are collected to assess the functional status of the new review system (3 to 6 months).

Phase 2: Evaluation. Data and experiences accumulated during the previous phase (system performance) are evaluated. Any redesign necessary to optimize the system is done at this time.

Phase 3: Maintenance. Changing the system to improve peer review operations or expand into additional needed review functions is now to be considered.

Phase 4: Impact. Evaluating the effects of the review system on the efficiency and integrity of the care system should precede the modification and publication of new operating instructions.

Organizational development

This section will examine the organizational aspects entailed with each stage of peer review as cited above. This discussion will be confined to a single hospital model, although the essential principles and practices involved are equally applicable to a regional or multihospital peer review system.

The rationale of choice

Any developmental endeavor of the magnitude of a medical peer review system requires a formal supportive commitment from the hospital's governing body (board of trustees). The responsibility to develop the system must be accompanied by the authority and the essential financing and manpower resources to get the job done. Anything short of total commitment, with the support of managers at all levels, can be expected to seriously jeopardize the successful implementation of an effective peer review system in virtually any hospital.

Basically there are three routes for introducing new operational procedures of peer review into an ongoing system of health care: (1) hire a consultant firm to develop, test, and supervise the implementation of the system; (2) use outside agencies (subcontractors) to provide whatever expertise is not available among the existing staff, while retaining inhouse the managerial aspects of the project; or (3) utilize existing hospital organization to complete the entire project inhouse while hiring on any additional personnel to accomplish specific assigned tasks. The third course of action is generally the most difficult, and the choice of approach is usually the second alternative, since some involvement of inhouse personnel is considered to be advantageous because it can assist in eliciting staff cooperation and acceptance of the peer review system once it is developed. Many managers consider this involvement an essential educational function as well.

Organizational concepts

The project manager concept probably provides the most useful organizational thrust in establishing the developmental program. This managerial position should probably be assigned to someone within the existing organization rather than to an outsider. Since systematic peer review is innovative, it requires more than the usual demands for organizational direction and supervision. This aspect most likely calls for a full-time project manager.

Organizational plan for development and implementation

An organizational manual (complete with an organizational chart, of course) should probably be prepared for the entire developmental project. Personnel recruitment for the project in most cases would capitalize on the abilities and skills of existing staff supplemented with whatever specially trained manpower needs to be drawn from outside consultants and part-time employees. These personnel comprise an effective task force charged with the responsibility to undertake the entire project.* The major organizational elements of this development plan are summarized below.

Advisory council. An advisory council or steering committee should be established to provide direction to the developmental effort and to assume responsibility for overall project supervision and monitoring. The major contributions of a supervisory body are (1) their expertise and objective counsel, (2) their service as a public relations board and as a communications link to the staff and the public, and (3) their assumption of institutional responsibilities associated with the accountability for public funds.

Project office. An undertaking of this magnitude merits a physical locus such as an office with sufficient staff to plan, organize, direct, control, and evaluate the

project. Appropriate staffing would likely include such personnel as the project manager, review coordinator, physician advisor, fiscal analyst, education and training coordinator, and secretarial and clerical personnel. Further, experience has shown that resource persons often function best when assigned to task forces that are given specific charges to undertake major project responsibilities. The following important activities are suited to be undertaken by task forces or ad hoc committees:

1. Criteria development (or adaptation of model criteria sets)
2. Data-base and medical records
3. Care system analysis
4. Education and training
5. Evaluation (of the review system)

The ultimate product of each organizational task force is the completion of a working document that describes a specific major component of an operating system. The specific foci of these task forces are described below.

Criteria development task force. The primary function of this group is to establish explicit review criteria and select the norms and standards for use in the hospital review process. Since model criteria sets are already available from the AMA (see Chapter 11) and other professional associations, the initial task of this group normally involves adapting model sets for local use and creating new criteria for clinical entities of local significance. Experienced personnel from the medical audit and utilization review committees of the medical staff are excellent candidates for this work group.

Data-base and medical records task force. The mission of this work group is to study and define the data elements needed to support review activities. Special emphasis is focused on procedures for gathering and recording a minimum of essential data to meet specified needs. This group should determine whether existing institutional forms, records, or data handling procedures need to be modified to increase

---

*The organizational concepts included in this chapter are based on experiences in installing a peer review system in four Ohio public mental hospitals under contract with the U. S. Department of Health, Education, and Welfare (HEW-OS-74-53). The project is titled "Design, Test and Implement a Model Medical Care and Assessment Program for Public Mental Health Hospitals" and is available through the Ohio Department of Mental Health and Mental Retardation, 30 E. Broad St., Columbus, Ohio 43215.

the efficiency and effectiveness of the review process and to ensure the confidentiality of the entire record system. Consideration should be given to the desirability of changing clinical record systems, so that they are more structured and uniform in gathering required review data and are more adapted to data security measures. The choice may be between converting to the problem-oriented system or optimizing existing source record formats to facilitate documentation. But the final test of any contemplated changes in records is whether they enhance clinical management of the patient. This is always worthwhile and should be the ultimate target as this group looks to data needs for review purposes. There is considerable overlap of review system data needs with those of clinical medicine. However, the review system contains some unique data elements also. Briefly, these additional data elements have to do with describing the peer judgments rendered with respect to inappropriate care or utilization of resources, how serious the deficiencies are, who is responsible for them, and recommendations regarding what should be done about them.

Care system analysis task force. A complete review and analysis of current institutional patient management procedures should be done covering admission policies, diagnostic and therapeutic practices, and discharge or patient transfer procedures before the definition of review procedures is attempted. The old cliché "don't automate chaos" aptly applies to the mission of this work group. Also the criteria, standards, and norms developed by the criteria group should be carefully examined by this task force to ensure that they take cognizance of practical realities and that the care system can reasonably be expected to conform to these standards and criteria in clinical practice.

Education and training task force. There are two major functions of the education and training task force. These are (1) to provide necessary education and training

for project and institutional staff on the operation of the peer review system and (2) to define and organize the appropriate mechanisms to carry out on a continuing basis the kind of education program needed to correct specific deficiencies identified by the evaluation process.

Evaluation and special studies task force. Formal evaluation is necessary to assure that the total review system functions properly. This involves the following: (1) evaluating the design of the review system, (2) establishing the mechanism for ongoing evaluation of the review process (that is, measuring the efficiency and effectiveness of the operational review system and its impact on the care delivery system), (3) specifying the scope and mechanisms of medical care evaluation (MCE) studies to supplement the routine surveillance of the care system, (4) specifying the scope and mechanisms of review system evaluation (RSE) studies to supplement the routine evaluation of the review system, and (5) evaluating the timeliness, frequency, format, and content of data summaries and statistics used to assess the functioning of the review system and to determine what policy or procedural changes are relevant and needed.

Planning process

Planning a peer review system begins with combining the results of the survey of existing surveillance systems with a systems analysis of current institutional care procedures. This is done to ensure that there will be an optimal fit between the care system and whatever review system is decided on prior to its implementation. Program readiness is a matter of applying the basic principles of management by objectives. Concurrent with or perhaps preceding program readiness should be a period of staff preparation. Implementation can begin optimally only when the institution and its staff are ready for the program and the program is ready for the institution. Comprehensive planning should therefore include a work plan, an implementation plan, and a financial plan or budget.

Work plan. A work plan listing all major development tasks assigned to each organizational entity is required. Tasks must be defined for individuals, standing committees, new committees, or special task forces.

Regardless of who assumes primary responsibility for a given task, each employee should have specific written instructions describing what is to be done and when it should be completed.

Implementation plan. An implementation plan containing a phased description of all major events that must be completed prior to making the system operational is the best insurance against a faltering start. A detailed plan highlighting sequence, setting completion dates, and with the identification of personnel involved and the methods for completing each task is probably a must, especially for larger installations.

Financial plan. The budget process includes three steps: planning, implementing, and controlling. The budget period for these procedures is likely to be the fiscal year, and the major steps in the budgeting process follow the usual practices for large projects. Underlying the entire budget process is a commitment to make scarce resources available for this effort, thus assuring the staff that it may proceed confidently with program development according to the approved plan.

Project evaluation

After the system is operational, a period of perhaps 3 to 6 months should be allowed to perform the initial in-depth analysis of the efficiency and effectiveness of the system to identify any pressing problems and to work out solutions. This may be considered the shakedown period. This initiates a period of optimization that should be planned with appropriate budgetary contingencies, so that the system can be brought to its most fruitful functional level before it is stabilized for routine operation. The scope and content of this evaluation is discussed later in this chapter.

Organizational plan for operations

Once the system has been developed, implemented, evaluated, and revised, the need for a large project staff no longer exists, so that temporary personnel should be reassigned and only necessary operating personnel remain on this budget. We conclude this discussion with the observation that the work on this phase of project development is not complete until a written plan has been provided for the design, implementation, and operation of the peer review system. It is clearly essential, moreover, that this plan include the provision of an executive committee assisted by standing subcommittees or that work groups be established to run the system.

DESIGNING AND DEVELOPING A COMPREHENSIVE PEER REVIEW SYSTEM
Conceptual base

For the sake of discussion the most comprehensive and all-inclusive model of a peer review system will be depicted. It should be noted that the same emphasis is given in this generic model to the quality dimension as to utilization review dimension. The rationale here is to present all components (subprograms) in a perspective of the overall scope of peer review so that comparisons can be made among them. The next step for the designer then is to identify those review subprograms that best fit local needs and institutional objectives.

Study of existing review activities

Most medical facilities have some form of medical audit and utilization review in place and functioning. Therefore it is best to start by analyzing the existing review activities for the following purposes: (1) to obtain baseline data, (2) to identify unresolved problem areas, (3) to establish necessary organizational relationships to expand review activities, (4) to document the need to adapt or modify existing administrative, clerical, or data-handling methods and procedures, and (5) to identify personnel, equipment, and other resources available to be utilized in the newer systematic approach to peer review.

Reducing the manpower cost of the new review system is extremely important, since both the expansion of functions and stepping-up of the intensity of review activities consumes manhours. Consequently it is essential to identify any personnel or functions employed in the old review activity no longer needed in the newly organized review system.

Once this is accomplished, alternative methodologic designs should be similarly analyzed and compared for efficacy, efficiency, coherency, and for compatibility of review operations with care operations. On completion of this analysis the actual design of the system begins. This consists of selecting and describing those alternatives best suited to meeting the goals and carrying out the objectives of the hospital. In short, the design phase consists of carefully describing the scope and dimensions of the optimal review system.

Dimensions of the review system

A comprehensive peer review system may be described from five different frames of reference, all of which relate in some manner to its design. Among those of importance are review system (surveillance) elements, medical care events, review strategies, the major review subprograms, and the levels of institutional review. They will be discussed in that order.

Review system components (operational and supportive). The design of a comprehensive model of the review process will likely be strongly influenced by the character of its organizational structure and by a mix of at least nine essential components. The first five of which are opera-

tional and the last four are supportive in character.

The operational components provide the building blocks of the basic audit process utilized in most any systematic approach to peer review, and the four supportive components convey the impact of the review process to the care process. This operational review consists of a five-step sequence[2] that is graphically displayed in Fig. 7-1.

For the purpose of this discussion the review process aims at the *assurance* of quality care to patients and not just the measurement of quality. Quality assurance pretty much commits the review procedure to include both process and outcome measures, since process measures alone cannot ensure that the four elements espoused by the U. S. Department of Health, Education, and Welfare (HEW)[3] (efficiency, safety, cost, and patient satisfaction) will be present to an appropriate degree in every episode of care. The basic audit strategy, whatever its stated purpose, should ultimately be capable of providing a reasonable basis for confidence that actions will be taken both to ascertain that the delivered care meets professionally recognized standards and that appropriate measures will be initiated through the supportive components to correct any deficiencies that may be found. It is more pragmatically thought of as an interactive process that is guided through some feedback mechanism to secondary changes that lead to an improved delivery of care. The operational components of the ongoing peer review surveillance process are discussed in the same order as represented in Fig. 7-1.

Criteria development. The first of the operational components is a set of valid explicit criteria (Fig. 7-1, *A*) permitting a responsible objective screening review of the care provided to all eligible patients. What is meant by valid criteria is that they should (1) be stated in measurable rather than in descriptive terms (meaning that they must be precise enough to

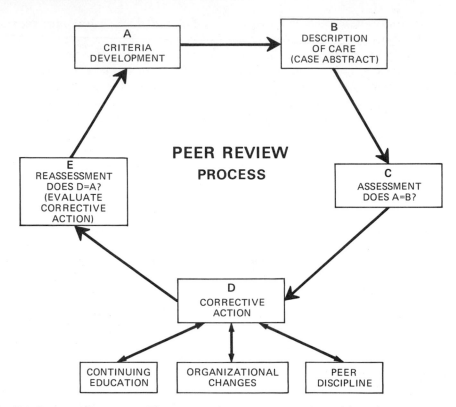

Fig. 7-1. Basic audit process. The peer review process consists of five elements: *A,* Consensus-generated clinical (and social) criteria; *B,* description of care as abstracted from patient's records by review coordinators; *C,* physician advisor judges care deficiencies and, *D,* refers deficiency reports for corrective action; *E,* reassessment determines whether corrective action was effective or whether new criteria are needed, *A.*

permit accurate observational measurement); (2) consist of statements of optimal achievable care; (3) include measures that validate the diagnosis, justify admission, surgery, or special hazardous procedures; (4) include a statement of expected patient outcomes; and (5) indicate the nature of ideal patient management under appropriate circumstances.

Description of care/case abstract. The second operational component (Fig. 7-1, *B*) provides a means for the assessment of care practices. This consists of describing and recording the actual care practices referent to the criteria. A well-defined and objective method for data acquisition is necessary whether the information handling system is automated or manual. Most surveillance systems employ a case-abstract method. Irrespective of

methodology, however, the essential thing is that consistency and accuracy characterize the data acquisition step.

Assessment. The third is the assessment step or a comparison of actual care to criteria. This is a simple analysis in which the criteria are compared against the abstract record for conformity (Fig. 7-1, *C*). If there are deviations or exceptions to the criteria in this screening phase, then those cases are sorted for referral to the appropriate peer for (1) identification to conformity to (or deviations from) explicit criteria, (2) case-specific justifications for all deviations from criteria that are found to be clinically acceptable, (3) the rendering of a peer judgment whether the given exception represents a true care deficiency (or inappropriate utilization of resources); (4) if it does, the peer reviewer must characterize the deficiencies as to cause and identify its source (why does component B not equal A and who was responsible for it?).

Corrective action. The fourth operational component is the action taken to correct the deficiencies (Fig. 7-1, D). Corrective action must be specific to the deficiencies identified and be effective in accomplishing the desired changes. Corrective actions must always be fully documented to reveal which contribute most to the improvement in patient care.

Reassessment. The fifth and final operational component is essential to assure that improvements in care have in fact occurred and once secured are retained (Fig. 7-1, E).

While the first five operational components of our model peer review system constitute the most basic review steps, they would not function as smoothly (if at all) without four additional supportive components to back them up, which are described below.

Peer management information system (PMIS). A management information system is the sixth component (the first of four supportive components). The PMIS captures and processes the data necessary for the monitoring functions that assess the utilization and quality of services rendered to each patient and reports all relevant results. Summary data, including profiles and statistics accumulated on patients, physicians, and institutions, are part of this latter function. The aim is to extract data useful to the peer review committees for revising criteria, norms, and standards for use in screening and in rendering peer judgments. Data must also be collected for managing the review system itself, and this is a component that cannot be overlooked in organizational planning if the system is to function smoothly.

Educational component. The seventh component is education. The review of performance data is widely held to be educational for those who do it. An organized approach to such a review will assist personnel in capitalizing on this learning opportunity. It is plainly obvious, too, that in identifying care deficiencies there is an implied commitment to mount an educational component to elicit clinical behaviors that rectify whatever deficiencies are detected. This function of peer review similarly requires the organizational support, logistics, and resources necessary to mount an effective and relevant educational program.

Evaluation component. The eighth (supportive) component is evaluation (review process monitoring), which comprises the set of procedures for evaluating the performance of the monitoring system itself as reflected by the data it generates. To state it another way, it is a proper function of peer review to assess how the monitoring system evaluates the care system. This vital feedback component should provide for the collection of performance data for managing the review system itself. Many managers overlook the evaluation function either in developing their organizational structure or in the initial design of the review system. This could prove costly, especially if much of the needed evaluation technology has to be developed at a later date—after the system is in place and running.

Organizational entity or structure. The last supportive component is the organization (and staff) essential to direct and perform the review functions. While the operational and preceding three supportive components form the building blocks of the review process, it is the integrity of its organizational structure (the ninth component) that holds the system together. Since this subject is covered in detail elsewhere (see Chapter 8), it will not be discussed here.

Medical care events. Since process-oriented peer review systems monitor the act of delivering medical care, it is necessary to obtain an overview of the spectrum of diagnostic and therapeutic events and the procedures that are to be monitored. This will assist personnel in determining the breadth of care events that the overall systems design should accommodate. Among the numerous approaches available, the one that appears the most practical at this time is to follow patients with differing diagnoses through the care system during a single episode of care (that is, through a single hospitalization). A macroanalysis of the hospital care process includes six generic events that can be monitored by the process-oriented peer review systems:

1. Preadmission
2. Admission

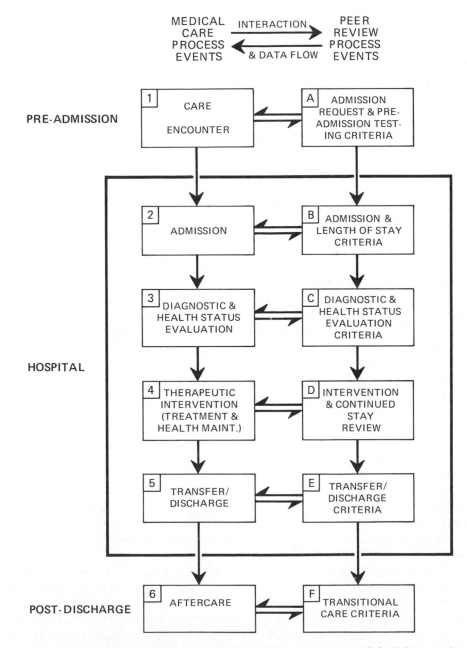

Fig. 7-2. Comprehensive adaptive control quality assurance model. Schema of integrated service delivery and quality assurance system.

3. Diagnostic and health status evaluations
4. Intervention (including treatment for illness, health, and maintenance)
5. Discharge or transfer
6. Aftercare or follow-up events

Medical care events are labeled *1* through *6* in the comprehensive adaptive control model (Fig. 7-2). The monitoring system that parallels the care system is labeled *A* through *F*. Conceptually this diagram illustrates the need for several reviews during an episode of care. The monitoring system (prospectively or concurrently) detects deviations from approved criteria and subjects them to peer judgment. In such a system the basic audit procedure described earlier (Fig. 7-1) is repeated for each review event (*A* through *F*) shown in the model and for each approved critical clinical criterion. The hospital is one of the most complex and sophisticated organizations in the whole world. Therefore it follows that an adequate monitoring system will certainly not be simple.

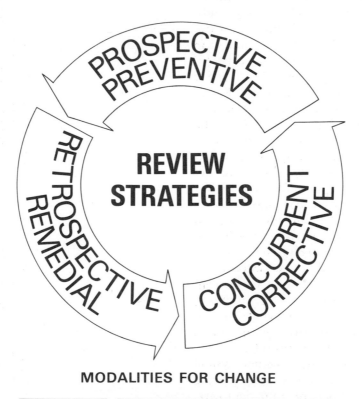

Fig. 7-3. Three basic types of time-related peer review strategies: *prospective* reviews are *preventive* in nature, *concurrent* reviews are designed to *correct* deficiencies in patients under care, and *retrospective* reviews are *remedial*, since they impact on care rendered to successive patients. The modalities for change are through continuing education, organizational change, or peer discipline. When viewed temporally, the action is circular in nature, moving from retrospective toward concurrent and prospective because patients admitted in subsequent months benefit from prospective changes in the care process resulting from the corrective actions taken in response to earlier concurrent and retrospective reviews.

Review strategies. Critical to the design is a clear understanding of the types, timing, and differences in review strategies.

Timing of review. A strategy that has a great impact on the design of a system is the timing of the review. There are three basic types of time-related reviews: prospective, concurrent, and retrospective. Each strategy carries a benefit to the care process that is unique unto itself (Fig. 7-3).

Prospective reviews are potentially capable of preventing an undesirable medical care from ever occurring in the first place. This is the foundation of individual (patient) quality assurance. Concurrent review provides for the initiation of corrective actions during a specific episode of care (that is, the capability of active intervention in the care process). Retrospective review, which is entirely remedial in nature, cannot impact directly on the studied patient cohort (because the review takes place after the receipt of care) but rather leads to improving the care delivered to future patient cohorts (which is the strategy employed in quality control). An example of what this interaction can mean is exemplified by the detection of patterns of deviant care on retrospective review that is found to be preventable. This can prompt changes in concurrent and prospective review strategies to monitor such unacceptable practices at an earlier time to correct them sooner or to prevent their occurrence entirely.

A fully comprehensive review system employs whatever review strategies bring the most practical benefits to patient care. Comprehensive systems would therefore aim at a mix of all three strategies in a dynamic review process that produces all three types of impact on the care process: namely, that retrospective review would be remedial in nature, concurrent would be corrective, and prospective would be preventive (that is, prevent care deficiencies from occurring). The major determinants in selecting the degree of emphasis each strategy should receive includes

Table 7-2. Comparison of major review programs: differences between cost, quality controls, evaluation, and continuing education

	Utilization review	Medical audit	Medical care evaluation studies	Continuing education
Purpose	Eliminate inappropriate utilization so that health care money will not be spent unnecessarily, and maximum use of health care dollars can be realized	Assure that health care services provided are of appropriate quality to an individual or group of patients	Pattern analysis that summarizes data generated from audit, utilization review, and medical evaluation studies into useful information to assist other peer committees to make better judgments	Meet educational needs of individual practitioners, based on the profile analysis

Method	Allocate units of health services to patients based on need	Assess provider performance to identify and correct inappropriate patterns of care	Analyze aggregate data and present in a meaningful way to review subcommittees and individual practitioners; prepare profile on patients, clinicians, hospitals, and recommend policies and procedures	Develop instruction programs to fit requirements of each individual or group
Concern	Cost: Preclude unnecessary payment for any unit of health care service unless medically necessary and not appropriately available at a lower cost elsewhere	Quality: Were the appropriate results of health care achieved? If not, why?	Identify possible causes of good and poor outcomes resulting from structure and process	Identify true educational needs of practitioners
Focus	Individual patient transactions; e.g., given patient's condition must require this unit of service	Patterns of care, based on patient cohorts of similar diagnoses or conditions	Seek improved ways to collect, classify, and analyze data to assist UR and audit committees in identifying outcomes	Develop educational programs to meet needs of individual practitioners
Measures	Process measures; e.g., does good care (care professionally recognized as appropriate to the problem) require that this service be provided to this patient in this setting?	Initially, outcome measures; uses process measures sparingly, as when relations between process and result known or when related to specific outcome problem	Structure, performance, and outcome measures	Decrease inconsistencies, decrease inappropriate admissions, and improve medical records
Time	Basically concurrent	Basically retrospective	Retrospective and prospective	Prospective, concurrent, and retrospective
Summary	Patient need Concurrent Individual patients Process measures Units of care Economic outcomes	Provider performance Retrospective Patient groups Quality measures Patterns of care Patient outcomes	Provides performance patterns Retrospective and prospective Patient groups Outcome process and measures Patterns of care Patient outcomes	Practitioner performance Prospective, concurrent, and retrospective Quality care Outcome measures Patterns of care Patient outcomes

1. The type of review most appropriate to the care provided
2. The existence of clinical opportunities to actively intervene in the care process
3. Acceptability of review activities or intervention to professional staff
4. Costs

The paramount issue in designing any monitoring system is to decide what time dimension or combination of the above review strategies will be utilized. To be discussed later are the equally important modalities for change, that is, continuing education, organizational changes, and peer discipline.

Major peer review programs. Understanding the differences among various peer review programs and a familiarization of how their major interrelated functions can be performed by the review system in an integrated manner is essential to design considerations. These functional relationships are best represented in a matrix as depicted in Table 7-2, which contrasts the difference between utilization review, medical audit (or quality review), medical care evaluation studies, and continuing education. It will be noted that while there is some overlap, each program may be independent and each possesses its own identifiable purpose. The purpose of utilization review and medical audit is routine surveillance of the care system. Medical care evaluation studies aim at mounting special studies of the care system, and continuing education aims at teaching the staffs of both the care system and the review system how to better do their jobs.

Types of reviews. The complexity of the health care system dictates that more than

Table 7-3. Inpatient medical care review strategies

Type of review	Applies to	Review screen	Decision at screening	Decision at peer review
Prospective Admission request (priority) Preadmission testing Safety clearance Discharge/transfer	One case	Criteria and standards	Refer possible problems to peer reviewer	Immediate correction of problems found/protection of patient safety
Concurrent Admission certification Continued stay Diagnostic and status evaluations Intervention (treatment, health maintenance)	One case	Criteria, standards, and norms (length of stay, etc.)	Allow admission/extension of stay or refer to peer reviewer	Allow or deny admission/extension of stay (refer for discipline if repeated pattern of abuse)
Retrospective Medical care evaluation studies (medical audit)	Group of cases	Criteria and standards	Probable/possible problem	Deny or confirm problem exists; correction of recurring problems through continuing education or discipline if repeated pattern exists
Claims review	One case	Criteria or norms	Pay or refer to peer review	Allow or deny admission of stay (for payment purposes)

one type of review strategy would be needed to monitor (or measure) both the quality of care and the utilization of resources. Conceptually the major types of review may differ in four basic ways: (1) the purpose for which the review is performed, (2) the organizational level at which peer review is performed and judgments rendered, (3) whether the review applies to one case or a group of cases, and (4) the timing of reviews in relationship to a given episode of care (prospective, concurrent, and retrospective review). Table 7-3 depicts timing strategies in use today. Understanding their characteristics will promote the recognition of possible alternatives that can be refined into solutions of logistic problems.

Major subprograms. A comprehensive model for a peer review program is depicted in Fig. 7-4. This model contains 12 subprograms and identifies which of them are appropriate to prospective, concurrent, and retrospective review strategies. This illustration encompasses all three major surveillance functions: namely, the daily monitoring (surveillance) of individual patients, the provision of summary data for use by peer committees for medical audit and utilization review, plus the structural framework for conducting medical care evaluation studies. The arrows depict the usual sequence of the review process for both quality assessment and utilization assessment and the general flow of information. The first seven programs are oriented toward individual patient monitoring, whereas the remaining five subprograms are based on aggregated data. At the outset it should be noted that all patients are not necessarily monitored by every program. For example, a patient discharged prior to the fiftieth percentile length of stay would not receive a continued stay review (Fig. 7-4, *4*). Further, special studies (especially MCEs) would be conducted on a sampling basis rather than a routine surveillance of 100% of the cases. Finally, the dividing line between them is not solid because concurrent review often uses the

accumulated past record (of a physician, for example) in rendering a judgment. Conversely, retrospective data can modify concurrent review by altering its criteria and so forth. The point is that strategies should and often do interact.

This model reflects those structural elements advocated and discussed elsewhere in this book or in the literature on peer review that collectively should be considered by those designing new systems or reexamining old ones. It should be noted, however, that a single comprehensive model which includes all these programs does not exist as an operational entity anywhere at this time to our knowledge.

The organizational levels of peer review. The last consideration in designing a model peer review system deals with establishing the organizational level at which judgmental decisions take place. Most authorities agree with the general concept that it is desirable to solve jurisdictional problems at the lowest possible level within the organization. Fig. 7-5 depicts an ascending order of functional responsibilities in the conduct of peer review, ranging from clerical duties to the establishment of policy directives, that effect the review system, the care system, and the entire institution. These functional responsibilities naturally cluster into four rather distinct levels so organized that each ascending level has an adequate, trained staff with authority appropriate to conduct its own prescribed range of review activities and a clear-cut access to higher levels of authority. Since the actual review functions to be conducted at each level will be discussed in the next chapter on operations, the present discussion focuses on a unified concept concerning how it might be possible to organize and structure the review process into a series of smoothly functioning entities that provide the decision-making machinery appropriate to each peer judgment.

Level 1. The unit most appropriate to conduct ongoing or routine review activities is what we choose to call the primary review team, generally comprised of a

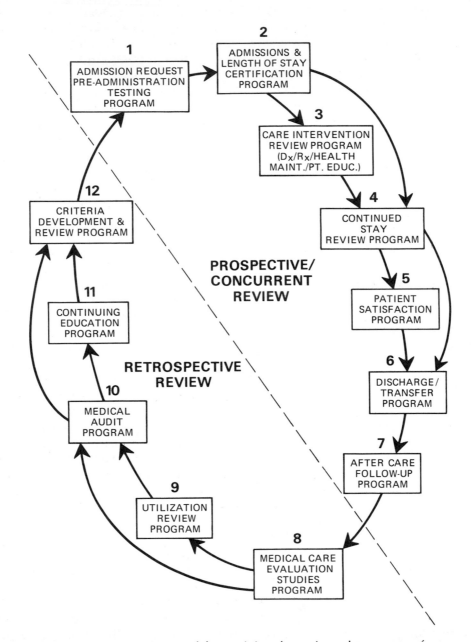

Fig. 7-4. Generic peer review model containing the major subprograms of a comprehensive quality assurance (peer review) program. Few existing programs include all the elements. The review process is depicted sequentially. However, not all process steps are used in the review of most patients. For example, a patient discharged prior to the fiftieth LOS percentile would not receive review step 5, but the review would proceed from step 4 to step 6. Steps 1 through 7 normally are employed in the review of individual patients and are prospective or concurrent review. Steps 7 and 8 may also focus on individual patients; however, steps 7 through 12 normally are conducted as retrospective reviews and deal with aggregate data (that is, profiles and statistics) on patient populations.

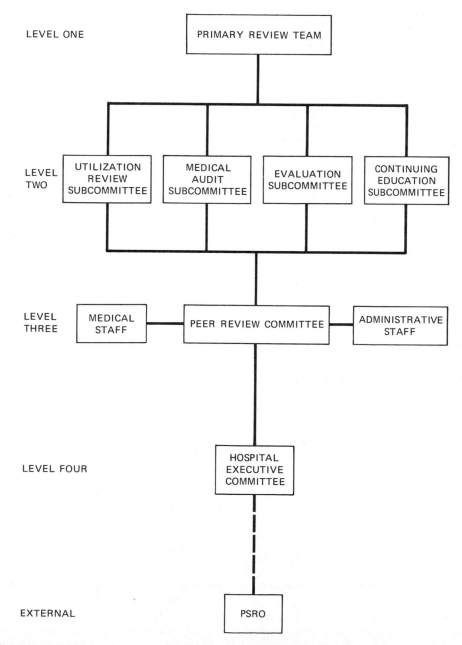

LEVEL ONE

LEVEL TWO

LEVEL THREE

LEVEL FOUR

EXTERNAL

PRIMARY REVIEW TEAM

UTILIZATION REVIEW SUBCOMMITTEE

MEDICAL AUDIT SUBCOMMITTEE

EVALUATION SUBCOMMITTEE

CONTINUING EDUCATION SUBCOMMITTEE

MEDICAL STAFF

PEER REVIEW COMMITTEE

ADMINISTRATIVE STAFF

HOSPITAL EXECUTIVE COMMITTEE

PSRO

Fig. 7-5. The peer review organization of a hospital and four levels of hospital review. The system operates on the premise that problems should be solved closest to the source.

physician advisor (PA), review coordinator, clerk typist, a records technician, and a continuity of care reviewer.* This team should be trained to conduct the initial surveillance of care. Typically this consists of the two basic review criteria. Any cases that demonstrate a variance between the record of care (review element in which case abstracts are prepared) and comparisons made to explicit criteria are identified and referred to the appropriate peer for a judgmental review.

The physician member of the team (the PA) is usually called on to render a judgment whether an actual care deficiency has occurred, and if so, who is the proper peer to handle the case. Should it be determined that the PA is also qualified to render the peer judgment, he does so and may elect to initiate a corrective action himself should that be within the proper limits of his vested authority. Should it be that some other reviewer is a more appropriate professional peer to judge the case, a formal delegation of responsibility must be made through established communication channels. In general the cases likely to be referred are the more serious ones requiring a higher review level for collective judgments and corrective actions.

Level 2. The titles appearing on an organizational chart are not very important, but review assignments and task definitions for level 2 are probably best organized around working units as permanent components (subcommittees) of the hospital's supervisory peer review committee. The reason for this arrangement is that it minimizes superordinate-subordinate conflicts when sensitive matters are involved. The workers who actually conduct various level 2 review activities also sit as supervisors who share the same policy-making power at review level 3. The utilization review subcommittee (URS) would review and act on referrals from the peer reviewer (level 1) of all cases that involve

inappropriate resource allocations (for example, inappropriate admissions), and the medical audit subcommittee (MAS) would act on referred cases that involve deficiencies in the quality of medical care. Other organizational units needed by a model system at this level are the continuing education subcommittee (CES), whose function is obvious, and the evaluation subcommittee (ES), which is responsible for maintaining and upgrading the data-handling procedures of the entire review system and lending assistance to all other working groups in data analysis and interpretation.

Level 3. The organizational unit of review level 3 consists of the full peer review committee (PRC). This is composed of all subcommittee members, representative peers of all other professionals subject to review, and representatives of the board of trustees, the hospital administration, and the public. The composition should be compatible with PSRO requirements for the directing body in delegated hospitals. The working tasks of the full committee are to evaluate the effectiveness and the efficiency of both the care system and the review system, to recommend any needed changes in policy or procedures, to provide direct supervision and guidance for all working review units, and to hear any appeals referred to it from level 3.

Level 4. The top policy-making authority of the institution comprises review level 4. This ultimate institutional authority may be analogous to the familiar executive committee, the board of trustees, or the joint conference that typically is a combination of both. It is this group that sets all internal guidelines for the conduct of both medical care and peer review activities. It is also the repository of all authority that deals with external matters such as the establishment of contractual arrangements with the third party payors and with the PSRO. Whatever the division of tasks or names by which working groups are known, an organizational plan for development and implementation of the review

---

*Those listed are for illustrative purposes only and would vary by type of hospitals.

system should explicitly communicate the composition of all working units at each level of review. It should also cite specific responsibilities, limits of authority, and the method of selecting membership in the groups.

Integrated hospital information flow

Any monitoring system intended to evaluate the full range of hospital-based care activities must conform to complexities of that kind of care. This does not necessarily mean that the review process itself needs to be similarly complex, but it does dictate that it be adaptive to complexities within the care process and that it be capable of monitoring what needs to come under routine surveillance without disturbing the natural flow of clinical information, neither of which are easily done.

Another aspect of the contemporary hospital environment deserving special attention is a wider cast of participants in the care process than has been traditional in the past. Fig. 7-6 depicts a model of the information flow between the five major participants in the interface between the care and surveillance process. It depicts which action step is required in both the care system and the review system in a running sequence (often in parallel) as the patient processes through the hospital.[4]

The participants in the data flow sequence are (1) the patient, (2) clinician, (3) hospital representative (clerk or administrator), (4) fiscal agent, and (5) peer review manager. The direction of the usual data flow is indicated by the arrows. The single point we wish to make with this diagram is that the logistics of data flow are complex and must be planned with care or bottlenecks will surely appear should a comprehensive surveillance system simply be imposed or grafted on a care-based data system.

To illustrate the many interactions and contingencies that actually take place between the provision of care and its evaluation, we will examine a typical hospital admission. This is a simplified model with only major decisions and actions depicted. To illustrate the complexity of even a single subprogram, the admission certification function has been selected to illustrate the data flow necessary to complete the transaction. Fig. 7-7 is a flow diagram depicting the hospital admission review protocol. This protocol is part of the utilization review process that has two stated objectives: the certification of appropriate admissions and the assigning of an expected length of stay (or the identification of inappropriate admissions).

Briefly, what takes place is this: once the admitting office is notified of an impending admission, the review team must also be informed (step *1*) to create a patient file and initiate the admission certification process (step *2*). On receipt of the admitting diagnosis, the review personnel will determine if there are established (approved) explicit criteria for this admission (step *3*). If there are none, a determination must be made whether explicit criteria are critical, that is, essential to conduct the review process (step *4*). If such is not the case, general review criteria will be used (step *5*). In either eventuality the review coordinator proceeds to complete a case abstract (as directed by either criteria set), and a determination is made whether general or diagnosis-specific admission criteria are met (step *6*). The first contingency in this review sequence may be encountered in step *4* where it may be determined that explicit criteria are essential to the conduct of review but are currently unavailable. All such cases are submitted to the physician advisor (step *7*) who reviews the case individually and renders an implicit judgment as to the merit of the admission request (step *8*). At this point a second contingency may be encountered. If he does not find the admission justified (in step *8*), he therefore disapproves the admission, that is, denies certification for payment (step *11*). All personally inspected cases he does approve (step *9*) are also certified for admission (step *10*). A length of stay is assigned for all approved cases

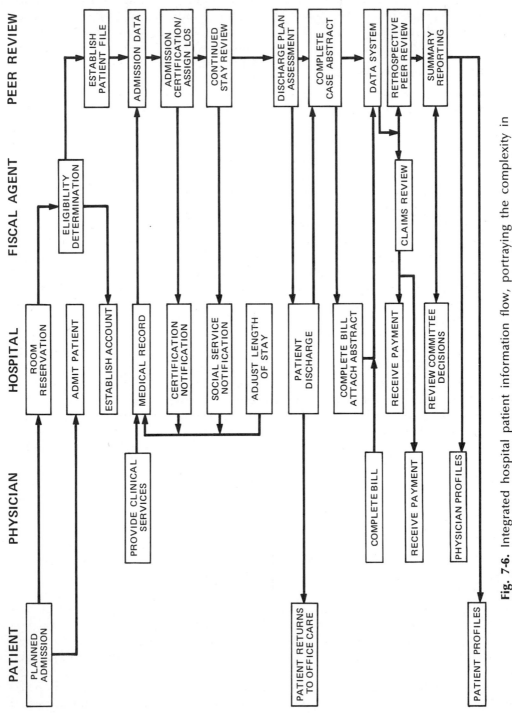

Fig. 7-6. Integrated hospital patient information flow, portraying the complexity in processing information for hospitalized patients. The five major participants in the care and monitoring processes are listed across the top. The personnel involved in the blocks represent those actions required as the patient progresses through the hospital care and review system and generates relevant data during an episode of care.

that pass the admission screening process (step *10*). On completion of the admission review sequence, the review personnel (through the data system) must notify the hospital admission office, the patient, and attending physician whether the admission was approved (step *12*). If it was not, it is up to the patient and his physician to make alternate plans for the care not considered justifiable for inpatient payment benefits.

It is intended with this illustration to

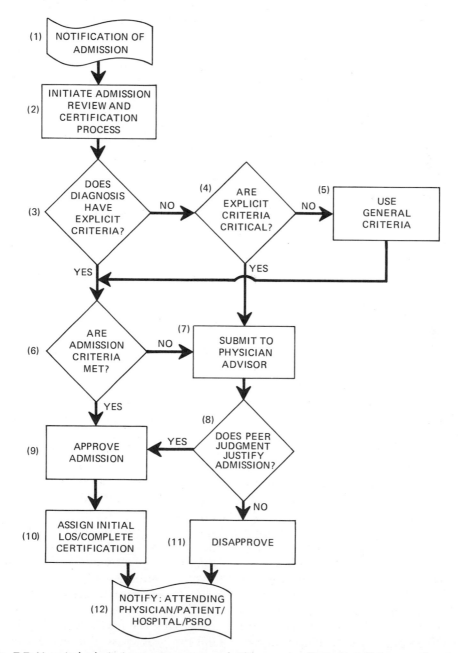

Fig. 7-7. Hospital admission review protocol. This process flow chart illustrates the steps for admission certification and assigning the initial length of stay for a hospital admission.

show that even with one of the more simple review procedures it is very important to plan for all decision contingencies to avoid organizational pitfalls in the design of review protocols that can interrupt communications and bog down the review process or, worse, interfere with the care process.

Peer review information system

This section will present some of the conceptual aspects of developing and designing an information system to support peer review. It should be recognized in so doing that many hospitals already have sophisticated data operations, and they may elect for economic reasons to utilize the same information system for peer review that supports other internal clinical and administrative functions. In any event the focus of whatever supporting information system is used must be oriented toward the collection of clinically useful medical care data to (1) monitor and evaluate the medical care delivered to patients (the care process), (2) develop statistics and profiles to assist peer judgments and to modify criteria, standards, and norms, (3) monitor, manage, and evaluate the effectiveness of the review process, (4) provide data for medical care evaluation studies, and (5) fulfill PSRO and other external reporting requirements.

The structural components of such a broad-purpose data system have been described by the American Association of Foundations for Medical Care with the suggestion that it be comprised of the following:

1. "The system should be fundamentally a data storage-retrieval system, capable of storing information for convenient retrieval in a variety of formats at later times.

2. "The system design must be flexible. While aimed at broad PSRO needs, it must leave each hospital or local PSRO capable of independent action in its daily activities, free to follow different philosophies of review and free to use local criteria for review decisions.

3. "Patient, physician, and hospital profiles must be available to support preadmission or concurrent decisions as well as retrospective analysis and medical care evaluation studies.

4. "The system should support model treatment analysis for each hospital or local PSRO designing it.

5. "The system must accept data from the fiscal intermediary or other sources such as PAS where the PSRO desires it. It must also accept data gathered directly to the PSRO and its delegated hospital review teams. It must be capable of combining all this data into a unified patient record.

6. "The system must be capable of extension to cover ambulatory care and prescription drugs and merge all forms of data together to obtain full patient profile.

7. "The system must be organized in such a way that protection of both physician and patient from inappropriate exposure is assured."[5]

Before allowing oneself to be driven by such descriptions of the ideal into concluding that all this has been achieved or that little remains to be accomplished in this field, we offer this reminder that Finagle's laws on information apply to peer review data systems. Finagle's laws state: "The information you have is not what you want; the information you want is not what you need; the information you need is not what you can obtain."

Unfortunately most existing management systems in the health field have evolved over time in opportunistic response to contemporary needs and without the benefit of the systems approach to long-range planning for future data needs. In the planning and development of the data system, user involvement is essential in development, testing, analyzing, and modifying the data system. But it is essential to look past the exigencies of the moment. The wise reservation of space for expansion should lessen the impact of Finagle's laws on data systems that are intentionally designed for the long haul to keep abreast of the peer review goals and processes that evolve over time.

Steps in planning the data system

The development of a data system proceedes through five discrete steps (Fig. 7-8).[5]

Step 1: Establishing objectives and defining them operationally. The first step in the planning and development of a peer review data system is the specification of data requirements and the establishment of objectives for operational information flow.

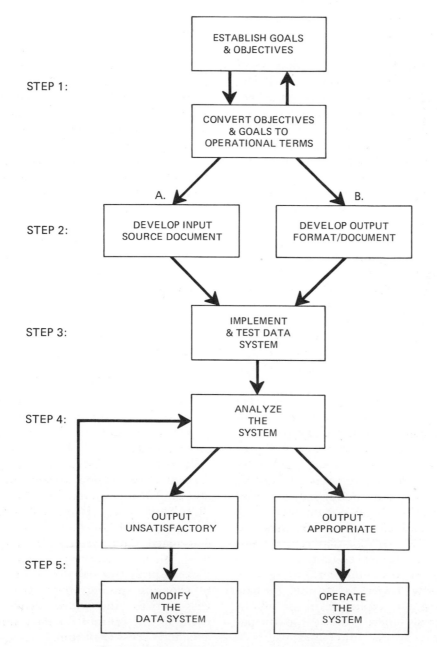

Fig. 7-8. Steps in planning the data system.

Step 2: Developing the input source document and the output format. The second step is to develop the input documents and the formats for all data reporting (output). The input document is generally a screening instrument, that is, an abstract or a component of the medical record. The form(s) for input to automated data systems are critical, since collected data are converted into machine-processable magnetic "blips" and eventually back into materials appropriate for human analysis and comprehension. All data items collected should support the objectives of the review system. Conversely, no data item should be collected that is not system justified. But it is not always obvious which data items are superfluous. Time and careful effort should be invested to determine which items are really essential to the system and which are not. Take, for example, the simple matter of the patient's age. Should this item be recorded as the birth date, which requires six digits at a minimum, or as the current age, which requires only two? The cost of processing a birth date is greater, but it need only be recorded once and can be used to extrapolate the present age at any time. It is also more accurate. The trade-off is between cost and flexibility plus accuracy. The designer must strive for the best configuration of data to serve needs of the system first and foremost. Further, displaying data output in a digestible form is an art and will save precious clinician time if properly formatted. Obviously the computer programs necessary for processing the data and preparing the profiles and other desired output reports must be planned, executed, debugged, checked again, then thoroughly documented.

Step 3: Implementation of the data system. An implementation plan is best developed by involving representative segments of the entire institution, including care providers and reviewers. An integral part of the plan is to capitalize on the educational process inherent in active participation of review personnel and principle

users in all developmental phases. The system will not run smoothly unless each user understands his part in the review process and how to make maximal use of the data system in meeting his own responsibilities.

Step 4: Analysis of the system. The fourth step is an analysis of the extent to which the system aids the review process. The relevant questions are: Does the data system function as designed? What changes are necessary to meet the design objectives? Does it produce reliable, valid results? Does it measure what it is supposed to measure? How sensitive, how specific, and how observable (available) are the data elements that have been chosen? Will the functioning of the data system meet institutional requirements for systematic peer review?

Step 5: Modification (optimization) of the system. The final step is whatever modifications of the system are necessary to provide more satisfactory answers to the above questions. Caution must be exercised at this stage, since a single processing change may precipitate problems in both input and output stages. It should be noted that since all changes cost something and consume valuable time, a thorough analysis should be made before any operational changes take place to be certain they are worth the effort.

Types of information systems

There is much controversy concerning what constitutes optimal information flow requirements and essential data management activity to support a peer review system. Major differences among the information processing systems now available for consideration can be clustered into three basic types: (1) manual systems, (2) semiautomated (abstract systems), and (3) automated data systems (interactive online). All are based on human decision-making processes, so this is not a factor in choosing among them. What largely characterizes the differences between them are the options for data input, storage, and access to output.

Manual system. This system contains most of the elements of the traditional retrospective audit approach, which has been operating in hospitals for a quarter century or so. Added to this approach fairly recently are admission and continued-stay certification processes. This simpler system depends on manually generated norms, profiles, and other statistics required in the conduct of review activities by physician advisors, review coordinators, and review committees.

Semiautomated system. This system normally contains similar manual operations for determining exceptions to admission certification, length of stay, and continued-stay criteria. However, the major difference is that after a case abstract is prepared and processed by machine (either by the hospital data equipment or by a data broker), computers are used not only to generate the profiles, norms, and other data for routine surveillance but often also to process data for medical care evaluation studies and as an aid to the management of the peer review system.

Automated system. Technically the automated model can vary considerably from a remote batch-oriented system to an online, interactive, real-time data processing system. There is much discussion these days as to which type of system is best for peer review. Any practical answer to that question for the average hospital will depend on the exact mix of review programs and subprograms that make up the total effect. Differences in what kinds of services these information systems can provide to assist this effort will therefore be discussed next. Fig. 7-9 depicts the information flow in an automated system that can be batch processed, handled on-line on an interactive mode, or developed as a combination of the two. It embraces the adaptive control mechanism for assuring quality. The sensor in this model *(1)* consists of the review personnel team (review coordinator and physician advisor, and so on). The function of identifying variances

between the record of care and the criteria can be performed by the computer as can notification of peer reviewer (effector) who renders a judgment and recommends corrective actions, both of which can be documented and reported to proper authorities through and by the automated system. One major difference the automated model introduces because of the speed of its automated data processing is that it enables the corrective changes to occur for the individual patient while he is still under treatment rather than settling for improving the care provided to patients subsequently admitted to the hospital. Since the volume of data handling that can be expected in most institutions will require computer technology to perform routine accounting and reporting functions efficiently anyway, an increased investment in automation is likely, which could probably be exploited to make the review process more efficient. This trend would favor an evolution toward prospective peer review strategies. The point we wish to make is that there appears to be a relationship between the peer review strategies, the degree to which automation is employed in the review process, and improvement in quality assurance. This relationship is graphically presented in Fig. 7-10.

As depicted, a trend can be expected away from the manual and semiautomated, retrospective and concurrent review strategies in use today and toward highly interactive prospective review strategies literally capable of operationalizing quality assurance and the prevention of inappropriate care to the degree that peer review is capable.

A further evolutionary trend that may grow out of interactions between the review system and the care system has to do with developing the capability for immediate intervention in care delivery. Sooner or later the concurrent review of the quality of care will encounter life-threatening circumstances or hazardous procedures while still in the planning stage

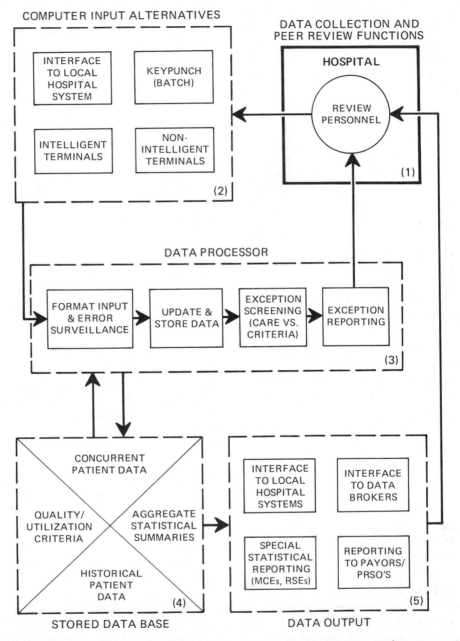

Fig. 7-9. Information flow of an automated prospective, concurrent, and retrospective peer review system. *1,* The review team monitors the care events; *2,* enters care deficiencies by one of the methods shown; *3,* the computer generates exception reports; *4,* stores the data; and *5,* generates periodic and special reports for use by the PA and the committees. Exception reports, *3,* are provided daily to review personnel for appropriate peer review action, *1.* Action taken is entered, *2,* and if appropriate, stored, *4.* If not, the cycle is repeated.

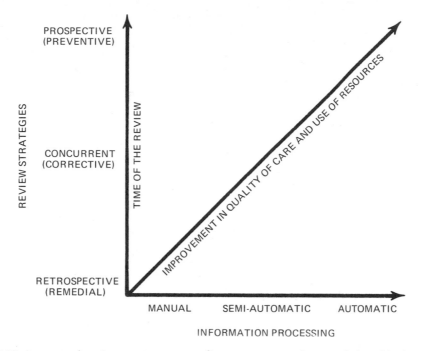

Fig. 7-10. Impact of review system on quality care, suggesting a relationship between degree of automation, review strategy (prospective, concurrent, retrospective), and capability to achieve improvements in the quality of medical care. (There is no empiric evidence to support this notion at this time, but the idea deserves study.)

(for example, ordered but not yet performed). Most hospitals develop special channels for immediate intervention to prevent patient harm under these conditions. This is prospective interaction. Is it likely to remain confined to this one application for long?

Assuming that there is a relationship between the degree of automation, review strategies, and the quality issue, what impact would the combination of these factors have on the cost per review? Fig. 7-11 presents a matrix with the cost variable added to the previous model for possible trade-off considerations. The model presents 27 possible configurations derived from the three covariables. On one extreme block *1* (manual-retrospective-low-cost process) offers the patient the least assurance of quality, whereas block *27* (prospective-automated-high-cost system) offers a patient the maximum quality assurance. It must be realized that peer review systems utilize a mix of these vari-

ables in some chosen combination, and it is only for discussion purposes that they are separated. The point to all this is that a conscious trade-off should be made in full recognition of all the available options and the implications of each with respect to the quality of the review process.

An expanded outcome model

It is generally found that the first priority in developing peer review systems is to implement and optimize process measures, but the validity of such measures probably depends on documenting improvements in patient outcomes, especially those attributable to changes in medical care made in response to review findings. The concept requires an expanded model of peer review that evaluates the status of patients both before and after their episode of care, which in the model we are discussing means prehospitalization and posthospitalization.

A conceptual framework for approach-

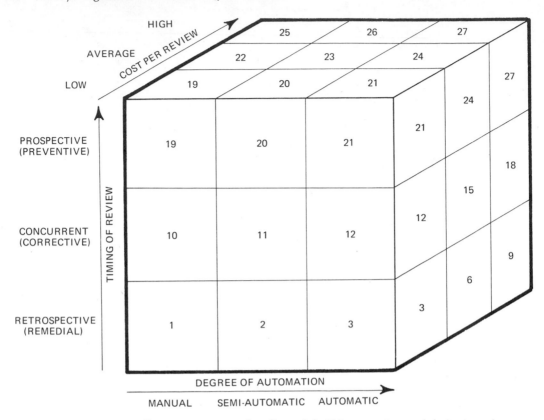

Fig. 7-11. Cost–quality assurance trade-off model. This generic model depicts three variables—timing of review, degree of automation, and relative cost per review. Two of these (timing of review and degree of automation) impact on both the degree of quality assurance and the cost of the review process. The model presupposes that block *1* offers the patient under treatment the least quality assurance for the least cost; whereas block *27* offers the best quality assurance for the greatest cost. A practical question to be addressed in evaluating a given review system is, To what extent does cost vary with changes in the other two variables?

ing this logistic problem was developed by Connell and Black[6] and built on the experience of others.[7-9] Fig. 7-12 is a model illustrating the distinction they make between "internal" and "external" validation of quality criteria in relation to current and expanded peer review models. As will be noted, the center section depicts the peer review process model used in most systems today. The expanded outcome model (dotted lines) evaluates both prehospital and posthospital patient outcomes (changes in health status and social function) for a random sample of patients. The potential for the further validation of criteria and refinement of review procedures

resulting from such external clinical outcome evaluations of inpatient care makes the expansion of peer review into the posthospital period especially attractive. One of the unsettled questions this strategy can answer is what happens to those patients who were denied continued hospital stays? Posthospital review may be the only way of detecting patient harm introduced by inappropriate review objectives or methodologies.

The expanded outcome model not only provides the feedback loop needed to validate process criteria but also can begin to provide the statistical basis for validating outcome criteria as well. Techniques al-

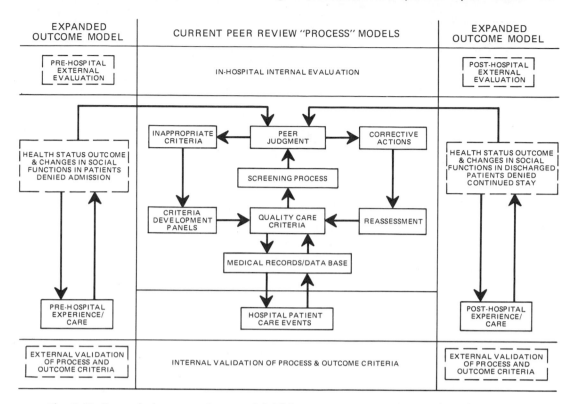

| EXPANDED OUTCOME MODEL | CURRENT PEER REVIEW "PROCESS" MODELS | EXPANDED OUTCOME MODEL |

Fig. 7-12. Expanded peer review model. This concept suggests expanding the current peer review process models (center) to monitor the patient's clinical outcome during pre- and post-hospitalization. The purpose of the expanded model is to establish external validation of process and outcome criteria.

ready utilized in clinical research have some application to outcome measurement. The randomized clinical trial (RCT) is one such strategy that can be adapted to the outcome review methodology in general and MCEs in particular. Beyond this, Bush,[10-11] Katz,[12] Ciarlo,[13] Brooks,[14] and Williamson[15] have demonstrated the feasibility of utilizing social function criteria for outcome evaluation. Unquestionably, further methodologic development will be required before adequate and appropriate social function measures can be applied routinely to systematic peer review, but the beginnings have been made, and the singular goal is more clearly visible. The overriding benefit of outcome information generated by the peer review mechanism is that it provides not only the feedback essential for advancing the care of individuals by discovering which mo-

dalities of care are optimal but also provides the feedback necessary for effecting secondary change in the overall delivery of services. That is the real challenge before peer review, and it must also be the measure of the effectiveness of the review process itself. This brings us to the conceptual basis for mounting medical care evaluation studies, which is to determine whether this ultimate goal is being realized.

Medical care evaluation studies (MCEs)

Research is needed to develop, test, and refine medical care evaluation studies for the assessment of medical management and its impact on the patient's health or functional status. A proposed model (Fig. 7-13) could provide an operational mechanism of retrospective MCEs dealing with care processes and treatment modalities

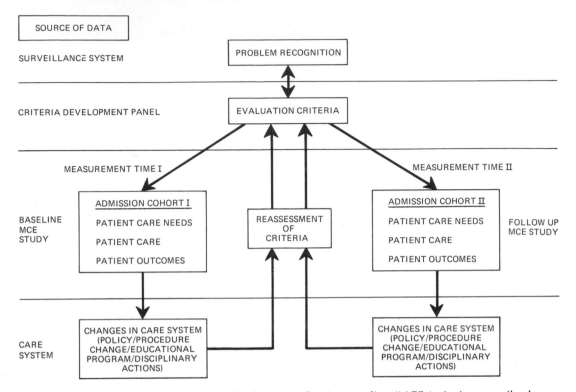

Fig. 7-13. Generic model for medical care evaluation studies (MCEs). A circumscribed clinical problem is studied in depth. Initial MCEs are usually based on an admission cohort of patients (cohort I) over a given time period, conventionally designated as measurement time I. If changes in care delivery are recommended as a result of the first study, new data are collected in a follow-up MCE (admission cohort II at measurement time II) to determine whether these changes have been implemented and what impact on care has been observed from the intervention strategies.

that would be useful to the refinement of criteria for admission, treatment, care transfer, discharge, and the follow-up of patients. This model suggests studying admission cohorts of patients both within and across hospitals.

These MCEs would attempt to answer questions relative to (1) the effectiveness and efficiency of different treatment modalities for a specific clinical problem, (2) whether a greater use of alternative services (extended care, home health, ambulatory care, and so on) provides a favorable outcome at a reduced rate of cost per episode of care, and (4) whether a greater sensitivity to planning posthospital care reduces readmissions. Provision of this type of design for periodic MCEs is the best way to obtain the answers to these kinds of

questions without encumbering routine surveillance activities to the extent that it loses cost justification.

Though most experts agree with the importance of such in-depth studies, few installations enjoy the financial backing necessary to make a serious effort to undertake many studies of great depth. This could change considerably if HEW can deliver on its proposition that a minimum 1% of annual budgets at all PSRO levels will be spent on evaluation.[16] Further, recent criticisms of the private health insurance industry regarding their alleged aloofness to require stricter surveillance of the medical care paid for by their policies has prompted the issuance of a position paper on the subject.[17] Member companies are now encouraged to provide start-up and operating costs for quality assurance programs. It has also been proposed that costs for quality assurance programs be separately calculated and financed through the hospital rate structure as a chargeable item. Thus from several sources the funding may soon be available to proceed with considerable review activity of this type, but one might question to what extent this is feasible.

Management audit program

Objective evaluation of the managerial performance of hospital administrators and other health care executives must not be overlooked because the review process would otherwise unjustly hold clinicians accountable for the impact of adverse administrative decisions on health care. The hospital industry must therefore eventually implement methods to determine how well its managers allocate financial, physical, and human resources to accomplish its objective of providing quality patient care at reasonable cost that is acceptable to the public, clinicians, the government, and other third party payors. A new viewpoint on the approach and mechanics of a management audit procedure is suggested by Gavin and Kessler.[18] The audit concept they suggest is intended to

1. Provide an effective evaluation tool for hospital management based primarily on hospital management outcomes
2. Provide a methodology for analyzing perceived problem areas
3. Lead to corrective action with accountability to the community through the governing body of the hospital
4. Satisfy likely future program reporting requirements for an audit of the management of hospitals participating in such government sponsored or financed programs
5. Act as a catalyst for planning the efficient allocations of community resources

It should be patently obvious by now that in concerning itself with medical peer review, this book is addressing a topic far wider than PSRO. It is recognized, however, that PSRO still occupies a focal point of interest, and so we will next place this form of review activity into organizational perspective.

Design strategies

Design concepts for hospital peer review systems are obligated first to reflect the priorities of the hospital and the priorities of those whose care is to be evaluated. If one of the established purposes of a hospital is to become delegated to conduct PSRO review, then the guidelines and objectives contained in Chapter 7 of the HEW *PSRO Program Manual*[19] becomes a part of the total institutional review obligation.

Preparing for the future

Although the focus of this discussion on peer review development has centered on the acute hospital care, one must not lose sight of the need for review of the other two important health care delivery components: namely, long-term and ambulatory care. A long-term commitment to develop the capacity for effective quality assurance for all patients may be realized over the next decade or so. Regardless of the organizational structure chosen to fulfill the leadership role in this development, the review process itself must include effective and continuing linkages between all major components of the health system. This is because cross-component review is critical to monitoring the delivery of quality comprehensive care to a patient over time as opposed to review strategies that monitor only the hospital component, which is but a cross-section that may not be representative of longitudinal care.

The point is that the developers or operators of existing systems may well wish to add long-term and ambulatory care components to the total review package at a later date and should therefore make allowances in their overall design for this eventuality.

IMPLEMENTING THE PEER REVIEW SYSTEM
Preparation

Peer review systems of the very best design can fail during the implementation phase if the wrong strategy or approach is followed in introducing it into the hospital environment where everything is of second priority to direct patient care. Gaining local PSRO approval of the program plan and negotiating for the options are necessary and meaningful, but they are also of secondary importance from the perspective of creating and maintaining a viable, effective, and efficient inhouse peer review program. A review program rejected by a majority of the staff cannot serve the purposes of the PSRO or any other purpose. Implementation prerequisites should therefore be of paramount concern to the hospital leadership. It is strongly recommended that implementation not be attempted until a thorough and successful preparation of both the review personnel and the clinical staff has been accomplished. Education and persuasion should be intensively used in this preparation effort; confrontation may to some extent be unavoidable, but coercion has little or no place among true peers. Under the best circumstances the sequence of staff acceptance moves from informed concession (often reluctantly given), through conversion and concensus, to cooperation. Once this level is achieved it must be continually reinforced by encouraging feedback from the clinical and administrative management to the care providers for the program to remain functional.

Caution in implementation should be the watchword from the outset. Following are some elements to be considered in a well-executed implementation program:[20]

1. A widely distributed (and read) executive order, directive, or an endorsement of the review undertaking by the hospital governing board.

2. A similar document of endorsement by the medical staff executive committee.

3. A formal commitment of assured continuing support by the hospital administration staff.

4. Written agreement by a substantial majority of the medical staff to permit an evaluation of their own patient care and a pledge of assistance in correcting obvious deficiencies.

5. Agreement by (a majority of) the medical staff to participate in the peer evaluation process and in the education program tied into it.

6. Favorable statements of support or approval by influential community organizations to establish credibility and enlist consumer participation and favorable media coverage if and when appropriate.

7. Approval by state medical societies.

8. Approval by medical specialty associations.

9. Review coordinators and physician advisors should be selected in a manner acceptable to the medical staff. The principal participants should be fully trained before commencing duties.

10. Review committee membership and leadership should be approved by appropriate peer bodies.

11. Nonphysician clinicians (dentists, podiatrists, psychologists, nurses, occupational therapists, physiotherapists, social workers, and so on) should be involved in developing review criteria for their own areas of care and actively engaged in its review as a part of the overall system.

12. A review of the program plan by the state hospital association, major insurance carriers, Medicare certification agency, and other accreditation agencies in addition to the PSRO can avert interface difficulties and prove helpful.

13. Legal assistance to the entire hospital staff regarding confidentiality and also assurance that no increased liability will befall those who consent to involvement in the review process.

14. Active participation from the initial planning and proposal preparation should include representatives of the medical staff, the governing authority, and ad-

ministrative staff. It must be remembered that implementation can only be achieved by a management team that is a working group and not an audience. Any advantage realized by broad representation and invited inputs of the uninterested or antagonistic are likely to be nominal and must be weighed against the possible disadvantages of opening sensitive negotiations to anyone who may complicate the difficult task of gaining staff acceptance, trust, and participation in the operational peer review program.

15. Major sources of anticipated resistance within and outside the hospital to the review process should be identified and a plan formulated to resolve problem areas.

Silent running

Following a thorough preparation of the environment in which the program must run, a period of silent running possibly might be preferable to launching directly into full-scale implementation. The rationale for this is to allow the review coordinators, physician advisors, practitioners, and others to become familiar with the peer review system logistics and associated data search requirements prior to full-scale implementation. If this is not accomplished, then a larger number of conspicuous errors that are virtually inevitable in any undertaking so complex as this could harass the care personnel and embarrass the review personnel. A positive benefit from a silent running period is reassurance for the clinical staff that effective peer review does not call for police state tactics.

Installation tasks

The installation of a peer review system into ongoing clinical operations of a hospital requires close coordination from top to bottom between the institutional governing board, medical staff, review team members, and key administrative staff. Critical installation tasks should have been previously identified during the planning stages. During the implemen-

tation stages a schedule with estimated time requirements will introduce each component in the right sequence for an ease of fit. This strategy will help avoid bottlenecks.

For the sake of discussion the installation tasks described below reflect a situation wherein the new review system is implemented in a hospital that did not participate in any earlier pilot program nor had previously conducted systematic review procedures. Furthermore, the use of a computerized review system will be assumed.

Administrative commitment. It becomes important to involve the professional and administrative leadership directly in the initiation and implementation of the system throughout the hospital. Their participation in the recruitment of the primary review team, for example, has met with success in a number of successful operations. Especially in the earlier stages, they can also provide valuable support to the primary review team as they encounter problems or pockets of resistance.

Implementation schedule. A schedule must be developed for implementing the system to assure the availability of resources when needed. A decision must first be made concerning the overall implementation strategy; that is, all at once or a phase-in schedule that establishes components one at a time. The phase-in schedule would require less personnel and resources dedicated to implementation at any one time, but of course it takes longer.

Staff preparation

The words *education, training, acceptance,* and *commitment* refer to crucial issues important in establishing an environment for the review program. Feelings generated within that environment can in great part determine the level of success that will be achieved by the review system irrespective of its basic merit. Considering the complexity of peer review programs and the numerous individuals who will be directly or indirectly affected by their implementation, the perceived threat of making substantial changes in the conditions of medical practice is of a significant magnitude in most hospitals. It is therefore best to assume the worst light will be cast on everything that occurs during the implementation phase. The only way to minimize the inevitable hassle if anything goes wrong is to anticipate it and to train all involved personnel in advance to respond tactfully and appropriately to any potentially provocative situation that may (and will) arise. A sample schedule of installation tasks is shown in Fig. 7-14.

Executive briefing. Formal briefing sessions to orient the entire medical executive and hospital administrative staffs to the peer review system is the first crucial task of the education and training program. This preparatory activity should initially focus on a group process strategy for achieving consensus, acceptance, and participation in the peer review program from key staff members. Rather than lead off with an explanation of what the system is, it is better to explain why it is needed. Specific information about the nuts and bolts of the review system can be effectively presented only after key administrators and physicians have already indicated a willingness to accept the system in the first place. Hesitancy on their part can be an obstacle just as their overt opposition can. The communication of vague fears of the unknown can be worse than those disadvantages of review systems that are real.

Staff orientation. Development of the orientation program for the institutional staff requires identification of several elements needed to formulate the training curriculum: (1) Who is the target audi-

INSTALLATION TASKS	NO. DAYS	5	10	15	20	25	30	35	40	45	50	55	60
I. Meet with Key Management and give general orientation package	5												
II. Meet with all physicians in facility for general orientation process	5												
III. Train the Quality Review team	15												
IV. Clinical staff briefed on peer review system	5												
V. Institution education coordinator prepares in-service training for review staff	10												
VI. Train Review Coordinators	5												
VII. Train non-professional review personnel	5												
VIII. Silent Running Period	20												
IX. Physicians and quality review team members review silent running period	5												
X. Review silent running period with professional and clinical staff	5												

Fig. 7-14. Tentative schedule for education and training.

ence? (2) What are the objectives for training? (3) What is the projected time of training (date and duration)? (4) What are the expected learner outcomes (behavioral responses)? and (5) What is the availability of training personnel?

When developing any specific-purpose curriculum module, one must remember that for differing target audiences, virtually the same basic informational content will have to be oriented differently when presented to audiences with differing needs and concerns. How the review system impacts on the social service department, for example, may be quite different than how it impacts on physical therapy, and orientation programs must reflect these differences. Each department's (or person's) position, level of training, leadership qualities, openness to change, and job status within the hospital will affect the manner in which he accepts the peer review system. The same considerations should influence how personnel are oriented to the operations and impact of the review system. When planning curriculum modules for these diverse groups, one may find it helpful to include each department head in an advisory capacity. Task preparation for all hospital staff members who will interact with the system must be begun early so that acceptance of and knowledge about the system proceeds before or concurrently with its implementation and certainly not after. The development of integrated curriculum modules to accomplish this will be discussed later in this chapter.

Procedural changes and personnel turnovers can occur with astonishing speed, and both necessitate retraining efforts. For both the above reasons the overall training program should be viewed as a continuum rather than an episodic instructional encounter requiring no further attention.

Primary review team training program. The one thing that cannot be afforded during the period of implementation is an inappropriate act committed by review personnel out of their own ignorance of how the system really works. All members of the review team (physician advisors, review coordinators, record technicians, computer terminal operators) need sufficient training that they not only become competent in their own tasks, but are also oriented to review operations generally. This group will then become effective in assisting with the orientation and training of the remaining hospital staff on all levels. Such a training program might consist of the following:

1. A general background orientation to the peer review system that covers its history, basic concepts, structure, and how it contributes to better patient care is the first order of business. An understanding achieved at the outset that any responsive peer review system is by nature an ongoing developmental effort minimizes the fear (and the reality) of arbitrariness and of stifling rigidity.

2. Orientation to the specific functions and the role to be assumed by each member of the primary review team is next in order. This would involve a thorough explanation of the input (abstract) forms used, where to find the data on hospital source documents, and the purpose that underlies each major review function. This portion of the training program should be expected to consume about one work week for most relatively broad-scope review systems. Task-oriented training should be interspersed with reading materials pertaining to hospital goals and to interrelationships established between the hospital's peer review system and the PSRO.

3. A general understanding of computer operations (if used) is always helpful, but specific knowledge of programming is not generally necessary for review personnel. This phase of the training program should include a thorough explanation of what the computer does but not necessarily how it does it.

4. If it can be arranged, a segment of training for the primary review team might include working with or observing

a review team at work in a hospital that has already implemented the same (or similar) review system. This is more of a convenience than a necessity though, as there is no substitute for familiarization with internal review procedures, medical charts, physical layout, and operational logistics of one's own hospital.

Practical training. Following general procedural orientation, the primary review team needs to develop its own proficiency in operating the system through in-service training. This is best done through a simulation of all review procedures. This drill and practice (silent running) period prior to full implementation has generally proven to require 2 to 4 weeks, depending on the scope and complexity of the system. The entire program of orientation and drill and practice should be accomplished in a period of 4 to 8 weeks, depending on the scope of the review program.

Continuing education for the clinical staff

The final task for the educational management team is the development of a totally new review-based education and staff development program at the institutional level. This calls for the preparation of curricula for continuing education of hospital staff members that address specific areas of demonstrated need. Individuals as well as groups of personnel in the care system need the kind of educational resource that is responsive to their own areas of care inadequacies as revealed by performance data. Frequent and consistent care deficiencies, for example, should be converted into an educational needs index to define the specific kind of instruction required to upgrade the care practices of individuals and groups of care providers.

Elements of the educational program. The types of training components that must be planned can best be defined by specifying the target audiences and assessing the training objectives in terms of desired behavioral changes. The matrix generated by specifying who needs what kind of

training provides a rational basis for pinpointing expected learner outcomes, for projecting training time-lines, and for allocating training resources most effectively.

Curriculum development. As alluded to earlier, the introduction of a major change such as the introduction of a new peer review system (or the changes it brings) can be expected to be traumatic for the entire organization. Therefore it is critical that training focus on the principles of planned change theory. It follows then that there should be priorities for the development of educational modules. While attention to review process functions is initially the most important aspect of the educational program, emphasis can be expected to eventually shift toward review content functions as staff acceptance of systematic peer review develops. Therefore orientation and overview of peer review is the curriculum module that will be needed first. It is also the most frequently in demand to train new personnel who enter the care system and the review program. Specific training activities and expected learner outcomes may vary in respect to the level of sophistication across the various target audiences, but the instructional approach is essentially the same for all.

Following is a listing of items that should be specified in a curriculum development plan for all training modules:

1. Module focus
2. Target audience
3. Training objectives
4. Training activities/modes
5. Expected learner outcomes
6. Evaluation plan
7. Project time-line
8. Resources needed (personnel and equipment)

Preparation of curriculum modules. Training modules should be prepared for at least six major learner groups: (1) hospital administration, (2) medical staff, (3) clinical and support staff, (4) the primary review team, (5) external liaison agents of third parties including the PSRO, and (6) patients and consumers.

The specific training needs of all these groups consists of some mix of the following components: (1) orientation and overview, (2) detailed review of the system's impact, (3) on-site training (for only those directly responsible for implementing the peer review system), (4) continuing education modules (which can only be developed after the system has been used), and (5) the nature and content of provider profiles and educational needs indices.

Summary of primary education and training tasks. Following is a summary of the tasks required of those responsible for training and education:

1. Gaining acceptance and participation from the executive medical staff and administration staff prior to implementation
2. Arranging for procedural and practical training of the primary review team
3. Developing in-service curriculum modules to train all hospital staff who interface in any way with the peer review team
4. Developing curriculum modules for continuing education of individuals as well as for groups of care providers based on demonstrated need (as evidenced by care performance documented by the peer review system)

Operating and maintaining the system

The next step is to operate the system, and the final step is to monitor its performance. The complexity of operating a comprehensive review system merits a full discussion, and the next chapter is devoted entirely to this subject, so we will now discuss how the peer review system can be evaluated, as this must be an integral part of structure of the review system itself.

EVALUATING THE PEER REVIEW SYSTEM
Conceptual base

The same triad of structure, process, and outcome applies to the evaluation of peer review systems just as it does in the evaluation of care systems. In the context of assessing peer review, *structure evaluation* refers to the compatibility of the system with the hospital environment, appropriateness of criteria, the organization and duties of review personnel and committees, qualification of the review staff, the adequacy of the training of review personnel, review procedures manual (rules and regulations), and the availability of resources for the monitoring system. *Process evaluation* includes the efficiency and effectiveness of the review personnel and other participants in accomplishing the tasks required of the review system. It embraces the conduct of all functions and activities pertaining to the nine major review components described on pp. 155 to 157. *Outcome or impact evaluation* measures the changes in behavior of clinicians and in the conduct of patient care brought about by implementation of the review system. An example of an impact question is, Did the system result in reduction in inappropriate admissions, length of stay, and care deficiency reports? Cost, patient satisfaction, improvement in a patient's functional status, and user acceptance are other examples of outcome measures.

Evaluation plan

It should be understood from the outset that there is no one best way to evaluate all review systems, and the approaches discussed here serve as points of departure rather than as representations of preferred methods. Evaluating the performance of a review system begins with development of a plan for data collection, processing, and analysis (as does the evaluation of a care system). A written plan serves not only as a general blueprint and reference but also as an instrument to maximize cooperation between the management of a review system and those who would evaluate it. This is important because the evaluation process is continuous during the life cycle of the project, which requires that there be coordination of assessment activities over time. There are four distinct periods in the development

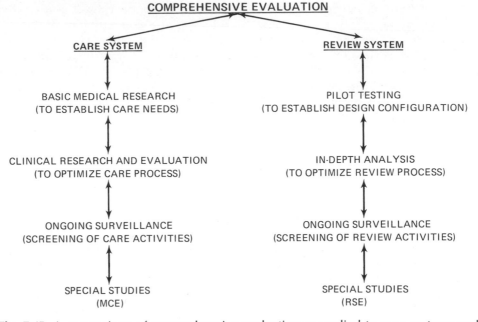

Fig. 7-15. A comparison of comprehensive evaluation as applied to care systems and to review systems.

and operation of peer review systems when evaluations of a given type are especially warranted and strongly recommended: (1) testing of the pilot system, (2) initial in-depth analysis of the review system soon after it becomes operational, (3) routine surveillance or monitoring of ongoing review activities, and (4) special studies. A comprehensive evaluation plan would include each type of assessment.

At this point it would be good to pause and consider all that comes under the term "comprehensive evaluation." As Fig. 7-15 illustrates, there is a very real parallel between what is involved in evaluating a review system and what is involved in evaluation of a care system. There are interesting differences, too, and these will be discussed briefly on pp. 187 to 192.

It is generally assumed in most discussions of peer review that a full complement of laboratory or clinical research stands behind new medical procedures or treatments before they are introduced into the care system. This is probably more true for procedures being introduced today than before, but many commonly used

contemporary practices were introduced years ago and have not been critically evaluated. While the scientific validation of medical care practices for the most part falls outside the scope of peer review, documenting what studies are needed may be its greatest contribution in the long run.

The kind of evaluation methodology devised for the ongoing surveillance (that is, the routine screening) of health care makes up the bulk of most descriptions of peer review systems. This is not to be confused with medical care evaluation studies. It is becoming increasingly clear that the proper role of MCEs[21] is to undertake the in-depth analysis of specific facets of care delivery that are more appropriate to periodic studies, cohort comparisons, surveys, or that in general require study methods impractical for routine surveillance activities. Ideally, MCEs would address specific problem areas that routine surveillance data indicate would likely be worthy of further investigation.

The two-headed arrows that link all the different types of evaluation in Fig. 7-15 signify that in a systematic approach, information feedback occurs not only between the review components but also between the care system and the review system. Properly utilized, this sharing of feedback can direct second order changes in both systems to the benefit of each.

Evaluation of the review system. Proper advance consideration in the planning of a peer review project can open two opportunities for evaluation of the review process that typically do not present themselves in the care process. The first of such opportunities arises during the trial period (pilot testing) while it is still in the design phase, and the second comes early in the course of operating the fully developed review system. Evaluation in the pilot test phase has already been discussed, and so it is the initial (in-depth) analysis of the operating system that will be discussed here.

Before doing so, however, it should be pointed out that the parallel between the evaluation of a review system and the evaluation of a care system includes the need to mount special studies in addition to the ongoing or routine monitoring of review activities needed primarily for management purposes.

Review system evaluation (RSE) studies are similar in nature to MCEs in that they are usually narrow in focus yet exhaustive in the depth of their analysis. Their purpose simply is to promote the effective and efficient use of the review system resources. They should solve specific problems in the ongoing surveillance of the operating review system. Plans for an indepth evaluation of an operating peer review system therefore must include plans for accessing and analyzing standard data items that describe the conduct of on-

Table 7-4. Evaluation of major review activities*

Clinical staff activities	Administrative activities	Review personnel activities
Minutes of Peer Review Committee	Hospital memorandum of understanding	Review of data on abstract worksheets and corresponding medical records
UR Subcommittee	Requirements for PSRO (review of completed delegation eligibility)	Coordination between review system, medical records, nursing departments, etc.
Medical Audit Subcommittee		
Medical/surgical staff committees	Information flow	
Actions of standing review subcommittees (reconsiderations, denials, sanctions)	Internal: among clinical, administrative, and review units	Clarification/concerns re: Hospital review/UR plan
		Discharge/transfer planning
Completed MCEs	External: between hospital and payors or regulatory agencies	Review coordinator
(criteria used, study design, recommendations, staff action, follow-up)		Workload
	Confidentiality policy and mechanism to ensure same	Meetings with PA/peer reviewers
Continuing education		Reconsiderations
(learning method, attendance, follow-up)	Data reports: forms of output, profile generation	Judgment decisions
Concurrent review	Administrative (nonclinician) review activities	Case reviews (percent referred to PA and to higher review levels, forms used, denials)
Extent of staff physician involvement in:	Admission/continued stay	
Admission certification	Denial notification mechanism, etc.	
Continued stay review		Professional interface activities
Development of care criteria	Clarification/concerns re: hospital review/UR plan	Completed RSEs (special studies of review system operations and impact)
Clarification/concerns re:		
Hospital review/UR plan	Hospital review costs and reimbursement	
Training of peer (e.g., physician) reviewers	Training for review personnel	

*Adapted from a presentation by Dr. Roy Miller at Physician Advisors Workshop, Ohio Peer Review Region X, Columbus, Ohio, August 1976.

going review activities and also of special data periodically captured during the course of conducting RSEs.

The overall evaluation plan presented here is organized around five areas of focus: (1) an evaluation of the major activities of key personnel, (2) an evaluation of explicit criteria (their development and performance), (3) an evaluation of the system design and its operations, (4) an evaluation of the efficiency and effectiveness of the information processing system, and (5) an evaluation of the impact (outcomes) of the review system.

Evaluation of major review activities

The approach to the initial evaluation of an operational peer review system is shown in outline form in Table 7-4. This summary illustrates a number of items that should be evaluated with respect to the major review activities to be conducted by key personnel such as the clinical staff, administrative staff, and review system personnel. This may require that a comprehensive questionnaire be devised to acquire in a valid and uniform manner the data elements suggested in Table 7-4.

Evaluation of criteria

Since explicit care criteria comprise the central component that triggers the entire sequence of the review system, a great deal of the evaluation effort should focus on them. Primary emphasis is on their appropriateness as measures of resource utilization and quality care delivery in the particular care setting. Secondary emphasis will likely be placed on the analysis of data pertaining to the validity and reliability of criteria to the extent that this can be scientifically established. The third concern is the comprehensiveness of the criteria (see following outline).

EVALUATION OF CRITERIA

A. Appropriateness
  1. Capability to discriminate appropriate from inappropriate care
  2. Impact of use in surveillance activities (influence on care)
  3. Compatibility with universal (e.g., national) standards of care
  4. Compatibility with unique care needs of individual patients
B. Validity and reliability of measurements
  1. Consistency in operational definitions for criteria items
  2. Appropriateness of criteria selection (for case evaluation)
  3. Accuracy of diagnosis coding and data entries
C. Comprehensiveness of content
  1. Admission and continued stay review
  2. Clinical intervention (health maintenance, medical or surgical, treatments, rehabilitation, patient education, etc.)
  3. Facilitation of discharge/transfer planning
  4. Capability to assess the adequacy of care follow-up

Appropriateness. To determine how appropriately the criteria measure care, it will be necessary to consider (1) content (problem definition), (2) development process (how and by whom), (3) statistical performance, and (4) outcome validation (clinical impact).

One of the leading questions to be answered regarding quality is whether the criteria generate enough variance among patients to discriminate good care from bad. A leading question regarding utilization is whether the expected duration of a hospital stay for a given condition under consideration is uniform enough (that is, is reasonably clustered) so that excessively long or short stays can be revealed statistically.

Data from the routine surveillance of a reasonable sample of patients should be analyzed first to provide preliminary (general) answers to questions of this kind. If problem areas are uncovered that would seem to be worth pursuing, then a full MCE study could be launched to obtain definitive answers. Such studies should constitute an unbiased review of an appropriate number of criteria to determine their sensitivity and specificity. All such study sequences proceed best if planned in advance to take maximal advantage of clinical data routinely captured in the process of care delivery.

MCE study procedures in general should begin where routine monitoring or surveillance procedures leave off, that is, should build on and expand the scope of the ongoing surveillance program. These evaluation procedures in general should be geared to deal with specific problems and to shift the focus away from the traditional chart review techniques toward a more systematic and objectively valid review for discerning patterns of care. Since MCE studies typically make comparisons of actual practices with preset criteria, they follow a strategy that differs from routine surveillance procedures more quantitatively than qualitatively. This difference can be found largely in the depth of detail of the review process employed, the degree to which clinical contingencies in the care process are studied, and the specificity of the study topics addressed by MCEs.

Studies that address the validity of deficiency reports should be undertaken when an excessive number of exceptions are reported to apparently otherwise valid criteria. A random sample of cases, which generated exception reports that initially were judged to be valid by the primary review team but later were not confirmed (or acted on) by the peer review committee, should be counted as false-positives. Conversely, selected cases in an adequate random sample that had not generated any exceptions should be reviewed by the same study group. Those cases found to actually represent inappropriate care (or require some corrective action) that had not been recognized by the routine surveillance system (that is, primary review team) should be counted as false-negatives. Excessive data trends in either direction should then trigger in-depth RSEs of the criteria.

Theoretically there is no limit to the number of conceivable circumstances or combinations of feasible conditions that could be construed as justifying admission to a hospital for any given diagnosis. But if criteria are permitted to become so all-encompassing, they lose their value as admission screening devices. This is but one example how excessive inclusiveness in the scope and content of criteria or in the flexibility of their format and structure can be overdone, with the result that they lose their power to discriminate and fail to have any impact on care practices. That is why false-negatives should be evaluated carefully.

Another of the issues confronting criteria development is: should criteria primarily reflect normative standards derived from professional goals (that is, expert opinions concerning what is optimal care) or empiric standards (based on statistical norms that reflect current practices)? The working approach taken by most criteria development efforts has focused on normative, professionally derived (consensus or universal) standards thought to be representative of ideal care (as exemplified by criteria that have been prepared by specialty societies and of course the AMA criteria discussed in Chapter 11). These typically serve as the models that local peer groups modify or adapt to reflect the conditions of practice in the community and that peer reviewers use as general guidelines in judging the appropriateness of care rendered to patients.

Validity and reliability of measurements. A critical issue that cuts across the entire review process is whether operational definitions used to guide review personnel in the conduct of review activities accurately reflect the content and intent of the original criteria. In other words, are review activities related conceptually to what is meant in the language of the criteria? Some criteria require explicit operational definitions of terms and concrete statements of review objectives to direct the search for relevant information from the hospital chart, for example. Thus attention should be paid to data that are indicative of the validity of interpretations based on these operational definitions. If the criteria for which formal operational definitions are required perform worse than do other criteria that require no such definitions, this would be indicated by a greater number of invalid exception reports.

Another question deserving of attention is whether diagnoses are uniformly abstracted from the clinical records and correctly coded. This question is closely related to the review process and therefore will be discussed together with reliability surveillance.

Built-in reliability experiments can be conducted periodically to provide data on the reliability of admission diagnoses, the appropriate selection of admission criteria, and the application of criteria for screening the quality of medical services.

Comprehensiveness of content. The completeness of a criteria set would be defined by whether it includes all the items necessary to achieve the purpose of the review effort. If the objective is to eliminate unnecessary hospital admissions, then it must contain reasonable indicators of which admissions are typically appropriate and which are not. The same principle holds for the inclusion of items that assess the quality of care if that is also an objective of the review system. Practical considerations that dictate how detailed or how extensive the criteria should be are defined by what is achievable (or affordable) in the given hospital. There is no point in insisting that certain types of tumors should receive cobalt therapy, for example, if no cobalt unit exists at the institution.

The content of comprehensive criteria should specify the scope of services that are clearly indicated or are unchallengeable from both a quality and utilization viewpoint and, in so doing, define those services that are not. Sufficient direction should also be provided to define the clinical circumstances (acuteness or severity of illness, complications, and so on) under which criteria items pertain, so that neither inappropriate deviations from the criteria (false-positives) are reported nor too many care deficiencies go undetected (false-negatives). The outline on p. 156 lists the four major content areas in which the above principles apply.

Evaluation of system design and operations (review process)

A comprehensive peer review system should be evaluated as an integrated whole rather than as an agglutination of separate parts (such as an information system plus a utilization review process plus a medical audit process, and so on). This holistic perspective calls for evaluating the operational adaptability of the review system within the hospital (that is, its ability to adjust to operating conditions) and the organization and structure of the review process. This prescribes two main tasks as illustrated in the following outline: (1) review of the hospital environment in which the review system functions and (2) review of the organization and methods of the review system. (NOTE: the peer review management information system is technically a part of this environment but for clarity will be discussed separately.)

SYSTEM DESIGN AND OPERATIONS (PROCESS)

A. System environment
  1. Compatibility with hospital environment (management policies and procedures)
  2. Records management (data base)
B. Review methods and organization
  1. Data collection and input procedures/on-site review activities
  2. Data output utilization/interface with review levels
  3. Thoroughness/adequacy of personnel training
  4. Direction and control of review system/personnel
  5. Efficiency and effectiveness of review system

System environment. Any peer review system must be compatible with the environment it monitors. The hospital environment is typically a labor-intensive organization with a division of labor that is characteristically extreme, requiring that highly specialized and independently functioning units coordinate their activities to provide quality patient care. The peer review organization is similarly labor intensive and dependent on specialized personnel including physicians and other health practitioners working in independently functioning units that require a high degree of coordination. Peer review is also subject to federal, state, and local rules and regulations and to the demands of third parties who pay the bill for their effort. The care monitoring system must be sensitive to all these requirements and yet work within these constraints with the independence that objectivity requires.

Hospital staff review committees and subcommittees make up a critical part of this environment. The interface of the peer review information system with these bodies should be scrutinized to determine how effectively they help or hinder the review process when relevant matters come under their purview. If, for example, there are problems in gaining access to clinical data on medical records needed for the review process or there are excessive errors in such data, this should be documented and referred to standing hospital committees that have the authority to rectify the situation. What is pertinent to monitor is whether the existing machinery that is responsible to act on matters of importance to review activities does so promptly and appropriately. Another issue is whether standard clinical data recording procedures are streamlined sufficiently to allow necessary documentation within the time frames demanded by efficient peer review operations and automation. The effectiveness and promptness of responsible hospital authorities and mechanisms in bringing about needed changes of this kind should be closely monitored, especially in the beginning of operations.

Review methods and organization. In evaluating on-site review activities, some of the more relevant observations include accuracy in the collection of data from the chart and in preparing the input documents, the appropriate utilization of criteria and reports generated by the information system, and the appropriate use of output.

The control of review activities and the direction given personnel can be evaluated by tracing the flow of data and case referrals through prescribed channels and sequences, and by the degree of compliance with stated procedural guidelines.

Efficiency in a review system can be revealed through a number of determinations: whether there is a proper personnel mix, whether an added burden to care delivery is exerted by data collection for review purposes, any duplication in data collection or review functions and activities, and unwarranted delays in completing any step in the review process. Its effectiveness, on the other hand, is observable by determining whether detected care deficiencies are promptly acted on and whether corrective actions are initiated that eliminate inappropriate care practices or remedy any negative consequences that might have already occurred. Effectiveness can also be manifested in the care system by improved diagnostic accuracy and specificity and in similar adjustments to review system impacts.

Once peer review data become available, the question is raised whether reports are used and acted on. It should therefore be determined whether physician profiles and other statistical data are read, evaluated, and taken into consideration when judgments are rendered concerning the appropriateness of care rendered by individual practitioners. It should also be determined whether the form and content of such reports facilitate the sequential conduct of review activities at all levels of authority.

The adequacy of the training of review personnel can be revealed through the error rates they generate as a result of the inappropriate selection of criteria sets, incorrect interpretations, improper data recording (the transposing of input data), and imprecise interpretations of output statistics and reports.

The above list of suggestions is obviously

far from exhaustive but should suffice as examples of the range of important topics appropriate for special RSEs. The presence of problems of this kind should be detectable by evaluating routine surveillance data that is readily available. All it really takes is the imagination to capitalize on using standard data in this fashion.

Efficiency and effectiveness of information processing system

An evaluation of the data-handling system can be undertaken independent of efforts to evaluate the functioning of the rest of the review process. However done, a complete evaluation of a computer-based information system should interrogate the documentation of its design configuration, user requirements, and operational efficiency.

The first step in answering such questions is to conduct a review of existing documentation. This review has three purposes: (1) to aid in gaining familiarity with the functions the data system is required to perform; (2) a comparison with what functions the system actually does perform; and (3) to determine if the system conforms to established operational standards. The review of documentation should include the following areas at a minimum: statements of scope and objectives, operational definitions, input and output specifications, data-base definitions, and file capacity and content.

Completion of the documentation review should provide a framework for making comparisons of user requirements against the performance criteria by which the system should be judged. Proposals for testing preliminary conclusions through operational analysis are part of the approach to evaluating the information processing system.

The second step in examining the data system includes a survey of user requirements. This generally requires personal contacts to determine whether users feel that system meets internal objectives. The user's feelings, attitudes, and dissatisfac-

tions (real and imagined, justified or not) are to be given equal consideration with objective data on system performance. A user's survey might address four broad categories: those relating to the usage environment, to client objectives, design specifications, and system implementation.

The third step is to assess any environmental instabilities that might alter user requirements. These might include actual changes in patient management practices, changes in managerial policies, shifts in personnel and other organizational factors, or shifts in external review requirements and specifications. Questions about the relevancy of the user's stated review objectives and the demands made on the system pertain to the attainability of these goals, their stability over time, and the appropriateness of performance criteria by which the user judges for himself whether his objectives are being met.

The fourth step consists of evaluating conformity to established operational standards. This refers to an assessment of the operational efficiency of the installed and working system. An evaluation of this type concentrates on the actual mechanical operations of the data system (as opposed to whether the system has achieved formal design objectives as described above).

The evaluation of operational efficiency should examine (at a minimum) the following parameters for each of its major operational processes:

1. Timeliness
2. Manpower requirements
3. Information quality
4. Controls
5. System structure
6. Equipment utilization

Each of the above parameters in turn should be evaluated from two points of view: the functional or user (external) point of view (that is, how well does the system service user requirements) and the data processing (internal) point of view (that is, how can the system be improved or made more efficient?). Specific questions to be considered for each of the

Table 7-5. Evaluation of data processing operational efficiency*

Operational parameter	Functional (user)	Data processing

1.0 Timing	1.1 Timeliness of results
	    Input delivered on time?
	    Turnaround time satisfactory?
		1.2 Schedules
		    Are they established?
		    Are they met?

2.0 Manpower	2.1 Is interface with DP satisfactory?
	2.2 Is the right level of technical assistance available when needed?
		2.3 Quantity
		    Are there enough (too many)?
		2.4 Ability
		    Education level and background
		    Performance measures (job return rate)
		2.5 Functional distribution of tasks
		    Does everyone have meaningful jobs that contribute to operational efficiency?
		2.6 Turnover
		    Too much or too little?

3.0 Information quality	3.1 File accuracy
	    Are there checks on this?
	3.2 Result accuracy and completeness
	3.3 Quantity of reports
	    Is volume of data delivered too much to read?
		3.3 Input error rate
		    Is it high?
		    What causes?
		3.4 Data security
		    Are data or reports being lost?
		    Is confidentiality of sensitive data protected?
		3.5 File security
		    Backups?
		    Ability to reconstruct?
		    Safekeeping of file copies?

4.0 Controls	4.1 User log
	    Does user keep track of jobs to be run?
	    What action taken when results not returned?
	4.2 Manual reconciliation
	    Does user make manual trial balances to check reasonableness of results?
		4.3 Computer files
		    Does computer run check totals?
		    Are there checks for reasonableness and lost data?
		4.4 Data transmission
		4.5 Contingency plan
		    Is there a plan to operate the system if computing facility were lost for extended period of time?

5.0 System structure	5.1 Are reports satisfactory?
	    Quantity
	    Content
	    Format
	5.2 How does user pay for service?
	    By report?
	    By time/resources used to produce report?
		5.3 Program design
		5.4 Is there any form of built-in performance monitors?
		5.5 Are there test programs plus test outputs?

6.0 Equipment utilization		6.1 Is hardware adequate?
		    More/different peripherals?
		6.2 Is hardware used efficiently?
		6.3 System load
		    Hours per day?
		6.4 Backup
		    What happens when machine goes down?

*From Black, G. C., Miller, R. R., Mougey, B., O'Dell, A., and Connell, K.: Implementation manual: peer review system for public mental hospitals, Columbus, Ohio, October 31, 1974, Ohio Dept. of Mental Health and Mental Retardation, p. 7-34.

operational parameters listed above are cited in Table 7-5.

Evaluation of review system impact (outcomes)

If demonstrable improvement in the actual clinical status of patients is the most important achievement of the care system, then it follows that clinical outcome assessment constitutes, as some suggest,[15] the most powerful and all-encompassing approach to the evaluation of that care. (The rising costs of care have assumed a significance that also is too great to ignore.) There is a close parallel to be drawn in assessing the impact of peer review on the care system. The only difference lies in the fact that a review system has its direct impact on care providers and the process of delivering care, whereas its impact on patients is only indirect. It is no less important to determine what costs are associated with peer review, and it is this aspect of impact evaluation that will be described first. Some suggested variables to include in evaluating impact/outcome are shown in the outline below.

EVALUATION OF REVIEW SYSTEM IMPACT (OUTCOMES)

A. Costs
　1. Cost of review system (developmental vs. operational)
　2. Impact of review system on costs of care
B. Impact on care providers and care process
　1. Staff acceptance
　　a. By those involved in peer review
　　b. By medical staff
　　c. By other staff
　2. Feedback
　　a. Education
　　b. Discipline
　　c. Changes in care standards (care criteria)
　　d. Changes in review standards (review criteria)
C. Impact on patients' (clinical) outcomes

Cost. Cost assessment has a dual thrust. The first component focuses on adding up the costs of developing, implementing, and operating the review system. The second focuses on analyzing the impact of the review system on the costs of delivering medical care (as calculated per admission or per patient day).

Definitive cost figures based on actual review operations should include the flat cost rate per admission for expenses incurred by the facility (salaries, equipment, overhead), automated data processing, and some method for amortizing start-up costs incurred by the facility (for example, in the effort to establish system specifications, initiate pilot operations, conduct staff orientation, and so on).

Development of a plan for an evaluation of the long-range impact of the review process on the cost of patient care must begin with setting specifications for essential or minimum (baseline) data requirements. For example, trends in the cost of care at that institution prior to implementing the review system should be determined and then compared with trends after its implementation, and perhaps even better, compared also to costs in like hospitals that have no comparable review system.

Evaluation of impact on care providers and care processes. The short-run and the long-run impacts (other than cost) of the peer review system on the care system fall under three headings: user acceptance, useful feedback to the patient care process, and positive contributions to the clinical outcomes of care. Again, it is essential to specify the kind of data elements and data collection procedures needed for an overall evaluation of the clinical impact of a peer review system.

A relevant impact assessment might be drawn from *objective data,* reflecting the care delivered to a control group of patients admitted or discharged from the hospital prior to implementation of the review system as compared to that received by a cohort of patients managed under full surveillance of the review system. *Subjective impacts* may be comparatively assessed by interviewing
　1. The primary review team

2. Members of the hospital peer review committees or its subcommittees
3. Random samples of physicians who practice in the test facility
4. Samples of patients admitted to the test facilities during the specified study period

Evaluating the level of understanding and acceptance of the review system by the medical staff will be more revealing if conducted in parallel with a like study among the peer review personnel. The collection of data from both clinical and review personnel would most reasonably be accomplished by a questionnaire supplemented by in-depth interviews.

Any good peer review system would be designed to have minimum visibility for the clinical staff of a hospital (that is, minimal interference in routine activities) while having a substantial long-range impact on their patient care practices. Essentially the goal of evaluating the impact of the review system on the care system is to see that this is true. If peer review is to have significant positive impact on standards of care delivery through a more relevant education of the medical staff, through peer discipline where necessary, and through upgraded standards for care, then these are the outcomes that must be documented. Making these kinds of observations, especially in an interactive system, is both a short-range and a long-range process.

Obtaining the impressions of review personnel in regard to these observations is based on the hypothesis that their assessments will reflect aspects of the system's environment that are most clearly affected in the short run. These would include such things as improvements in patient management procedures, in admission procedures, in diagnostic and treatment services, and the like.

The impacts of peer review are dynamic, since both the care process and the review process are constantly undergoing change as directed by feedback. Therefore long-term observations are essential to determine trends over time.

Thus this discussion ends much as it began—with a reminder that systematic peer review is a dynamic continuum; yet, unavoidably, any discussion in the printed medium is static, while the evaluation activities discussed above ideally will undergo change as a result of the findings they uncover.

Impact on patients (clinical outcomes). Longer term follow-up evaluations are generally also needed to detect improvements in patient (clinical) outcomes in terms of shortened hospital stays, reduced durations of morbidity, and the enhancement of patients' social functioning and occupational capabilities. To perform evaluations of this kind requires long-term follow-ups and calls for a commitment to continuing data collection beyond the hospital period.

Obviously the real payoff of feedback of this kind is that it will have the positive effect of encouraging the greater use of care practices that create improvements in patient care and the abandonment of those alternatives that do not.

SUMMARY

This chapter addresses organizational issues in planning, designing, implementing, testing, and evaluating a peer review system. It also explores the functions of project organization for managing the effort to develop a peer review system.

Some thoughts are offered on how to structure and manage the peer review system once it is operational. Further, the chapter contains methodologic suggestions for evaluating the review system itself; that is, an approach to assessing the performance and cost of the evaluation technology that aims at improving the effectiveness and efficiency of care delivery and maximizing health benefits to patients.

Hopefully some insight has been provided into the integrated planning, organization, and conduct of systematic review activities that have thus far not been fully developed or conceptually integrated in the literature on medical peer review. This chapter makes explicit the theoretic basis for those organizational processes essential for successfully operationalizing systematic peer review.

REFERENCES

1. Bennis, W. G., Benne, K. D., and Chin, R.: The planning of change, New York, 1961, Holt, Rinehart and Winston, p. 33.
2. American Hospital Association: Quality assurance program manual, Chicago, 1972, The Association, sect. 6, p. 1.
3. Forward plan, publ. no. FY1977-1982, Washington, D.C., June 1975, U.S. Dept. of Health, Education, and Welfare, p. 142.
4. Miller, R. R.: Peer review systems: applications in mental health services, Paper presented at the National Association of State Mental Health Directors PSRO Workshop, Boston, March 2-3, 1976, p. 5.
5. American Association of Foundations of Medical Care: Key issues in PSRO data support (working paper).
6. Connell, K., and Black, G. C.: Patient outcome project: utilization and medical care assessment plan for public mental hospitals, Columbus, Ohio, 1974, Ohio Department of Mental Health and Mental Retardation, Division of Mental Health, p. 4.
7. Miller, R. R., Black, G. C., Ertel, P. Y., and Ogram, G. F.: Psychiatric peer review: the Ohio system, Am. J. Psychiatry, December 1974, pp. 1367-1370.
8. Black, G. C., Miller, R. R., Mougey, B., O'Dell, A., and Connell, K.: Implementation manual: peer review system for public mental hospitals, Columbus, Ohio, October 31, 1974, Ohio Dept. of Mental Health and Mental Retardation, pp. 7-9 through 7-14, para. 7.6.6, and p. 7-34.
9. Clausen, G. T.: Some problems of design and inference in studies of community tenure, J. Nerv. Ment. Dis. **155**(1):22-35, 1972.
10. Bush, J. W.: Health index project, La Jolla, Calif., University of California at San Diego, Department of Community Medicine Health Index Project.
11. Bush, J. W., Franshel, S., and Chen, M. M.: Analysis of a tuberculin testing program using a health status index, Socio Econ. Plan. Sci. **6**:49-68, 1972.
12. Katz, M. M., and Lyerly, S. B.: Methods for measuring adjustment and social behavior in the community. I. Rationale, description, discriminative validity and scale development, Psychol. Rep. **13**:503-535, 1963.
13. Ciarlo, J. A., Lin, S., Bigelow, D., and Biggerstaff, M.: A multi-dimensional outcome measure for evaluating community mental health programs, NIMH research grant no. 5Ro1MH20954, Denver, University of Denver and Denver General Hospital Mental Health Center.
14. Brooks, R. H.: Quality of care assessment: a comparison of five methods of peer review, publ. no. HRA-74-3100, Washington, D.C., 1973, National Center for Health Services Research and Development, Public Health Service, U.S. Dept. of Health, Education, and Welfare.
15. Williamson, J. W.: Outcome assessment for implementing quality assurance systems; quality assurance in medical care: a monograph, publ. no. HSM-73-7021, Washington, D.C., February 1973, Regional Medical Programs Service, Health Services and Mental Health Administration, U.S. Dept. of Health, Education, and Welfare.
16. Public law 94-63, sect. 205(a), (4), p. 18.
17. Goodwin, J.: Quality health care programs—development, financing and evaluation—a private sector view, Paper presented at MAI/PSRO symposium, Columbus, Ohio, November 24, 1975.
18. Gavin, M. P., and Kessler, P. R.: The development of a management audit program for hospitals, Hosp. Health Serv. Admin. **20**(4):21, 1975.
19. Office of Professional Standards Review, U.S. Dept. of Health, Education, and Welfare: PSRO program manual, Washington, D.C., March 1974, U.S. Government Printing Office.
20. Black, G. C.: Ohio's computer-assisted psychiatric peer review system, Paper presented at annual meeting of American Psychiatric Association, Anaheim, Calif., May 1975.
21. Goran, M. J., Roberts, J. S., Kellogg, M. A., Fielding, J., and Jessee, W.: The PSRO hospital review system, Med. Care **13**(suppl. 4):15, 75, 1975.

8

An operational model of systematic peer review

PAUL Y. ERTEL
GORDON C. BLACK

INTRODUCTION

Planning eventually evolves into doing, and it is then when theory gives way to practice and good intentions must be tempered by what is achievable. The output of the developmental sequence described in Chapter 7 is the achievement of a peer review system capable of sustained operation within the hospital. But this is not to say that there is a sharp cleavage between the planning and developmental stages and the operational stage. Rather the latter is really a starting point in yet another revolution of the creative cycle that involves continuous evaluation and modification to effect continuous improvements in the system. This is often termed the **optimization** of operational efficiency and effectiveness.

From the above it should be clear that the central goal of all the organizational activities is not the development of **the ultimate** peer review system[1] but rather a functional one that has sufficient expandability and adaptability in its design that it can eventually be molded through continuous feedback and research[1] into the best achievable system for the operational setting in which it is placed. With that definition in mind, this chapter will explore those key features of peer review systems that contribute the most to these objectives. These are the features too important to overlook in planning a peer review system.

The following describes in almost outline form those major operational steps to be performed at various hierarchical levels in the functioning of a model systematic peer review system. This then is a discussion of peer review operations in the abstract and not an expression of methodologic preference.

Relationship of operations to other theoretic considerations

Since no preference will be presented here for any one review method over any other, we will offer no formulation of "dos" and "don'ts." In keeping with this posture, neither will any attempt be made to define each step in the review process to the level of detail that involves precise task descriptions. While recognizing the critical nature of all such considerations in real-world applications, the reader is referred to the Practice Part of this book where he can find illustrations of task descriptions in several of the chapters.

The common clinical thread

The first purpose of this discussion is to identify a conceptually unifying common thread that is woven through most operational peer review systems irrespective of their methodologic approach. That common strand, in our opinion, has its origin in the natural sequence of clinical events that begin at the time of a patient's admission to a hospital and typically proceed in an almost inexorable manner throughout the hospital stay until discharge. For the vast majority of hospitalizations (that is, for routine admissions) these events typically unfold in a uniform and often preplanned sequence,[2] and it is this sequence that shapes the operational concepts presented here.

Irrespective of the precise diagnoses involved, personal demographic and financial data are collected on each patient at the time of admission. This may have been preceded by the collection of clinical data from preadmission laboratory or other investigations that are standard procedures at many institutions. In any event the remaining elements of the clinical data base, which includes the routine medical history, physical exam, and basic laboratory profile, as recommended by the Joint Commission for Accreditation of Hospitals (JCAH),[3,pp.105-112] are normally obtained immediately after admission. All this typically precedes the initiation of special diagnostic or therapeutic services related to the specific condition that prompted the hospitalization in the first place. Further, the sequence of postadmission diagnostic investigations typically precede therapeutic interventions, and both are triggered by the natural history of the disease process. Thus for most patients clinical services are provided in a rather predictable cadence until discharge. Even discharge procedures themselves exhibit commonalities in the sequencing of aftercare planning, patient education, and billing procedures.

Because the provision of the great bulk of clinical services does follow the same general pattern in most cases, the generation of most care-related data (and its subsequent availability to care assessment reviewers) will also follow a predictable

pattern. It only makes sense to accommodate this sequential generation of essential data through the establishment of a logical sequence and pattern in operationalizing whatever peer review process is ultimately implemented. To do otherwise is to interfere with or unnecessarily complicate the care delivery system.

The process of conducting comprehensive* peer review thus segregates into an integrated sequence of discrete activity levels, which we referred to in the previous chapter as the four levels of peer review. Each level in the sequence should be staffed and organized to carry out an ascending hierarchy of responsibilities as suggested in Table 8-1. The review functions to be conducted at each of the four levels are described below in the context of their usual temporal sequence along with an indication of the types of personnel most likely to be involved at each step.

REVIEW LEVEL 1 (PRIMARY REVIEW)
Conceptual base

The step that initiates the entire review process typically consists of data acquisition for the purpose of screening out cases that have a high probability of deficient care for a more intensive subsequent review by a professional peer. Thus review level 1 typically consists of a screening phase and a judgmental phase, and the personnel involved in both phases must work together closely as a team.

Organizational structure of the primary review team

The primary review team is a term by which we designate the single functional unit organized and held responsible for conducting the primary (or initial) level of review.

---

*Comprehensive peer review, in the context that applies to the following discussion, is defined as that systematic review process which adequately performs at a minimum the seven functions cited by Aldridge in Chapter 4. See Glossary for a more formal definition of this term.

Table 8-1. The four levels of hospital-based peer review

Level 1	Primary review team			
Level 2	Utilization review subcommittee	Medical audit subcommittee	Evaluation subcommittee	Continuing education subcommittee
Level 3	Peer review committee	Medical staff	Administration staff	
Level 4	Hospital executive committee/board			
External	PSRO			

Activities of the primary review team can be generally divided into surveillance, information processing, data correction, and the usual peripheral (clerical) and supportive functions. Detailed descriptions of the activities of the primary review team may be found in several of the practice chapters, so it is the overview that will be discussed here and not the specifics. The flow diagram for level 1 (Fig. 8-1) provides a stepwise model of the major surveillance processes in their usual sequence and also identifies the personnel usually involved. Because most review strategies rely on an ongoing screening or surveillance procedure for initiating virtually all subsequent review transactions, the success of the entire system often depends on this team meeting its responsibilities.

For purposes of presenting the most inclusive scope of discussion, it will be assumed that a single interdisciplinary review team is to conduct both medical audit (quality assessment) and utilization review within an acute care hospital that utilizes a case abstract methodology and uses some type of computer-based data processing system. Those steps in which the team would be involved primarily with interactive computer systems will be described in italicized print.

Function of the review coordinator

The review coordinator is usually a full-time position often filled by a nurse, and it is this person who generally serves as the operations manager of the primary review team. Among the many functions and duties of this position, the selective abstracting of clinical data from medical charts is often the most critical, and this is listed as step 1 on the flow diagram. Additional duties include error surveillance and correction, detection of deviations from quality criteria, preparation of exception reports, maintaining liaison with the clinical staff, and assisting the physician advisor in his duties. The ongoing screening operations of level 1 review is typically the primary responsibility of the review coordinator.

Functions of medical records specialist

There are essentially two areas in which the functions of the review coordinator could be complemented by medical record specialists when warranted by case loads or by the type of review strategy employed. Providing assistance to all review levels in the preparation, use, and interpretation of aggregated data (profiles and retrospective statistical analyses) is one such area. Another is a direct involvement in the review process in a role of what is currently labeled "continuity of care review." Because the natural difference in clinical expertise of these personnel as compared with nurses coincides closely with systems distinctions between periodic and episodic (or aperiodic) surveillance encounters, the review coordinator should focus on periodic clinical assessments. This suggests that it may be expedient for a continuity of care reviewer to perform episodic monitoring activities such as

1. Certification of admission
2. Documentation of recorded progress notes
3. Documentation of recorded treatment/discharge plans

4. Confirmation of aftercare planning and so on

NOTE: Social service planning and follow through and the monitoring of patients' rights would also be appropriate aspects of care to review in a mental hospital and similar settings. Obviously a social worker

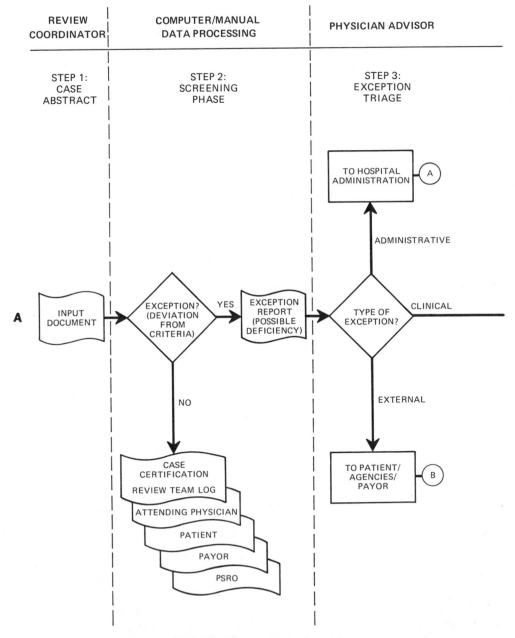

Fig. 8-1. Flow diagram: level 1.

may be the most appropriate person to do this.

Functions of the clerk-typist

The primary review team's informational needs and data-handling requirements typically involve a large number of daily data-handling transactions in most hospitals of any size. These and the majority of the associated clerical tasks can and probably should be performed by a clerk-typist who would work under the direct supervision of the review coordinator. Typical tasks may include as-

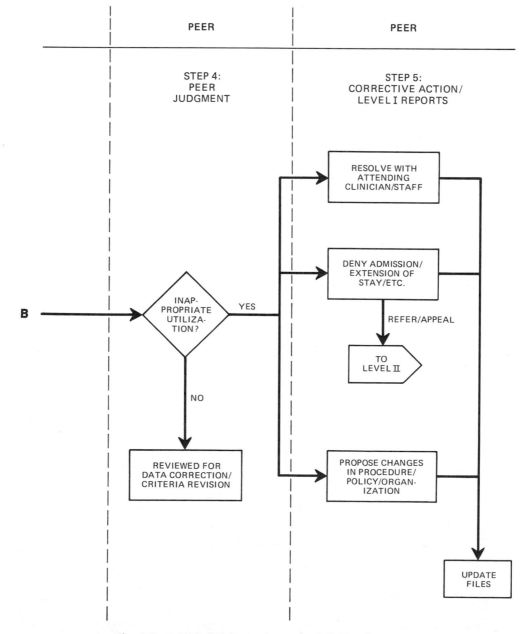

Fig. 8-1, cont'd. For legend see opposite page.

sembling and labeling of the data forms and documents, data input into computer, filing, workload management, report dissemination, and other clerical functions.

Computer operations (step 2)

Although computer operations in reality constitute a discrete subsystem, this particular subsystem is conceptually inseparable from all the others. Consequently electronic data processing will be considered collectively with the primary review team as a single functional unit. The potential applications of computer technology that review personnel might conceivably find useful are endless but for present purposes can be summarized as supportive or interactive. Supportive applications are passive operations that take over the bookkeeping functions such as aggregating data and generating profiles or reports in a retrospective fashion as do data processing service organizations. Interactive applications, on the other hand, are involved in review transactions as they occur in real time (on-line mode) or nearly so (remote batch mode). In addition to supportive functions, interactive systems introduce possibilities of screening cases on the basis of branched or conditional criteria and of intervening in the actual delivery of care rendered to the individual patient (individual quality assurance). This discussion will cover both types of computer applications.

For the present discussion, though, computer data processing is construed to mean an item-for-item comparison of case-abstract data with the explicit criteria stored in its memory banks (Fig. 8-1, step *2*). Where a deviation is detected between the record of care and the criteria, an exception report is generated that represents a potential care deficiency (or inappropriate resource utilization). It is this document which signals that review by a professional peer is indicated, and a report of the specific exception encountered is forwarded to the physician advisor for triage.

Functions of the physician advisor

Peer involvement in the review process begins with the physician advisor (PA). His primary duty is to act on exception reports, which in reality are the output of the screening phase. Whether prepared by the computer or not, these reports are generally presented to the PA by the review coordinator along with supporting data including the medical chart.

Evaluation of review data. The PA's first specific task is to determine whether sufficient information has been made available to him to render valid determinations. If so, the next step is triage.

Exception triage (step 3). The PA must then decide whether he has proper jurisdiction as a peer. If he determines that he is not the professional peer of the one who caused the exception, he should refer the case to someone who is of the same professional category or specialty training. This step is referred to as exception triage because it is a judgmental process in which a sorting decision is made as to the proper peer to judge the case.

Peer judgment (step 4). Assuming the PA is the appropriate peer (as in the preponderance of cases), the PA renders a decision whether the exception report resulted from an actual deficiency in clinical care or misuse of clinical resources. If such be his judgment, he must then characterize the deficiency in regard to who was responsible for it, what caused it (if determinable), and to whom this should be reported.

Corrective action (step 5). Assuming a true care deficiency did occur, the PA must decide (1) whether to initiate corrective actions himself or (2) to refer the case to a higher review authority either to undertake a more thorough review or to initiate corrective measures beyond his authority (referral).

Immediate intervention. *In interactive systems intervention in the care process is possible, and the PA must also decide if immediate action is necessary (for example, to save a patient from harm or death) or whether the subsequent review* *can proceed in a routine manner.* (NOTE: This potential capability is not represented on the flow chart).

Reporting. The full and precise reporting of all judgmental decisions and resulting corrective actions forms the keystone of efforts to prevent leakages or a dissipation of the effectiveness of the review process. It is essential that proper persons be notified to complete the requirements of public accountability.

Administration. There is also an unavoidable minimum of administrative duties for the PA to perform as the responsible director of the primary review team.

Activities of the level 1 review process

It is one thing to spell out who does what in a model systematic review process, but it is quite another thing to state why they should do these things, in what sequence, and how the different review functions interact with each other. That is the purpose of this section, and in pursuing these points unavoidable repetition will be minimized.

The place to begin of course is with that natural sequence of events that characterizes the care process and dictates the sequence of level 1 review operations. This description will be independent of which strategy, methodology, or data system is used to implement the peer review process, whether sampling is done or all cases are reviewed. (Only those steps that are **major components of the review process** are the ones depicted in the flow diagram.)

1. On admission of a patient to the medical care facility a completed patient demographic and fiscal (payment source) record that meets both review system needs and institutional needs should be made available to the primary review team.

2. Clinical data from preadmission testing or direct admissions of emergencies (if applicable) should be abstracted from existing medical documents and also made available for review.

3. On receiving demographic, fiscal, or preadmission data from the admitting office the clerk-typist normally enters the data into permanent review files *(or into the computer terminal).*

4. The clerk-typist also prepares case-abstract documents by filling in case identification headings and makes them available to the reviewers.

5. A reviewer then examines the patient's hospital chart (usually within 24 hours) and abstracts information relevant to the admission of certification status (step 1 on the flow diagram). (NOTE: The chief review coordinator should be alerted to investigate any information that appears medically questionable, and an attempt should be made to obtain prompt clarification before the physician advisor is consulted.)

6. The review coordinator examines the records of all (or selected) patients for indicators of compliance with quality care standards. These indicators may consist of a panel of routine review (screen) items common to the care of all patients and items specifically pertaining to the admission diagnosis. All such data requirements are usually contained on a case-abstract document that is based on explicit disease-specific quality criteria such as those prepared by the AMA Criteria Task Force.[2] In actual practice both the general and disease-specific quality criteria are simultaneously abstracted in a single chart review (step 2).

7. Diagnoses are verified and appropriately coded[3,pp.105–112] by the review coordinator.

8. A reviewer inspects the entire case-abstract document to spot and correct any recording or coding errors prior to the screening operation (either a manual comparison with criteria items or computer input for automated data processing). *Interactive systems can take advantage of real-time automated error surveillance techniques to automatically scan data for determinable accuracy and to request immediate correction when entries are beyond acceptable parameters.*

9. An exception report may be generated whenever a disparity is detected between either general or the disease-specific criteria items and the record of care as abstracted from the medical chart at the time of review. This report should specify which particular criteria element was not satisfied to be of maximum use to the peer reviewer. Exception reports may be considered the output of the screening phase of the review process, which really amounts to the **selection of cases that should undergo a subsequent judgmental review by peers.** The usefulness of this output is maximized when it specifies a particular problem in care or resource utilization that should be investigated.

NOTE: The following definitions of terms are of extreme importance to understanding the next steps in the peer review process:

exception an apparent (unestablished) inconsistency or deviation from approved criteria for quality patient care as detected by a comparison of the case record abstract against explicit criteria items (screening process).

exception report a report from the screening phase that contains one or more case-specific exceptions that have not yet undergone analysis by a peer reviewer.

medical care deficiency a judgment rendered by an authorized professional peer that a given exception was valid (established) and does represent inappropriate or inadequate medical care. NOTE: An "inappropriate use of medical resources" is analogous to but not a synonym of a care deficiency.

10. On receipt of the exception report the PA first must decide whether he is the appropriate peer to render a judgment. When, for example, available facts indicate that a given exception report was caused by a delay in the typing of a patient history and physical exam or a delay in placing the workup in the chart, then the real problem is not attributable to an attending physician but to the clerical staff. Clerical problems would not normally be handled by the PA but would be routed to administration for action. The investigative process that attributes the exception to its human source and identifies the proper peer to render a judgment is called exception triage (step 3).

Another triage concept that should be discussed has to do with separating relatively minor exceptions, meaning those with low clinical (or fiscal) risk, from those that are more serious and worthy of immediate attention by a PA. A minor exception is typified by the unperformed routine urinalysis or rectal exam (when no pathology is suspected) or some neglected routine item in the medical history and so on. A review system that fails to filter out such minor exceptions but forces them all through a single investigative channel is not only inefficient and expensive, but it will soon lose credibility with professionals. This is why a triage step should be inserted in comprehensive review systems that investigate at this level of detail before a time-consuming and detailed investigation is launched into every exception report. The paradigm of an ideal system would call for an optimum sequence of selective steps that places into the hands of the ultimate review authority all those cases on which it should render a judgment and none that can be rendered at a lower level of authority. The ideal is rarely fully achieved in the real world, of course, but it can be approached.

In Fig. 8-2 we have illustrated this process of selection as occurring through a series of three screens. The first screen is physically performed by a computer (as envisioned by the framers of the PSRO law[1]) in the data-processing step that compares the record of care against the criteria. It has been our experience (which others seem to have shared) that the criteria-screening phase of combined quality and utilization review systems will identify on the average about 15% of the total number of cases reviewed as exhibiting some deviation from explicit criteria. Of these, about two-thirds (that is, 10% of total input) are likely to be minor or noncritical in comprehensive systems. This

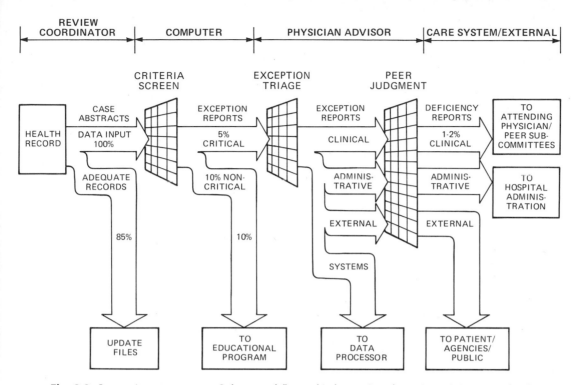

Fig. 8-2. Screening sequence. Schema of flow of information from its origin in medical record, preparation of a case abstract for input into the data system (computer processing), reporting of an exception (deviation) from preset criteria, rendering of a judgment by a physician advisor that a true care deficiency has occurred, ranking of these deficiencies as to type and origin, and referral of these deficiencies from level 1 to level 2 peer groups. Progressively fewer cases are passed through the screens, as there are data sinks at each step.

signifies some deviation from standards in which patient care is not seriously threatened or resource utilization was not grossly inappropriate, although the identified practices are still undesirable. *Interactive data systems can have the critical versus non-critical triage step built into the automated data processing sequence.*

Minor exceptions are best handled by aggregating them statistically for analysis of performance trends. Should the accumulation of minor exceptions indicate persistent or recurring problems for either individuals or groups of care providers, then the continuing education subcommittee should be notified, derive an educational needs index, and design appropriate remedial education programs to deal with the problem.

Roughly 5% of the cases can be expected to signal potentially significant problems in either the quality of care or the utilization of resources. However, the exception triage step will identify that from this group of cases a certain fraction will reflect administrative rather than clinical problems, and still other problems will be attributable to external sources (as discussed below). It has been our experience that in most of the hospital settings we personally investigated with mature (stable) review systems, it was usual for about 1% to 2% of the total cases to actually be presented to the physician advisor for his review as critical exceptions worthy of appropriately prompt attention (either immediate or within 24 hours).

It should be unequivocally stated, however, that this is a **target** percentage that can be adjusted up or down, depending on the desired stringency of the screening and triage steps.

There should be no mistake either about the very consistent finding that the initial experience with the review system in all hospitals we studied generated several times that percentage of exception reports for the PA to examine. Wise planning will take into account that adjustments will be needed (and will be made) in the care system to conform to criteria and to improve documentation, while trivial criteria elements will need to be eliminated and errors in the screening process must be weeded out of the review system. All this takes time, of course, but the greater the commitment of the hospital leadership to this effort, the shorter the adjustment period will be.

Before departing from the topic of triage we wish to point out that an important benefit to the institution comes from the identification of exceptions that are attributed to factors **external** to the hospital's own control. A classic example (and one that is not at all uncommon) is typified by the patient who has received maximum clinical benefit from the hospitalization and whom the attending physician's notes clearly indicates is medically prepared for transfer to a long-term care facility only there are no beds available to place the patient. All such cases of forced inappropriate utilization of acute hospital beds should be scrupulously documented and properly attributed to external agencies or unmet community obligations. Such cases should not be absorbed in the hospital's inappropriate stay data. Only in this way can the documentation be accumulated to prod the community or the payors to look for long-term solutions to long-term problems.

11. Once the PA determines that a given exception is a clinical one and that he is the appropriate peer (rather than a nurse, dentist, psychologist, and so on), he must then evaluate whether he possesses sufficient information to render a valid judgment.

In some cases the exception report may contain all the information necessary to render a peer judgment, but frequently it does not, and other information must be made available. In conducting his review the PA may utilize such diverse data sources as

1. Exception reports
2. Provider profiles (record of past performance)
3. The original case abstract
4. Patient's chart
5. Guidelines for criteria interpretation
6. Consultations with care provider
7. Patient interviews or examinations

Having assembled the information essential to rendering a judgment, the PA must of course conduct a systematic and thorough review of it.

12. Should the peer reviewer determine that a care deficiency has occurred (step *4*, Fig. 8-1), it should next be characterized as to type or underlying cause, and depending on the problem encountered the peer reviewer either recommends a course of corrective action or refers it to some other appropriate authority for further review.

A point to be made here is that the PA sits in judgment not only of the care process but also of the review process. Should he find, for example, that the data presented to him are in error, it is his duty to see that appropriate data corrections are made by those review personnel responsible. If he finds the criteria are medically irrelevant, he so notifies the criteria development authority, and so on.

Thus we see that the peer judgment step is multifaceted. On the basis of the evidence before him the PA must judge whether a true care deficiency has occurred (or an inappropriate utilization of resources) or whether the exception report itself was for some reason inappropriate and, in any event, who was responsible and what should be done about it.

13. The point is that by the time the PA

becomes involved in the review process, **some action on the part of some one was inappropriate and by definition requires that some corrective action must be taken (step 5).** *Interactive systems can respond promptly.*

14. It is essential to the integrity of the review system that when a care deficiency is encountered, the PA must either fully document what corrective action he has recommended or indicate to what higher review authority and for what reason he has referred the case. This action is vital to fix responsibility and maintain an intact chain of accountability. To assist in this, some sort of report validation mechanism is then needed to systematically record all decisions made. Properly designed, this should represent a basic mechanism for reporting medical peer judgments with maximal precision to those who need to act on them and also to document through the data system where the exception report was sent (and how long ago to detect inordinate delays). The documentation of this decision complex is referred to as a deficiency report and differs from an exception report in that it carries a peer judgment.

Where the reporting mechanism operates in conjunction with a computer-based screening device that utilizes explicit criteria, the exception report resulting from step 2 merely serves to identify potential care deficiencies requiring review by a peer. *Interactive systems, on the other hand, can utilize a special version of the exception report itself as a turn-around document for reporting peer judgments (which then become deficiency reports).* The linkage of peer judgments and corrective actions taken in response to specific exceptions then assures a full record of accountability. All those responsible for monitoring the review effort can thereby evaluate the effectiveness of the entire integrated process. Since the generation of the initial exception report is involuntary as far as either the review personnel or the care personnel are concerned, it is what happens in response to them that becomes a measure of the institutional commitment to peer review. Thus the audit trail that is essential for full public accountability must forge a direct and traceable linkage between the screening process (exception report) and the corrective action (deficiency report).

There is a substantive yet seemingly confusing difference between taking an action and the consequences of that action. Before proceeding we will attempt to clarify that point. To begin with, the mere reporting that a corrective action has been recommended by the review system is not equivalent to a confirmation that the correction has in fact taken place in reality.

All recommendations for corrective actions made by the physician advisor should be thought of as having two end-points and therefore require two reports. The first is the deficiency report itself, which signals the peer reviewer's recommended action in the case. In reality this is a **request** for corrective action that is to be transmitted to the management of the care delivery system for implementation (see step 4 of review level 3). Subsequently there should also be a final-final action, which is a **confirmation** of the eventual outcome of that recommendation. In short the act of recommending some corrective measure on the part of the physician advisor requires a subsequent report that the problem has actually been rectified by the attending physician (or by whomever the deficiency was attributed) or a confirmation that some other remedial measure such as continuing education or disciplinary action has in fact been initiated and carried out.

To illustrate how the review system can be subverted if this is not done, consider the situation where the screening phase produces an exception report that indicates some critical (that is, required) data are missing from the patient record. If the PA determines in step 4 that this probably represents substandard clinical charting on the part of the attending physician, the final action he is likely to recommend is that the missing data be supplied. What the PA cannot know, however, is **whether that very information was deliberately missing to obscure the fact that substandard care was given** or that the entire admission was inappropriate in the first place. If the PA's deficiency report merely requests more data, and that is allowed to terminate the review transaction, there will be no resolution to many of the potentially more serious problems that might be hidden by poor documentation as in the case illustrated.

What should happen instead is when the PA requests more data, a reviewer should subsequently return to that particular medical chart and ascertain that the missing data are now present and in the process ascertain that the new data also conform to all explicit criteria. That is the only substantive way to be sure that there are no underlying problems. Naturally, if the follow-up chart review reveals that the requested data are still missing, then a problem of persistent noncompliance or of willful obstruction has been uncovered, and this in turn should trigger a wholly new peer transaction. All it takes to subvert any review system is for clinicians simply to not record data on the chart. Given the opportunity, experience will soon teach them how to avoid generating exception reports.

Clearly the final-final report cannot be written until there is documentation of resolution of the problem detected. The closer such evidence reflects actual corrections in deficient care rendered to the individual patient or reflects actual behavioral changes on the part of involved clinicians, the stronger is the evidence that the peer review system is working properly. This second confirming report is a critical part of the surveillance process, as it is another essential ingredient of public accountability.

15. With regard to the frequency of review, the individual patient may be sequentially monitored from admission to discharge when concurrent or prospective review systems are employed. At a minimum the hospital charts of most patients would be reviewed by such systems on admission (24 to 48 hours after admission), at or near the average length of stay (based on norms determined by disease or condition), and reviewed again at the time of discharge (or immediately before or after it). *Interactive systems possess the capability of continuously monitoring specific items of services that connote appropriate medical care or any resource utilization that is illogical on a longitudinal basis.* Both of these time-dependent capabilities are obscured by retrospective summary reviews that by definition would collapse the sequence of events and report them after the inpatient care process had been terminated and the patient discharged.

Exact review procedures will vary substantially from one method to another and from hospital to hospital. Flexibility and selectivity in adapting standard procedures to a specific peer review program are features to be highly valued irrespective of the methodology employed. Prudence also dictates that tempting revisions should be postponed until the program has been fully implemented and matured (operationally stabilized).

REVIEW LEVEL 2
Conceptual base

It is the purpose of this section to discuss the nature of the next higher level in the review process, the division of responsibility among review work groups, and the conceptual base or the logic system that determines the sequence of level 2 operations (Fig. 8-3). As was proposed in the preceding chapter, major peer review activities can (and probably should) be performed at level 2 by some mix of standing peer groups derived from the membership of a single supervisory peer review committee. The structure, organization, and relationships of these discrete but interdependent working groups may be determined wholly or in part by hospital staff bylaws, by the PSRO or JCAH requirements, or by some other influences. Irrespective of these factors, the description that follows is concerned with the functional units and their activities organized on the basis of purpose and not on the chain of command or methodologies that might be used for achieving that purpose. This operational description should therefore be applicable to any review method. Since function is dictated by purpose, we pause here to consider the basic objectives of peer review.

Objectives of peer review

It follows that each institution, by defining its own peer review objectives, will be defining what is for them unique functional units. In actual practice the universality of the broader objectives of peer review lend similitude and a comparability among institutions. These common objectives are

1. Assurance of necessity in patient care (admission and continued stay review)

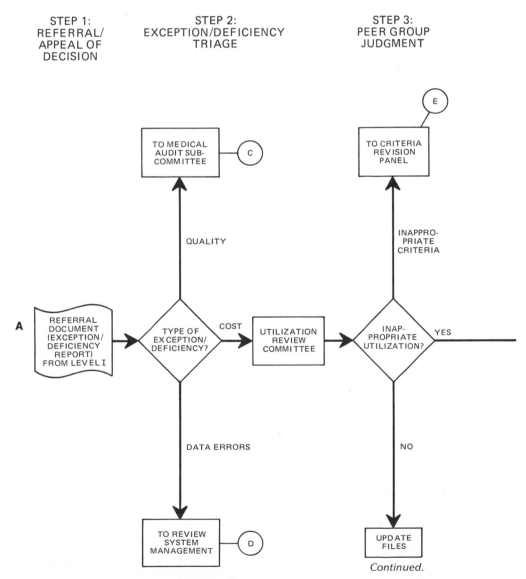

Fig. 8-3. Flow diagram: level 2.

2. Assurance of quality in care and services (for all patients, not just federal beneficiaries)
3. Assurance in the quality of practitioner decisions and technical proficiencies
4. Assurance of quality education for both patients and practitioners based on needs

Review functions and activities

In describing the activities necessary to carry out the above basic functions of comprehensive peer review within a hospital, it would prove useful to first define a "transitional philosophy" for clarifying what organizational changes might be needed in the usual existing hospital review structure to bring unity to the func-

STEP 4:
CORRECTIVE
ACTION

STEP 5:
LEVEL II
SUMMARY REPORTS

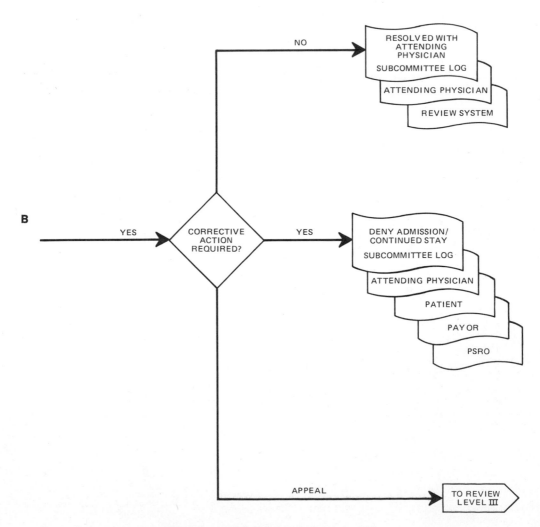

Fig. 8-3, cont'd. For legend see p. 209.

tioning of the system as a whole. As discussed in Chapter 7, for most hospitals this unification concept would call for changes not only in how review work groups are structured but especially in how their separate functions are coordinated to achieve both efficiency and thoroughness in review activities. In actual practice there may be any number of organizational structures that can undertake the four major objectives (only basic structures to fulfill basic purposes will be discussed here), but the one-purpose–one-peer-group rationale would call for a minimum of four subcommittees to be created from the membership of the peer review committee (PRC). While the names assigned to these work groups are immaterial, the rationale for their existence is not.

Utilization review subcommittee (URS)

Structure. This workgroup would become an adaptation of the usual freestanding utilization review committee.

Function. This particular committee substructure would be concerned exclusively with conducting review designed to optimize and maximize the efficient use of hospital facilities and resources.

Medical audit subcommittee (MAS)

Structure. This subcommittee can be thought of as a single replacement for the usual variety of committees that traditionally conduct fragmented quality review activities such as the medical audit committee, tissue committee, mortality review committee, and so on.

Function. This particular peer group would be primarily concerned with combining, condensing, and streamlining all quality review activities into a single-focus, quality-centered review operation.

Evaluation subcommittee (ES)

Structure. This subcommittee really constitutes an expansion of the whole peer review concept and will need to create its own identity in being responsible for the mechanics of all evaluative processes.

Function. Its primary function will be to establish and optimize all review procedures needed to meet present and future internal expectations (institutional goals) and to assure compliance with external regulations and contractual obligations (for example, PSRO).

Continuing education subcommittee (CES)

Structure. This subcommittee will consist of those who are directly concerned with meeting the educational needs of the entire hospital staff, which includes the specific needs of individual practitioners as revealed by their own particular profile analyses in addition to groups.

Function. This is no longer merely a good idea; in the state of Ohio, for example, it has become law that continuing education is an obligation of continued licensure. Gone are the days when continuing education merely means the occasional attending of medical staff meetings or clinical conferences. Gone too is reliance on the standard lecture-discussion format as the primary educational resource for the continuing education of an entire hospital professional staff. Obviously there will be common educational needs shared by many staff members that might be met by traditional continuing education programs, but it is the specific educational need of individual practitioners for whom this subcommittee assumes an entirely new functional responsibility. That is where the future effort of this subcommittee will need to be focused.

Common responsibilities

There are purposes common to all working groups that call for them to act collectively as authoritative agents. For example, all are concerned with the application of and compliance with quality criteria in the hospital setting. As the line between an inappropriate use of resources and inappropriate care can be a thin one at times, this should be jointly determined. All groups are also charged to provide continuing direction, support, and guidance to the primary review team in keeping with the areas of expertise and interest represented by the group membership. The conduct of these shared functions would be facilitated by joint meetings to periodically assess criteria, for example, and to iron out common problems.

Divided responsibilities

The operations of these four basic subcommittees and their related enabling activities are separable, but there is also a minimum of unavoidable overlap. It therefore follows that all four audit processes must be closely integrated and connected generically. Indeed, it is even conceivable that a single properly managed committee would undertake to pursue all four purposes in a small hospital, but the work load would probably be unmanageable in a larger one. In any event the work of all these subcommittees can be made easier by their having direct contact with those most intimately involved with the review process, namely the primary review team. To assure this contact, individual members of the primary review team can serve as subcommittee assistants or resource personnel in such assignments as indicated below (NOTE: the PA is discussed separately):

1. Continuity of care coordinator: assist the utilization review subcommittee
2. Nurse reviewer: assist the medical audit subcommittee
3. Medical records technician: assist the evaluation subcommittee

Before we discuss the scope of activities that come under the purview of each subcommittee, three generalizations are in order. The first of these is that two of the subcommittees (the medical audit and utilization review subcommittees) become directly involved with the review of individual cases, while the remaining two (the evaluation and continuing education subcommittees) do not. The latter two function in support of the first two. The second generalization is that while it is convenient to discuss the activities of the several sub-

committees separately, in practice they perform no function wholly independently because the personnel of all subcommittees interact with each other at the policy-making level as they jointly participate in the peer review committee. The third generalization is that the review functions and their sequential steps are essentially the same for both quality assessment and utilization review.

Level 2 review sequence

As seen in the flow diagram for level 2 (Fig. 8-3), all major discrete steps in the review process are virtually identical with level 1 review activities and differ chiefly in that they involve the collective judgment of a group rather than that of an individual (PA).

Since there are no essential differences in the sequence of reviewing quality or cost factors in the individual case, for illustrative purposes we chose to trace the review sequence involved with an inappropriate admission because it is easier to describe.

Unlike level 1 review, a judgmental decision has taken place in the initiation, that is, the act of submitting a case for review at this level. Either there is a reason in someone's mind for appealing the decision of a PA or it is the judgment of the PA that there is a good reason for referring the case to a higher authority.

Step 1: Referral/appeal of decision. In some cases a PA refers a case precisely because he is unable to render a determination whether a care deficiency has occurred or, as in our illustration, if he is unable to decide if an admission was justified. Thus either an exception report (which identifies a specific deviation from explicit criteria) or a deficiency report (which conveys a PA judgment in the given case) is transmitted to the subcommittee along with the medical record or other pertinent data.

Step 2: Exception/deficiency triage. It is as appropriate that the subcommittee should first determine whether it has jurisdiction in the case before proceeding further with an investigation as it is for the PA to do this. In our example the URS should determine whether it is dealing with an uncomplicated case of an inappropriate admission or whether there are grounds to suspect that the admission was the product of inappropriate care to begin with. If so, this should prompt a transfer of the case to the MAS.

Step 3: Peer group judgment. Assuming it was a proper referral, the URS will then render a judgment on the basis of the evidence whether the admission was inappropriate or not.

Step 4: Corrective action. When it is clear that an admission was inappropriate, the corrective action usually deemed necessary is the denial of certification for payment. Often along with this goes a request to the attending physician and patient that either alternative care arrangements or alternative financing arrangements be made.

Step 5: Reporting. It is vital to promptly communicate such actions to the patient, to third parties such as the payor and the PSRO, and also to channel provider performance information to the continuing education subcommittee, which will determine whether the given case is part of a pattern that justifies the launching of an educational program to counter it.

UTILIZATION REVIEW
Conceptual base

With anything even resembling the degree of reorganization of functions proposed in Chapter 7, the utilization review and medical audit subcommittees would likely share a common conceptual problem. That problem is engendered either by a forced marriage or by the rather artificial separation of utilization review from medical audit functions. Typically these level 2 functions are either overly combined with little or no conceptual distinctions or they are overly separated by a gross oversimplification of definitions. The reader is referred to the JCAH *Accreditation Manual for Hospitals* for an in-depth analysis of these vital concepts and how

they relate to each other. Suffice it here to provide an abbreviated statement from the manual:

It is, therefore, evident that the definition of *quality of care* includes consideration of the utilization of services and facilities. In this context, high quality can realistically be expected to depend upon efficiency in the logistical aspects of the delivery of patient care.[3, p. 184]

We distinguish the cost function from the quality function by designating the former **utilization review,** and we find several terms acceptable for the latter: namely, **medical audit, patient care audit,** or **quality assessment.** It is not within the scope of this discussion to resolve the conundrum as to whether or to what degree the boundaries of the resource allocation and quality care review should be separated or combined at the operational level. It is germane, however, to point out that this issue will not go away, and it therefore must be addressed deliberately and forthrightly irrespective of the methodologic option taken.

Areas of activity

Utilization review subcommittee functions are best defined from the perspective of the types of activities with which it will become involved. Using this approach, there are three principal identifiable utilization review activity areas:
1. Appropriateness of admission
2. Appropriateness of length of stay (continued stay)
3. Effectiveness of discharge planning

Classes of activity

Within each of these three review activity areas are contained the following identifiable and discrete subcategories or classes of activities:
1. Individual case review: a case-by-case determination of inappropriate care or utilization (peer group judgment) and the recommendation of corrective action in referrals or appeals
2. Profile analysis: the identification of undesirable patterns of accumulated

exceptions or deficiencies (patterns of abuse) in the profiles of care providers individually and collectively

3. Evaluation of the effectiveness of corrective actions in aggregate (by type of deficiency or provider group and so on)
4. Evaluation of the efficiency of the primary review team
5. Evaluation of the usefulness of explicit utilization criteria

Although theoretically this design of five classes for each of the three activity areas would presume a minimum of 15 discrete utilization review functions, in actual practice most of these activities can be (and are) combined in various ways contingent on the unique needs of the hospital or of the clinical situation. Further, the first of these functions obviously relates to continuous (concurrent) review of an individual patient, while others are periodic in nature and more closely related to the retrospective review of aggregated cases. Obviously the relative importance of these differing review activities would be a function of the review methodology used. Specific tasks and defined procedures for the URS should of course be developed by each individual hospital to adapt to its own organizational structure and operational patterns.

Individual case review functions

To be discussed briefly here are utilization functions that are generally the most common or essential to most review strategies and thus have value as nuclear paradigms. As the sequence of individual case review activities at this level has already been presented in the discussion of the flow diagram, what will be discussed here are the most likely reasons for case appeals and for referrals to level 2 review.

Physician advisor referrals. As their experience grows, most PAs independently arrive at similar conclusions regarding which types of exceptions they feel they can handle themselves and which types should be referred to the next level of peer review

for further action. Following are some components of the most likely consistent pattern of referrals from level 1 review to the URS:

1. Inappropriate admissions identified by profile analysis to be part of a recurring pattern or to be a persistent deficiency on the part of an individual physician or patient
2. Disallowed length-of-stay extensions in hardship cases
3. Disallowed major services or procedures
4. Inadequate or unrecorded transfer or discharge plans, especially those that involve inadequate community facilities or agency support

Appeals. An established and effective in-house appeals mechanism must be available to all care providers and patients affected by the program. Fair decisions are of course essential but may often be difficult to achieve in the area of utilization control because of the fear of setting restricting precedents. Justice would appear to be best served if the hospital URS acts as the court of first appeals and routinely transmits all decisions rendered in appeals to at least one additional review level beyond itself, namely to the full peer review committee (level 3). This is the best insurance against complaints or suspicions of prejudicial treatment whether justifiable or not.

Examples of especially difficult utilization appeal issues with considerable potential to perplex the URS include disallowed extensions of hospital stays that are not attributable to any single person or factor; the question of the legitimacy of disallowing length-of-stay extensions when a patient has already been declared medically prepared to leave but there is no place outside the hospital that will accept him; the nature of staff responsibility and accountability when external forces (such as unresponsive social placement agencies) are the major factors causing inappropriate admissions, unacceptable lengths of stay, and inadequate discharge plans. There are many more difficult judgment calls that assure sufficient challenging appeals cases for even the most active and aggressive URS to handle.

Profile review function

The URS must assume the responsibility for developing a multifactorial approach to deal effectively with recurring and cumulative utilization abuses perpetrated by individual care providers. Involved here is the identification of chronic offenders and of underlying causes through profile analysis. The real causes of persistently inappropriate utilization of hospital facilities, as was pointed out earlier, may well extend beyond the control of attending physicians or hospital administrators and actually be attributable to patients themselves or to failures of the community to meet its social obligations in providing less costly care alternatives. In such an eventuality the most effective corrective action may be that of mounting education programs aimed at reorienting the demands of patients or restructuring the priorities of the community.

Integrative activities. Integrating review functions with standard hospital operating procedures relative to utilization is another responsibility of the URS. Appointing the hospital medical records librarian as secretary to the URS may prove to be a most useful organizational strategy to achieve results in this area. For the foreseeable future the medical record will likely remain the basic informational source document, and the usefulness of the data it contains to peer review is absolutely related to the organization, form, content, and accuracy of the record itself. More efficient utilization review may well be a function of more efficient record keeping.

Reporting activities. Summary statistics and computer outputs need to be discussed in conducting the ongoing work of the URS. Periodic statistical summaries and pattern analysis reports such as cumulative utilization profiles by physicians or specialty services must be reviewed at least on a monthly basis by the URS. Each official review requires an activity report sufficiently explicit to reveal the proficiency of utilization review procedures. This requires informational linkages that document exactly what corrective activities are taken in response to each pattern of inappropriate resource utilization identified. The more promptly the reviewers detect a delinquency, the greater the likelihood of effecting change. *Interactive data systems would allow even a daily monitoring of utilization review.*

The preparation of specific reports required by PSRO contractual agreements also is the responsibility of the URS. While such reports will most likely be automatically generated by computer, the URS probably should retain the responsibility to supervise how such reports are to be compiled and interpreted.

Revision of reports. At regular intervals, perhaps annually, a complete review of all reporting requirements should be done for the purpose of combining and eliminating those utilization reports found to be essentially duplications or of little real value. Unnecessary paperwork can be eliminated through finding ways to reduce the number of reports such as by making them broader in scope so that they can serve multiple applications. There is, however, a limiting factor to broader reporting formats that is the hazard of breeching confidentiality through the inclusion of sensitive case-specific information in widely circulated reports, so this can only be achieved with aggregate data bases.

Role of automation

The report-generating capability of an automated data-processing system makes it a mixed blessing where any large-scale utilization review activity is concerned. However, the evaluation and translation of these or any other reports into worthwhile actions remain committee tasks. Stated another way, data are generated by the review system (computer). Information is generated by an alert peer group. To remain alert the subcommittee must periodically ascertain that it is receiving useful reports with which to work.

MEDICAL AUDIT

As previously described, it is the medical audit subcommittee (MAS) that addressed itself specifically to considerations involving the quality of care.

Conceptual base

Evaluating the quality of care, like utilization review, requires both a direct involvement in individual case review and an indirect involvement in level 2 support operations. Unlike the assessment of resource allocations, however, there is a great deal more at stake than just money.[4] Quality assessment not only asks what was done for the patient (process) but also what happened to the patient that was beneficial or otherwise (outcome) as a result of that care.[5] Thus quality assessment has many more facets than does utilization review. Yet parallels do persist between the activity areas of hospital medical audit and those already described for utilization review. This is because both are bound by the same thread of clinical continuity. It follows that both the quality and the utilization of inpatient resources will be influenced by events that precede and follow the hospitalization. It is essential therefore that the period of hospitalization be viewed as but a cross-sectional episode in a continuum of care rendered to a given patient. The explanation for why this is particularly germane to quality assessment is simple. Hospitalization all too often represents a failure of outpatient diagnostic acumen or therapeutic care or both. It follows that the MAS will need to focus considerable attention on ambulatory care rendered in the immediate preadmission period to ascertain if the hospitalization was the product of inappropriate care rather than being medically unavoidable. Similarly, high-quality inpatient care often may be dependent on the thoroughness and quality of discharge planning and the rehabilitative

effects of follow-up ambulatory care to achieve a satisfactory clinical result.

Wherever lines might be drawn on either side of the hospital care segment to limit the scope of medical audit, they would be artificial. Yet practicality (chiefly in the form of limited funds available to support review activities) dictates that most hospitals must draw such lines somewhere. For reasons of space restrictions this discussion must observe pretty much the same limitations, but this is not to be construed as condoning a tunnel-vision conceptualization of peer review. Indeed, one might go so far as to predict that time will likely reveal that it is a short-sighted disservice to both physicians and patients to permit critical programmatic decisions to be made on the assumption that the overall quality of medical care is accurately revealed by auditing only the hospitalization period, which is but a narrow segment of total care.

Areas of activity

With the above disclaimer understood, the areas of activity for inpatient medical audit may be described as follows:
1. Admission preparation
2. Diagnostic assessment
3. Therapeutic intervention
4. Discharge planning

Classes of activity

The parallelism between medical audit and utilization review holds to the extent that virtually the identical classes of activities are common to both, as is seen below. There the parallel ceases, however, as the kinds of judgmental decisions to be made concerning the quality of care and the types of information needed to make those decisions differ markedly from those involved in utilization review:
1. Individual case review
2. Patterns of deficiencies
3. Effectiveness of corrective actions
4. Efficiency of review team
5. Usefulness of criteria

It is unnecessary to discuss here all the

complexities of quality care review, as many of these classes of activity are discussed elsewhere in this book. It is appropriate to point out, however, that there are at least 20 major aspects of quality review to be evaluated.

Suffice it to say the MAS becomes involved in an ongoing medical audit of the individual case just as the URS does through appeals and referral to it by the PA. The MAS also participates indirectly in the review process through its creation, revision, and modification of explicit quality criteria and its other review support functions.

Individual case review

Medical audit functions at review level 2 are often defined by the data base needed to support the review activities employed. Primary data sources may include physician advisor case referrals, provider profiles, patient profiles, MCEs, diagnosis and procedure profiles, and other retrospective summary statistics. The real purposes of the audit process at this level are first, to confirm the PA's judgment in especially serious or persistent care deficiencies, and second, to respond to the need for direct or remedial intervention that will eliminate these types of deficiencies in the quality of care.

An implicit assumption is that the authority will be granted to initiate and enforce the remedial actions called for above. Therefore two conditions for effective medical audit need to be mandated from the very beginning. First, the subcommittee must have access to any information it requests at any level of confidentiality. Second, the actions taken or recommended by the subcommittee must be binding on the hospital administrative and professional staffs alike. There are no hidden agendas or intervening variables in medical audit such as often contaminate utilization review activities. It would be less than candid to suggest that cost containment is not a major consideration in utilization review or that only physicians will comprise the

peer group that sets utilization standards and enforces them. Medical audit asks whether the care was acceptable to peers, and the sole agenda before the MAS is to improve the quality of care provided by physicians. It is obvious, however, there has to be a recognition of "quality at what cost?" as there are finite resources involved in addition to human cost in terms of anxiety, safety, and dignity.

The focus of MAS review appears to be determined by the type of case referred to it. This in turn determines the scope of information or data base that must be made available to the MAS for it to participate effectively in any given deliberation. While the above statement is certainly not stated as an axiom, it nonetheless provides a convenient classification for dividing subcommittee functions.

Categorical referrals. As was noted in the discussion of referrals to the utilization subcommittee, it probably is not necessary to set fixed guidelines for referrals by the physician advisor to the MAS, since it is usual that a reasonable pattern spontaneously manifests itself in referrals from the primary review team. Generally physician advisors tend to refer to the MAS those categories of cases they are uncomfortable about because they appear to involve practices that could pose critical threats to good patient care. Critical exceptions are usually those that involve potentially life-threatening deviations from accepted care practices, those capable of other serious long-term harm, or those that entail unwarranted distress to a patient.

The nature of the responses invoked by these referrals pretty well defines the working relationships that develop between the first and second peer review levels. The subcommittee may occasionally overrule the PA's interpretation of the facts in a given case or settle on an alternative recommendation for corrective action, but in practice we find it seldom does. What usually happens is that the MAS confirms the PA's judgment that the exceptions reported were actual care deficiencies and usually also validates both his judgment as to who was responsible for them and what ought to be done to correct or prevent them from happening in the future. As a practical matter, however, there is another factor that should be recognized, which is the observation that the impact of subjective judgments can be much greater when they represent the concurrence of an entire subcommittee rather than the opinion of a single individual. Referrals can also be used by the PA in a deliberate effort to avoid implications of prejudicial treatment in especially sensitive cases. This rendering of a collective judgment could be crucial to effecting desired results.

In the interest of review efficiency the MAS should concern itself with and be responsible to only those deficiencies that are both critical (serious) and attributable to an identifiable physician care provider. Whenever, in the judgment of the MAS, patterns of deficiencies that are relatively minor in singular occurrence but if repetitious or persistent are not reflective of high quality care, they should be referred to the continuing education subcommittee to serve as indicators of staff educational needs. Those deficiencies not attributable to a physician should be transmitted to some other staff member, perhaps on to the full peer review committee for disposition as was described on p. 212. However, the hospital may choose to structure the referral, a similar kind of intensive individual assessment would be performed by the professional peers of whatever nonphysician is responsible for the suspected substandard care.

There is an ethical imperative involved in the auditing of professionals irrespective of how it is conducted. Any care providers judged by peers to have rendered deficient care have the right to expect that they will be fully informed regarding all aspects of the judgmental processes and that there may be an exchange of views prior to the consequences of such judgment.[6]

Action referrals. A special category of cases the MAS should handle includes those in which there is an assumption that the remedial action indicated is of such magnitude or severity that it either merits consensual validation or requires authority beyond the PA's power to act. Following are examples of anticipated actions that might be more appropriately taken by the MAS:

1. Assignment of an individual to a required remedial education program
2. Clinical supervision
3. Professional censure or reprimand
4. Revoke specific clinical privileges
5. Conditional staff probation
6. Staff probation
7. Termination of staff appointment

Appeals. The types of cases that come to appeals usually involve critical exceptions in which justification for a given clinical action is contended by the attending physician but denied by a refusal to grant an exemption by the PA.

Unlike the utilization review subcommittee, the MAS is not just the first level of appeal but the only level of appeal in cases dealing exclusively with physician's services. There is substantive justification for this on close examination. Medical audit and peer review describe much the same process when only physicians evaluate the care provided by other physicians. (This is not the situation that usually pertains in utilization review, as nonphysicians typically participate in the review process.) The issue of confidentiality is a poignant reason for restricting exposure to professional colleagues in the auditing of quality care, as the potential exists to inflict unwarranted damage to professionals through the mere knowledge of the existence of an appeal in a contested case, regardless of what final judgment is rendered. For it to become known that the quality of a physician's care is being questioned will in all probability do harm to his reputation, which is an injustice to all those whose care is found to be appropriate. Because of this risk any possible advantage to the attending physician from the objectivity gained in referring an appeal beyond this subcommittee (and especially outside the hospital) would be offset to some degree by the danger of a wider exposure to illicit disclosures. Any attempt to offset the exposure risk by a protective reduction of specificity in the data supplied to the appeal body (in an attempt to eliminate sensitive information from falling into the wrong hands) carries with it the danger of deleting the depth of knowledge needed to render a justifiable decision.

Any injustice that might be inherent in this proposal to limit the appeal structure could be offset by the staff physician's right to binding review by an acknowledged expert in the particular specialty or clinical area in contention.

Finally, there are those who would question whether the physicians-only composition of the medical audit subcommittee might not violate the spirit of the so-called "sunshine rule" by insulating the medical profession from public accountability. Either a positive or a negative answer to this question is dependent on the hierarchical disposition of the reviewing authority and on the review methodology employed. If explicit quality criteria are used, then objective ground rules for both the conduct of care and of the review of that care will have been laid down, which can become a part of the public record. If the screening of medical care is then tied to these criteria and the chart review is performed by persons independent of the control of physicians, and if all deviations from the criteria (exceptions) are also a part of the public record, then **there is no way to avoid accountability.** If judgmental decisions are inseparably linked to each reported exception, **there is no way to duck the responsibility to act.** If the power to act is shared by public representatives, **there is no insulation.** If corrective actions must be confirmed by the same independent agent, **there is no way to suborn the review process.** Conversely, **if judgmental review is done by anyone other than pro-**

fessional peers, it is not peer review. But if all the above conditions are met, the public interest will be served by peer review, and confidentiality of the review process will also be preserved.

Persistent deficiencies. These are cases with persisting problems in which previous citations and corrective actions initiated by the PA did not result in improved care and that were once again detected by a follow-up review on the same patient (applies to concurrent review systems).

Profile reviews. Understandably, because there are human limitations connected with both the care delivery process and the review process, it would seem a safe assumption that occasional exception reports will be generated and at least some of these confirmed as care deficiencies for nearly every practicing clinician. It is the dual purpose of the level 2 profile review to ascertain whether excessive numbers of or unusual patterns of deficiencies emerge from the cumulative profiles of individuals that may not be apparent on case-by-case surveillance. If so, a determination must be made whether such patterns reflect unacceptable care practices, inexact review procedures, or medically irrelevant review criteria. The responsibility to periodically review the profiles of all individual care providers to search for problem areas is conveniently fixed with the MAS. The profiles of individuals may be compared against norms and standards derived from like data accumulated by specialty type, institution, or by region, but the focus of profile review at this level remains on individual care providers.

In actual practice MAS activities tend to be either disciplinary or mediating in nature when dealing with profiles. To generalize, the usual primary objective of profile analysis is either the detection and remediation of knowledge deficiencies, the elimination of performance deficiencies by improving physician skills through education, or the imposing of restrictions on clinical privileges if necessary. This latter, more drastic, alternative should be reserved for only those cases in which performance impairment is not merely contingent on inadequate knowledge or skills, but rather is the product of uncooperative attitudes or other personal failures.

Integrating activities. The greatest potential for improving the quality of medical care, irrespective of the corrective method chosen, must be based on an objective needs assessment that effectively directs the initiation of relevant corrective actions. If this effort is invested in providing a better education program, for example, a more relevant curriculum could be derived from the objective evidence of real care deficiencies than can be presently done without any such hard data. Medical audit and staff development (continuing education) activities are thus linked in a continuum as demonstrated in Fig. 7-4. Obviously the long-range impact of medical audit activities will to some degree be dependent on the capability of the educational effort to mount programs capable of changing staff behavior in the direction of compliance with medical audit directives. If the institution has a director of medical education (DME), it is probably desirable that this person serve on or be responsible to the MAS, as the position of DME can be viewed as an implementor of remedial education programs that are defined by the medical audit.

Criteria reviews. Indirect audit activities involve the evaluation of explicit quality criteria and the recommendation of revisions. At regular intervals (at least yearly) the committee would probably wish to solicit formal recommendations from the medical staff regarding the usefulness and appropriateness of all quality criteria employed at that institution. Summary printouts that document actual criteria performance, a master list of contested criteria, criteria panel outputs, exchange data from other hospitals, current PSRO rules and regulations, and all other available relevant material would all probably need to be reviewed and analyzed for the expressed purpose of maintaining criteria current

with recent enhancements of medical knowledge and skills. This formal review of the criteria by the MAS in no way substitutes for direct challenges to the criteria mounted by attending physicians caught up in the review process or for informal information exchanges between the CES and the clinical staff during data-reporting sessions.

A report on the conclusions from formal criteria reviews along with committee recommendations should be prepared for inspection by the medical staff after it has had the opportunity to react to the data and make input to the interpretations. For permanent reference and public interest this report would contain a narrative summary of how the review process was conducted along with copies of relevant source documents, an abstract of general recommendations, and an analysis of any proposed changes in each criteria.*

Audit reports. Medical audit reports are generally less of a preoccupation than are utilization reports. Regular reporting would include the amount of review effort performed on individual staff physicians' profiles, criteria reviews as discussed above, preparation of the educational needs profiles, and periodic reports to inform the medical staff or the local PSRO on the status of referrals or appeals as discussed below. Any requests for additional reporting should be carefully considered, as there is little of the routinely retrievable information that is not already incorporated into one or another of the reports described above.

Activity reports. For full accountability the activity records of the MAS should log every PA referral to higher levels and document the specific committee response made to each (and how long it took). It should formally document that proper

---

*This task is not as overwhelming as it might seem. A complete presentation can reflect the status of all criteria packages by using one of the following notations behind each item: *C, U, D,* or *N.* Depending on the letter code, the status of that particular criterion would be Changed, Unchanged, Deleted, or New.

notification was sent to the attending physician of any referrals or any actions pending.

For illustrative purposes the following items might be suggested for the MAS activity report:

1. Number and type of deficiencies confirmed
2. Method or basis for confirmation
3. Attribution of the exception (identification of the care provider responsible)
4. Remedial action recommended/initiated (with adequate justification)
5. Fixing of responsibility/accountability for accomplishing the recommended remedial action
6. Communication of all actions taken to the attending physician, the medical director, or any of the following: immediate supervisor, medical staff administration, hospital administrator, or hospital board of trustees
7. Notification of rights to the involved care provider (including rights to appeal and to expert opinion)

EVALUATION SUBCOMMITTEE

So far we have seen that other subcommittees are responsible for conducting direct and indirect review activities, but it is the evaluation subcommittee (ES) that focuses on the methods or the actual mechanics of the review process. The purview of this work group centers on developing and maintaining those review procedures routinely used to assess the overall care delivery patterns of the entire hospital. In short the ES is responsible to oversee the development of all basic (mostly retrospective) review procedures that employ summary data.

Conceptual base

While it cannot be argued with any force that there is some mysterious and compelling reason why it is so uncommon for any but a handful of members of most hospital medical staffs to exhibit any detectable interest in statistical reports, that neverthe-

less seems to be the way it really is. In recognition of this phenomenon it only makes sense that the supervision and analysis of all the various statistical summaries and profiles be done by those who are both interested and prepared to understand them. It is essential, however, that there always be adequate clinical representation on this subcommittee, as it is dangerously easy to draw overly simplistic explanations and conclusions from aggregated clinical assessment data.

Areas of activity

The statistical approach to patient care evaluation shifts this subcommittee's focus away from the care of individual patients as the center of the review activity and toward the broader overview of how care is delivered to groups or to all patients in a total hospital effort. Actual (observed) practices patterns can be compared with preexisting explicit consensus (performance targets) criteria, which makes the review process more uniform and objective.

By analogy the functions of this working group may be compared to that of law clerks in the judicial system who gather data and analyze it for the prosecuting attorney (utilization review committee) and the trial judge (medical audit committee). Perhaps apologies for this analogy to judicial procedures are due those who have been burned by the latter. The central truth is, however, that if the review procedures described above are conscientiously applied by and within the medical profession, there may be less malpractice work for the legal profession to do.

Review support functions

Devising and maintaining the effective retrospective review procedures, as modeled in Chapter 7, entails the following support functions:

1. Specifying the report formats for both aggregated data and for access to review data on individual patients *(especially in interactive concurrent review systems)*

2. Analyzing the utility of all profiles, summaries, and statistical outputs
3. Providing assistance in interpreting statistical output to support the needs of the medical audit, continuing education, and utilization review subcommittees, the full peer review committee, and the executive committee
4. Providing assistance with the design and conduct of medical care evaluation, pattern-of-care studies, and outcome analyses
5. Making recommendations for changes in review methodologies or in the policies that regulate the review process

CONTINUING EDUCATION SUBCOMMITTEE

At this point the discussion leaves what has been the singular theme of review operations and touches briefly on another topic so intimately associated with the purposes of peer review as to be literally inseparable from it. This of course refers to integrating the program for continuing medical education into the peer review corrective process as an instrument of effecting changes in practice behaviors.

Conceptual base

Until recently there would have been little purpose served in questioning the justification for mounting continuing medical education programs. It has long been a given not only that such programs are inherently a good thing but also of necessity they constitute the chief medium for correcting whatever happens to be wrong with medical care as currently practiced. However, studies by Williamson et al.[7] have now raised a serious question as to whether formal instruction employing case conferences or lectures can be relied on to effect significant changes in clinical judgment and thus correct care deficiencies. Since, however, there does not appear to exist at this time convincing evidence to the contrary (namely, that continuing medical education is of no value in

correcting the care deficiencies that are detected by peer review), it will be assumed that this activity does have its proper place in the overall peer review picture.

Areas of activity

It should be conspicuously obvious what continuing education is all about, but in the connotation that peer review will demand objectively tailored independent study programs, it really is not. The standard lecture-discussion format aimed at some predetermined topic selected by popular demand just is not relevant anymore for today's hospital staff. Even if it were, the standard selection of topics probably would be shown to be inappropriate. When a truly effective peer review system is installed in a hospital, probably the first thing to be discovered will be that the care rendered for some conditions is better than anyone imagined and the care rendered for others is unexpectedly far worse. It is really only toward the latter group of medical topics that economy dictates educational programs should take priority. The present experience, however, tends to show that there currently exists almost a random relationship between the topics popularly chosen for traditional continuing education programs and those which objective performance data would dictate that the staff really needs. Thus the CES should actively seek to provide relevant educational experiences of whatever kind it takes to meet the demonstrated needs of individuals as well as group programs aimed at the collective staff.

Educational functions

The first relevant function for the CES therefore is to invest the time to familiarize itself with whatever objective data the peer review system can provide, which will identify the most common and important care deficiencies prevalent among the staff individually and collectively. Then the CES must translate such care deficiency data into educational needs profiles.

Educational resources/programs. Next the

CES must either develop or obtain those instructional resources and materials required to meet specific educational needs that have a priority to effect improvements in care delivery. Maximum uses should certainly be made of whatever regional education facilities exist, such as medical schools and other teaching centers, to conduct group-oriented training programs that are demonstrably viable. But a much greater effort will have to be made in the development of new independent learning resources to meet the documented educational needs of individuals than has been done heretofore. Independent learning resources, programs, and materials, like library books, can be shared to effect cost reductions and to build subject matter inventories.

Outreach function. The outreach function of the CES is one that has been sorely needed for years yet is technically unapproachable until systematic peer review systems are in place and operating. It is time that the care delivery institutions provide constructive feedback to educational institutions as to what kinds of training are relevant and needed[8] to improve the performance of their graduates. After all, teaching centers can hardly be held accountable for what or how they teach unless they are informed how well or how poorly their graduates are prepared to care for patients in the clinical practice. The initiation of this outreach function begins with abstracting cumulative data from the educational needs index that reveal patterns of educational deficiencies. Little else could be of such immediate value in planning the curricula for undergraduate and postgraduate training programs. The more medically precise (based on patterns of health care deficiencies) the educational needs profiles can be reported, the more compelling will be the motivation to change how clinicians are taught. To be successful in this effort is to reduce the need for catch-up or remedial education among practicing physicians for that neglected part of the learning that should

have been a part of their formal training programs in the first place.

Peer review training. There is no historic precedent for externally imposed peer review systems in this country, and certainly most everyone currently in pactice needs to learn much more about the evolving requirements of the PSRO type of review and how they will be effected by them. The staffs of most all hospitals obviously need to be informed about their obligations under this mandated program. Many also need to be specifically trained for active participation in the peer review process in general and PSRO in particular. Clearly both introductory and periodic update programs of instruction on peer review scope and procedures must be devised and kept current.

Staff performance reporting. Active participation in peer review functions, including the development of explicit criteria, has often been cited as having an intrinsic educational value.[5,6] This general principle can be extended to the entire hospital staff when the effort is made to regularly report to them current and relevant performance data derived from peer review activities. There appears to be a strong positive force in the basic desire of individual health care providers to conform with what their peers identify as high standards of conduct (care practices). To harness this force it is first necessary to depict in understandable terms just what kind of care health care providers are actually delivering and where their performance is demonstrably suboptimal. Shakespeare described this kind of educational service as "holding the mirror up to nature as 'twere.'" This is not, however, something that should be done casually or thoughtlessly lest it invoke negative responses. Educational strategies of the highest order should undergird every effort to appraise the staff of where the level of care is less than desired. To avoid negativism the reports should be balanced and the staff should also be informed where care is optimal or superior as well. Reams of data may be available for reports of every description, but the highly judicious selection of only the most relevant data is of considerable importance to avoid overkill (intimidation by printouts). Those who address the staff must be responsive to the prejudices of key individuals and the personality and herd instincts of the group. Rising to this particular educational challenge may effect the most penetrating of desirable behavior changes and thus be the most rewarding single endeavor of the CES.

Educational feedback loop. No continuing educational effort can be assured of success without completing the educational feedback loop. The CES must therefore obtain tangible evidence from the care reassessment step (described in level 3) that the original care deficiencies that shaped its educational programs have in fact been eliminated. This will require periodic reviews of summary statistics on patients, diagnoses, and clinical performances prepared by whatever data system is employed to provide the documentary information that can demonstrate the efficacy of remedial education measures. The objective is to document whether desired behavioral changes that occur also persist over time. It is only through documented changes in actual clinical practices which persist that a successful educational impact can really be said to have been mounted. Surely the positive reinforcement from the recognition and reward of excellent care deserves a similar trial and evaluation.

REVIEW LEVEL 3

The following discussion represents a hypothetical model for review level 3 review operations.

Conceptual base

While discussions of the first two review levels dealt with the process of peer review, neither actually dealt with its product. The product referred to is a set of summary statistics that depict the overall pattern of medical care delivered by the hospital as a whole. In short the tasks reserved for this level (besides the review of appeals) are to review and interpret overall performance statistics that reflect the level of care provided by the hospital as a whole and how well the review system serves this end. The main objective is to make appropriate broad-scale recommendations in response to persistent broad-scale deficiencies or malfunctions of the review system that would have an anticipated effect on the entire institution or its large components.

Organizational structure

Since the rationale for the multidisciplinary make-up and high-level membership of this all-important committee was fully discussed in Chapter 7, it will not be repeated here. Suffice it to say that its internal organization must be so geared that persons who are knowledgeable and vested with policy-making authority are placed in supervision of both the care delivery system and the peer review system. Actual review functions may be performed either by the full committee or by its designer(s).

Corporate review responsibilities

The full peer review committee (PRC) has the undivided responsibility to review all aggregated profiles and summary reports that deal with the corporate performance of the institution as a whole. This corporate responsibility embraces the overall assessment of not only how well the care system is functioning but also how well the review system is functioning. It is a fundamental conceptual point of immeasurable importance that the same policy-level group be responsible for both systems. Only in this way can there be a full appreciation of the applicability and limitations in utilizing peer review performance data in the definition of policies and problems that in anyway affect the care of patients.

Participating review responsibilities

Participation in the actual review of individual cases is limited to a (second) hearing of appeals and to referrals for review by clinical specialists or nonphysician peers who may not actually serve on subcommittees. The concept that is critical to an understanding of the boundaries existing between the responsibility to conduct review activities at levels 2 and 3 is that the utilization and medical audit subcommittees of level 2 deal exclusively with performances of **individuals,** whereas the full PRC reviews the combined performances of the **entire hospital staff or recognizable groups within it.** An example of this is in assessing the results of MCEs.

Areas of activity

Specific activities of the full peer review committee include

1. Coordination and integration of all subcommittee activities
2. Review and analysis of institutional summary statistics and activity reports prepared by subcommittees
3. Preparation of final reports and recommendations to hospital departments, specialty disciplines, and hospital administrators regarding resource allocations, professional task assignments, service deficiencies, special service needs, in-service education needs, assessments of community service alternatives, aftercare service needs, and so on
4. Plan and oversee the development of medical care evaluation studies (see *PSRO Program Manual,* Sect. 705.31 to 705.36).
5. Overall administrative responsibility for the entire peer review system including the assigning and directing of support staff as needed.

Level 3 review sequence

The sequence of hearing appeals and referrals in individual cases at level 3 is identical to that of level 2, and thus the same flow diagram pertains to the review of individual cases. The only real difference is that a larger review body with broader interdisciplinary representation is available to conduct the review. For this reason the flow diagram of level 3 emphasizes the corporate review functions (steps *1, 5,* and *6,* Fig. 8-4).

Step 1: Analysis of reports. Except for the appeals mechanism (no longer to be discussed), the input for level 3 generally consists of aggregate data of two types: those reports that deal with the care system and those that deal with the review system itself. These reports either originate within routine surveillance activities or result from special studies from time to time.

Care system reports. The routinely generated reports of most interest to the PRC are those that depict patterns of resource utilization, patterns of care practices, and patient outcomes. Examples would include aggregated data that characterize the level of compliance with care criteria met by certain groups of care providers (for example, by specialty areas) or that characterize patterns of overstays by diagnosis, and so on.

Special insights into care practices and patient outcomes are provided in the findings of MCEs. Perhaps one way to think of MCEs is that they generally begin where the routine surveillance system leaves off in fact-finding about the care process. Typically they examine aspects of care that only need periodic assessment. Properly designed, these nonroutine and episodic studies should probe topics at a depth of detail or in a manner unsuited to regular (daily) surveillance procedures because of complexity or expense. This is not to say that each MCE should be expected to call into existence its own separate data-collecting instrument in mounting such studies. Indeed, efficiency demands that in-place channels of data flow, both within the care system and the review system, be used to the extent possible. This not only would help contain the cost of MCEs but also would set into motion follow-up studies of similar types that can utilize virtually the same investigative machinery. Further, the closer MCE and routine surveillance methodologies approach one another, the more readily routine surveillance can screen for and identify problem areas that merit

MCEs and that are likely to produce worthwhile results.

Once the study topics are chosen, it would be the option of the PRC to set the criteria and conduct the study itself or delegate these responsibilities to one of its subcommittees, which the full committee would then supervise.

Administrative actions. Depending on the exact nature of the needed policy or procedure definition, implementation may be carried out by managerial-level personnel of the medical (clinical) staff, the hospital administrative staff, or the review system management.

Disciplinary actions. It should be obvious

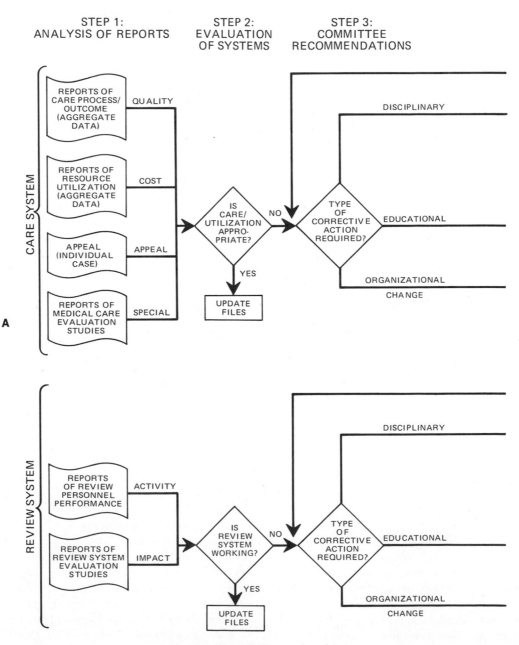

Fig. 8-4. Flow diagram: level 3.

that when any disciplinary measures are contemplated, the responsible supervisory personnel in either the care system or the review system must be participants in determining what disciplinary measures are needed, as they are inevitably responsible for carrying them out. The principles of due process must prevail, and the views or explanations of all personnel involved must be heard. The right of appeal applies to collective actions as it does to individual cases.

Irrespective of the kind of problem encountered, full documentation necessary for the reporting step (to be discussed later) must include not only the decisions

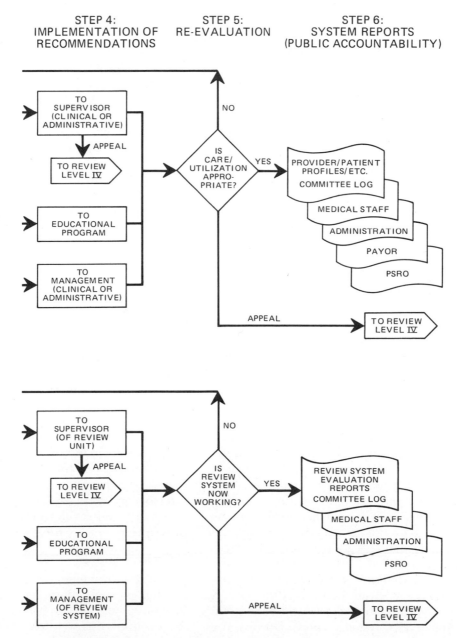

Fig. 8-4, cont'd. For legend see opposite page.

made and corrective actions recommended but also who was responsible for implementing them and, finally, confirmation that the corrective action was carried out.

The important area of coordination and integration of subcommittee activities occurs prominently with this particular step. An effective interface of the medical audit and continuing education subcommittees, for example, really requires a joint effort in the translation of medical audit data into educational needs data as had been described previously. This is in actuality one of several needed interpretive conversions of data into useful information[9] commented on earlier. It is a step that involves a high level of judgment on the part of the continuing education subcommittee, but the peer review committee still should provide the guidelines to expedite the process of interpreting profile analyses and educational needs assessments. In the process of doing these things, it also provides the direction and leadership to insist on consistency in the recording as well as the reporting of data in uniform and useful formats.

Step 5: Reevaluation. This is the step most easily ignored, for some reason, yet it is also the most crucial single step in assuring success of the whole review operation. It is the step that says: "Now that we have located a problem and tried to correct it, the question is whether we have succeeded." Essentially this consists of once again applying the same assessment methodology after the implementation of corrective actions that previously detected the existence of problems in care delivery or in the review process in the first place. It is, in short, the point at which follow-up MCEs or RSEs should be performed. As indicated on the flow diagram, this step involves a feedback loop to the PRC itself. It is not until the PRC is satisfied on the basis of systems performance data that things are working better that the issue is resolved and final reports can be written.

Step 6: PRC systems reports. On final determination that all steps at this review

level have been completed and properly taken a summary report must be prepared to appraise the medical staff, the review system staff, the hospital administration and the highest institutional authority of the status of the care system, the review system, and the PRC's stewardship of these broad responsibilities. In addition, these reports must provide the institution full coverage of all the informational reporting requirements of the PSRO.

REVIEW LEVEL 4

This is conceived as the highest level of review within a hospital. The responsibilities at this level direct downward to oversee the hospital's entire peer review system and direct outward to meet societal expectations including PSRO.

Conceptual base

Just as the PRC is vested with the power to make recommendations affecting the entire hospital, review level 4 is the functioning component vested with the power to order that they be carried out.

Organization structure

The functioning structural unit at level 4 for some hospitals might be their executive committee or their board of trustees or some mix thereof. The basic membership of the group would include the usual supervisory-level persons who typically populate such committees and boards. The membership of the level 4 review authority, however, probably will have to be expanded to include not only the mandated representatives of the public but also key review system personnel, including its director and representatives of all categories of care-provider personnel who are subject to review by their peers.

Ultimate responsibilities

The responsibilities of this highest functioning internal committee are to render final judgments in any matters affecting the institution as a whole. Following are some of the activities involved:

1. Final institutional appeals adjudication
2. The initiation or authorization of hospital-wide policies and procedures to improve the quality of care rendered to patients
3. The initiation or authorization of hospital-wide policies and procedures to redirect the conduct of the peer review system
4. Serve as the vested hospital authority in the negotiation of external (for example, PSRO) contracts
5. Assume ultimate responsibility for compliance with contractual review obligations to payors and comply with all statutory requirements
6. Create and maintain the environment and working conditions in which both the care providers and the care evaluators can do their work well

Positive reinforcement is always preferable over punitive measures as a constructive force to encourage the best performance from all those associated with the hospital. It may become progressively more important even to professionals that they be made aware of appreciation for the good work that is done and that recognition or reward is accorded those who provide exemplary care. This is because effective peer review by definition must exert pressure for change, and this is something easily misinterpreted as being coercive and negative. To counterbalance this an overtly positive contribution of incentive and reward must also be attributable to peer review. It is good to be able to end our discussion on such a positive note.

This is more than enough to occupy the time and resources available to this otherwise very busy policy-making group. We would not presume to detail here how it should structure itself or proceed in conducting its business. Thus we offer no flow diagram for level 4.

OVERVIEW

The structure, function, and activity of the four review levels described in this chapter were intended to provide the reader with a reasonably inclusive overview of the operations typically involved in a total peer review process and a hypothetical structure for carrying out that review. Greater operational detail and clarification of specific tasks and functions are described in various chapters of Part Two. It should be understood that the structures, functions, and procedures described here are offered as models and that for the individual hospital, variations in the model will require corresponding changes in specific operations at the local level.

REFERENCES

1. Report of the Committee on Finance: social security amendments of 1972, Washington, D.C., 1972, U.S. Government Printing Office, pp. 254-268.
2. Elsom, K. O.: Elements of the medical process, J.A.M.A. **217:**1226-1232, 1971.
3. Joint Commission on Accreditation of Hospitals: Accreditation manual for hospitals, Chicago, 1973, The Commission.
4. Fried, C.: Rights and health care—beyond equity and efficiency, N. Engl. J. Med. **293:**241-245, 1975.
5. Williamson, J. W.: Evaluating quality of patient care, J.A.M.A. **218:**564-569, 1971.
6. Donabedian, A.: Promoting quality through evaluating the process of patient care, Med. Care **6:**181-202, 1968.
7. Williamson, J. W., and McGuire, C.: Consecutive case conference, J. Med. Educ. **43:**1068-1074, 1968.
8. Stearns, N. S., Getchell, M. E., and Gold, R. A.: A systematic approach to developing education programs in community hospitals. In Continuing medical education in community hospitals: a manual for program development, Boston, 1971, Postgraduate Medical Institute, pp. 7-71.
9. McNeil, B. J., Keeler, E., and Adelstein, S. J.: Primer on certain elements of medical decision making, N. Engl. J. Med. **293:**211-215, 1975.

9

Design and content determinants of systematic peer review

PAUL Y. ERTEL

The how and the what of systematic medical peer review are inextricably tied together. The goal of this chapter therefore is to elucidate what is involved in relating the conduct of review activities (the review system) to what ought to be reviewed in the first place (the review content). There are many options a hospital might take in determining what the design configuration of its peer review program ultimately will be. By contrast the hospital exercises virtually no control over the fundamental disease processes that basically determine what kind of medical care is appropriate for its patients. Thus we see that the design of a review system is largely a matter of rational choice, while the content of review activities is wholly determined by the care process[1] and is in that sense not a matter of choice.

The most useful way to bring these concepts together is to relate them at the level of their determinants. In doing so it will be possible to show how the purpose of the review process influences the design of the review system and dictates how the review process will be conducted, but it will also be shown how clinical factors dictate the content of the review process.[2]

The point is simply this: given limited hospital resources for mounting a peer review program, some trade-offs have to be made between the completeness of a review system and its complexity (that is, cost). It is best that alternatives be chosen with full knowledge of which determinants are realistically subject to conscious choice and which are not.

CHOICE OF REVIEW PROGRAM

Institutional review objectives determine the choice of review programs and the basic methodology used to conduct peer review in most acute care hospitals. The selection between utilization review and quality review programs depends on whether the hospital's principal interest (objective) in mounting a peer review program stems from concerns about controlling the cost (utilization) of medical services or the quality of medical care or both.[3] These programs are illustrated in Table 9-1 and will be further discussed separately.

Utilization review program

The most commonly implemented subprograms of utilization review are admission certification and continued stay review (which are intimately associated with PSRO).[4] The surveillance of major services and discharge/transfer surveillance are two additional subprograms discussed

Table 9-1. Determinants of hospital-based peer review

Determinant	Example	Features	Relevance (basis of choice)
Review program	Utilization review	Cost control	Institutional review objectives
	Quality review	Quality control	Institutional review objectives
Review activity	Program evaluation	Management of care system	Institutional resources/capability
	Case evaluation	Management of individual case	Institutional resources/capability
Review strategies	Retrospective	Remedial intervention	Institutional review objectives
	Concurrent	Corrective intervention	Institutional review objectives
	Prospective	Preventive intervention	Institutional review objectives
Review content	Diagnostic plan	Diagnostic decisions	Clinical presentation
	Prognostic estimate	Functional assessment	Pathophysiologic variables
	Therapeutic plan	Therapeutic decisions	Clinical management objectives
	Care participation	Patient involvement	Patient motivation

in Chapters 7 and 8 that are of potential interest. The important thing to note here is that the selection from among the various utilization subprograms is one of conscious choice that ideally is the product of careful study and thought on the part of the hospital leadership.

Quality review program

More diversified subprograms fall under this heading, since quality review is much wider in scope and more complex in aggregate than is utilization review.[5] This is simply a function of the fact that quality determinations involve a more complex matrix of care elements to be monitored, as will be shown later.

CHOICE OF REVIEW ACTIVITY

In large part the choice of the review activity will be determined by the level of intensiveness or thoroughness of monitoring activities that are within the hospital's economic resources and staffing capability and that are also compatible with its service program. The two main divisions of review activity are referred to here as *program evaluation* and *case evaluation*. Specific choices among strategies will be directly related to the content of review activity undertaken.

Program evaluation

Generally speaking, review systems that aim at program evaluation are less complex and also less expensive to conduct. The most familiar forms of program evaluation are generally termed "cost control" and "quality control" programs. The objective of program evaluation is to assess and to help manage the system (or the process) of delivering care to the population served by the institution.[6] It is the kind of evaluation by which a PSRO, for example, may wish to compare the performance of one hospital against another. Performance data are obtained from all (or from groups) of patients and care providers in aggregate. Statistical norms are calculated from this accumulated experience, and standards are derived by defining the ranges of acceptable deviations from the norms. The review process consists of comparing hospital performance data against these standards.

Case evaluation

In contrast to the above, if case evaluation is the strategy chosen, it must be based on the assessment of care delivered by an individual care provider to a given patient. It is the objective of this kind of review program to evaluate or to influence the act (that is, the specific process) of delivering care to a single patient. Because of the focus on care delivered to a single individual, the rendering of a peer judgment is by definition situational,[7] and therefore the closer its proximity in time to the actual delivery of care, the more sensitive it can be and the greater impact it can have.

CHOICE OF REVIEW STRATEGY

Institutional review objectives typically dominate the selection of the main strategies for conducting whatever kind of review program the hospital has chosen to develop. The selection to be made is between retrospective, concurrent, and prospective review strategies, or some combination of the three. The basis for this choice will be the degree to which the review system is involved with case evaluation in contrast to program evaluation.

Retrospective review

Since program evaluation is entirely statistically based, retrospective review is the strategy most suitable to conducting this type of review activity. Some retrospective review component is also appropriate to generate the statistical data from which norms and standards of case evaluation may be based or its screening criteria modified, but this does not affect the mechanics of conducting the case review,[7] which is basically concurrent.

Concurrent review

This may be described as the strategy of necessity in case evaluation for both utilization and quality review programs. Its contribution to case evaluation derives from the need to give immediate attention to any serious problems detected in care in order for the individual patient to derive any benefit from corrective measures. While retrospection is useful to improve the future care of patients with similar problems, there is no such thing as improving the care of a given patient with a specific medical problem by retrospection and hindsight.

Prospective review

This may be described as the strategy of the future. It uniquely offers the capability to monitor and to intervene in the care process before a patient experiences harm from his care or before the hospital bill mounts up.[8] While some clear-cut applications of this strategy are currently practical (for example, the advance clearance of patients for elective surgery, and so on), a great deal more needs to be known about the delivery of care and the impact of review programs on it before this strategy will find widespread use (or acceptance).

SCOPE OF REVIEW CONTENT

Once it is determined which type of review activity and which programs are to be conducted and what basic strategies will be used to carry them out, the content of the review process must be defined in operational terms.

Unlike the first three selections, which are largely matters of institutional choice, the content of the review process is largely determined by care objectives and the actual demands of clinical management rather than by review objectives or policy decisions on the part of the hospital leadership. This is because the content of a review program nearly always must reflect the basic care elements, that is, "three arts" of medical practice.[9] These care elements in turn are dictated by medical needs that arise from disease processes in patients.

Among the care objectives consistent from one clinical condition to another and therefore relevant to peer review are (1) to establish the correct diagnosis, (2) to assess the prognosis, (3) to institute appropriate therapy, (4) to deal with the human needs of patients as individuals, and (5) to institute a plan for establishing continuity in ongoing personal care. Relevant comprehensive review systems would thus be obliged to monitor key care elements in each of these objectives of clinical management. They must also be responsive to the unique individuality of each patient, to the natural forces that direct his disease

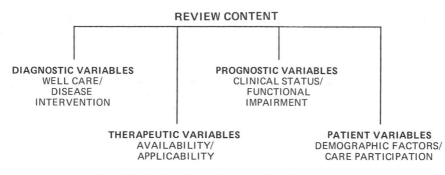

Fig. 9-1. Major determinants of review content.

and healing processes, and to the milieu of hospital practice. Consequently the major factors that determine the content of peer review (that is, the care elements or services to be monitored) can be cited as follows: diagnostic variables, therapeutic variables, prognostic variables, and patient variables (Fig. 9-1). A closer examination of these variables reveals how they can influence review strategies, define data requirements, and shape the design of the review method.

Diagnostic variables

What constitutes appropriate care is most always dependent on the patient's specific mix of problems—medical, emotional, and social, since care must relate to all facets that impact on the patient's condition. Expressing this thought through an example, a total body cast is as absurdly inappropriate to treat diabetes as an insulin injection would be to set a broken bone. Also, we can readily see that the care of the healthy consists of clinical measures that are essentially unrelated to any disease state. The relevance of this concept to peer review is that the specific set of services appropriate to monitor the care of a patient when he is well differs conceptually from that set appropriate to monitor his care when sick. This is because well person care is largely predicated on the minimization of risk factors, the detection of subclinical diseases, and the initiation of general preventive measures that are reasonably appropriate to a population defined on the basis of age, sex, and other characteristics. In contrast, disease intervention aims at determining the nature or cause of complaints and physiologic disturbances that already exist in a particular patient and then to initiate treatment that is as specifically effective as current clinical capabilities will allow.

Well care. What constitutes quality health care is definable by peer consensus in terms of not only which specific services are appropriate but also their optimal sequence. To cite just one example, recommendations for specific items of well child care and their timing (precise ages when most appropriately done) have for years been recommended at the national level by the Joint Committee on Health Problems in Education.[10] Where there is broad staff acceptance of such recommendations, the hospital's review system can be highly specific in specifying particular items of service to be monitored in all patients and in what sequence (age adjusted, of course) the patient should receive them. This shows that where there is agreement in what peers can accept as minimal (or optimal) standards for the care of the healthy, there can be greater uniformity in how it is monitored than is generally applicable for disease intervention.

Disease intervention. In contrast to the above, what constitutes appropriate care of the ill is more uniquely tailored to the individual and his diagnosis than it is generalizable (uniform) from patient to patient. There may be some commonalities or similar patterns in the care of closely related conditions, but inherent diversities in medically indicated services are great across the entire diagnostic spectrum and unique to individual patients. That is why considerable latitude must be allowed in the review methodology to monitor a wide range of medical and clinical observations. It is of course a practical necessity that the explicit standards or criteria on which the review of disease intervention is based should consist of generalizations that are descriptive of appropriate care in the majority of cases or a typical patient with a given condition. But it must also be recognized that averages are derived from extremes and that individual clinical courses may require care alternatives in clinical management that deviate considerably from what might be described as average. Flexibility must therefore be built into the monitoring system to accommodate commonly occurring clinical variants.

Prognostic variables

This heading brings to bear those factors related to how seriously ill and how severely incapacitated the patient with any given diagnosis is likely to become over time. If a disease process is a relentless one leading inevitably to invalidism or premature death, the objective of management is directed toward patient comfort and support. A more benign disease process would have a circumscribed physiologic impact, and the objective of management would probably aim at a cure. There are all gradations in between. The importance of this to the review process is that distinctions must be made concerning what constitutes appropriate care on the basis of prognosis in addition to the diagnosis. For example, the proper management of in situ carcinomas or localized Hodgkin's disease should aim at cure, while the management of metastatic or disseminated forms of the same diseases would aim at palliation.

Clinical status. This term refers to the pathophysiologic variants of a disease process or injury as manifested in the duration of its clinical activity. What constitutes proper care in the acute form of a disease state (or intoxication and so on) may differ markedly from the care appropriate to its chronic form or long-term effects. Gross differences in management are not infrequently called for in the acute versus the chronic forms of polio, rheumatic fever, gall bladder disease, or lead poisoning, for example. Beyond this, management objectives may also differ, depending on how mild or severe the disease process itself might be and what influence host factors might play. An acute disease process that is also severe in its clinical manifestations is likely to be an emergency type of case that may even call for lifesaving techniques. In general the more acutely and seriously ill the patient is with a given condition, the more pressing it is to establish a diagnosis and the more intensive the therapy must be. There are often both qualitative and quantitative increases in the demands of medical management under these circumstances.

What all this means to the design of review methodologies is that both in the criteria used and in the review process itself there must be allowances made for variants in the clinical status or natural history of the disease process in the individual patient.

Functional impairment. Often a part of the overall management plan is directed specifically toward rehabilitation in the sense of getting the patient on his feet again. That may require anything from simple advice to formal and extensive programs of medical, physical, or mental rehabilitation with or without the utilization of mobility aids, mechanical devices, home care, and a variety of other community services. Which of these rehabilitative services are medically appropriate depends not on the patient's diagnosis but on the degree of impairment of his social activities, mobility, activities of daily living, and self-care capability. Where self-care is critical to the outcome, it should also be monitored.

Therapeutic variables

There are usually legitimate options in what constitutes appropriate medical or surgical treatment of a given condition (though there are exceptions of course). Where there is a choice among acceptable forms of therapy, the selection will be affected largely by factors of availability and applicability.

Availability. The availability of a care service implies that a professionally accepted (validated) treatment modality exists in the medical armamentarium and also that this specific service can be made available to a particular patient. Factors that determine whether an acceptable therapeutic service is realistically available to the patient include access to essential treatment materials (drugs or other expendables), necessary equipment, appropriate physical facilities, professional personnel who are properly trained, and support personnel who are essential to the conduct of the given procedures. If any of these are unavailable, then that fact should be documented in the review process, since it is the root cause of care inadequacies or inappropriate resource utilization.

Applicability. Given the physical availability of a therapeutic modality, it is then necessary to consider its medical applicability (that is, clinical appropriateness) to patient care in both general and specific terms. General applicability pertains to those treatments considered medically appropriate for the given clinical entity as typically manifested in the average patient. It is this level of applicability at which explicit criteria are aimed. It is also the level at which quality control programs operate. Specific applicability, however, pertains to the treatment regimen determined to be most appropriate for the given disease entity in the individual patient. As we have seen, this involves taking into account the diagnosis, prognosis, clinical status, impairment level, and the fact that the patient is being treated in the local milieu with whatever resources exist there. This is the level at which implicit judgments of knowledgeable peers must be operative. The focus on the individual case is also the essence of due process and the key to the preservation of humaneness in the surveillance as well as in the delivery of medical care.[11] When care delivered to an individual undergoes this kind of quality assessment and is backed up by an affirmative program for taking any and all needed corrective actions, this constitutes that form of peer review we believe is best described as individual quality assurance.

Patient variables

There are some personal characteristics of patients that are also sometimes of clinical significance and therefore of relevance to peer review. These characteristics relate to their risk factors. Risk factors signal probabilities of developing certain diseases and constitute a group of items that may actually impact on the management of patients in a direct manner.

Demographic factors. Age is once again a demographic characteristic of significance to the monitoring of care. For example, infants are often more seriously ill from a number of common diseases (for example, pneumonia) than are adults and even older children.[12] What constitutes proper care of patients at either age extreme may therefore call for more vigorous therapy or earlier hospitalizations than might be considered medically necessary for other patients. The patient's sex may determine the expression of disease (as in hemophilia) or its seriousness. Racial and ethnic factors may also relate to the expression of some diseases. Personal habits such as smoking[13] and drinking[14] or physical characteristics such as obesity are frequently of great importance.[15] Variations of this theme are endless, but before leaving the topic there is a problem area that should be mentioned. The management of difficult, complex, or unstable conditions in patients where geographic isolation is involved can pose all kinds of impediments to rational management.[16] Geographic obstacles to the provision of quality care or to the conservation of resources are examples of factors external to the care system that need to be monitored by the review system. The review system is obliged to recognize and account for all such legitimate exceptions from care standards that are imposed by significant demographic factors.

Care participation (personality factors). The clinical importance of personality factors can vary enormously among individuals of course and range from virtually no influence to a total negation of the care management plan. Personality factors tend to become more relevant to peer review as the opportunity increases for effective patient participation in his or her own care. Conversely, the patient who refuses to cooperate in the care plan or who refuses to care for himself must be recognized by the review system for limiting management options, for redirecting the utilization of resources, for altering the quality of care received, and for being responsible in some measures for the outcome achieved. Newer approaches to self-care strategies have emphasized more independence on the part of individuals to care for themselves. "Self-care distinguishes itself from other medical activities in that the process leaves the individual with specific knowledge and skills for self-evaluation of his health status across time."[17] This calls for incorporating into the review process some method of detecting when the patient's involvement in the care process has been less than optimal and why. The importance of building into peer review some mechanism for encouraging patient participation and self-care is derived from its relevance to the evolution of a care system that is more responsive to the ends and desires of patients and of society at large.

We have previously seen how a host of variables can influence the choice of the type of review program to be instituted and the strategy to implement it. The content of what should be subjected to review, on the other hand, means taking a close look at the care process the review process is designed to evaluate.

SURVEILLANCE OF THE CARE PROCESS

The contemporary medical care process that peer review is obliged to monitor would most closely fit what has been described as the engineering approach to medical care.[18] It is the surveillance of comprehensive care that is technologically oriented (irrespective of its setting) that is the subject of this discussion. Reduced to its fundamentals, a correspondingly comprehensive surveillance program would monitor all elements of the care process that can influence the clinical effectiveness of management objectives and all clinical outcomes that can influence the well-being of patients. While this generalization applies to both utilization review and quality review, there are more care elements and clinical outcomes applicable to quality assessment than to utilization review.

Scope of the care process

In the interest of brevity, key elements of the care process that relate to clinical effectiveness are presented in summary form in the following outline. This listing may prove useful in two ways. First, in defining the scope of care activities that potentially could apply to any given case, it defines the potential scope of comprehensive peer review. Second, it can serve as a checklist to make an inventory of how many care elements are covered by any given review program under evaluation. For example, we have indicated by an asterisk all those care elements that might be considered for inclusion in a comprehensive program of utilization review.

SCOPE OF THE CARE PROCESS (ELEMENTS OF CLINICAL EFFECTIVENESS)

A. Diagnostic decision process
    *1. Prepare appropriate diagnostic plan
     2. Obtain and properly interpret data from clinical history, physical exam, laboratory and special studies
     3. Arrive at accurate diagnosis and prognosis

B. Therapeutic decision process
  *1. Properly assess the therapeutic need, risk, cost, and available options
  *2. Arrive at appropriate treatment plan (that is, medically indicated treatment type, amount, duration, and care facility)
C. Conduct of care
  1. Skillful performance of diagnostic procedures
  2. Skillful performance of therapeutic procedures
  3. Proper surveillance and management of clinical response or complications
  4. Optimal patient rehabilitation
  *5. Clinical preparations for discharge or transfer to other (for example, less costly) treatment facility
D. Preventive intervention
  1. Screening for health problems
  2. Establishment of definitive diagnosis(es) or risks
  *3. Initiate appropriate measures of prevention, intervention, and education
E. Patient (community) involvement in the care process
  1. Prepare patient and family to participate in and share responsibility for care
  *2. Arrange for ongoing personal care and involve community as indicated
  *3. Fulfill obligations of accountability to patient and public

Sequence of the care process

The care process is with few exceptions a dynamic one, and the sequence in which clinical services are provided can be as important as their proper selection. The natural course of the disease process and the objectives of medical management determine the appropriateness of the timing and sequencing of services. Thus for surveillance purposes it can be critical to monitor in which order the items of service were provided. The four principal care sequences a review system may monitor are presented in the following outline as a simplified summary that highlights the leading characteristic of each.

SEQUENCE OF THE CARE PROCESS
A. **Acute care intervention** (self-limited conditions)

1. Iatrotropic stimulus (for example, patient concerns or symptoms)
2. Action to seek care (by patient)
3. Participatory involvement of patient/family/community in management
4. Initiation of diagnostic services
5. Initiation of therapeutic services
6. Follow-up (to assure diagnostic validity, therapeutic response, and resolution of problems)
7. Ongoing personal care plan (initiated/continued by care system)

B. **Chronic care intervention** (long-term conditions)
1. Iatrotropic stimulus (for example, patient concerns or symptoms)
2. Action to seek care (by patient)
3. Participatory involvement of patient/family/community in management
4. Initiation of diagnostic services
5. Initiation of therapeutic services
6. Assess response to therapy
7. Monitor for progression/complications of disease or therapy
8. Manage complications/progression of disease
9. Rehabilitate patient to maximum achievable functional status
10. Integrate health maintenance measures with therapeutic intervention
11. Institute ongoing personal care plan (if none provided elsewhere)

C. **Disease control program** (subclinical or presymptomatic conditions)
1. Identify specific population at risk to treatable conditions (by care system)
2. Educate population at risk to detect early signs of illness
3. Promote patient action to seek early diagnosis (or screen population at risk)
4. Institute early definitive diagnostic services
5. Initiate early therapeutic services
6. Assure follow-up care (if needed)

D. **Preventive care program** (conditions at risk)
1. Action to identify preventable conditions to which general population is at risk (by care system)
2. Educate general population to need for preventive measures against these conditions
3. Promote patient action to seek preventive services
4. Institute preventive measures

As the outline above shows, what constitutes an appropriate care sequence is defined by the objectives of the care program and the type of clinical condition being managed. Perhaps the sequence that comes most readily to mind as a model care episode would be typified in the management of a patient who develops chest pain or a sore throat, that is, some symptom he considers serious or annoying and for which he seeks medical attention. The sequence of care initiated for acute conditions is in part a direct response to the patient's symptoms or worries (that is, the iatrotropic stimulus), and in part it is related to the diagnostic or therapeutic management plan the clinician may think appropriate. An important aspect of managing acute conditons is that they place a finite limit on the duration of both care and surveillance responsibilities. Chronic diseases, on the other hand, create a longer-term surveillance obligation and are usually also of broader scope and complexity, since they are more likely to involve rehabilitative needs, interdisciplinary care, problems in care logistics, or in the continuity of care over time. (These generalizations are presented for illustrative purposes only, and it is recognized that exceptions exist to each.)

But any care model that begins with an existing disease in a sense represents a failure in disease prevention. As one moves away from the management of a symptomatic clinical condition into early disease detection and especially to disease prevention programs, one is moving from management objectives directed toward a personal care of sick individuals to management objectives aimed at healthy populations. With this change in goals comes an overall shift in emphasis from the specifics of remedial care to the principles of disease prevention (hygiene, prophylactic measures, public education, and responsible self-care). There is also an accompanying shift in the sequence in which care services are delivered. Since care processes are likely to be structured in any number of different ways, they may follow different patterns as a function of management objectives. Review processes must have the capability to do likewise.

One final point: The old adage that an ounce of prevention is worth a pound of cure is just as relevant for the review system as it is for the care system. Just as disease prevention is preferable and less costly than disease treatment, it is better to prevent the delivery of inappropriate care than to deal with its consequences. The long-range implication of this principle with respect to peer review is that it favors an evolution from retrospective toward prospective review sequences.

SURVEILLANCE OF CARE (PATIENT) OUTCOMES

If surveillance of the care process looks at what was clinically done for the patient, then surveillance of the clinical outcome seeks to answer questions about patient benefits of the care. An overview of what is involved in the ongoing monitoring of patient outcomes reveals that there are several kinds of outcomes that could be monitored and a variety of circumstances under which certain of them become more clinically relevant than others. Just as with the care process, it is when alterations in patient outcomes are of clinical significance that they become relevant to peer review. The relevancy of patient outcomes to the evaluation of care is dependent on four key factors: the review strategy employed, the timing of review activities, the objectives of clinical management, and the objectives of the review program employed.

Review strategies

As with process review, outcome review also centers on whether a program evaluation strategy or a case evaluation strategy is employed. Program evaluation by definition examines aggregated statistics on the outcomes of care as manifested in the entire population served by a hospital (or among selected subgroups). Case evaluation, on the other hand, examines the clinical outcome of individual patients one at a time.

Time frame

The natural course of a given disease process largely determines what is the most appropriate time frame in which to monitor the care outcome in patients (just as it determines when to monitor the care process). The relationship between the choice of review strategy and the potentially relevant time frames to conduct outcome assessments is depicted in Fig. 9-2. While the very best time for conducting outcome reviews may need to be determined on an individual case basis, there are nevertheless some useful generalizations or patterns suggested by this model that are useful as guidelines. Those clinical conditions that are either relatively brief in duration or require only limited intervention generally call for a short-term outcome evaluation (either at the time of hospital discharge, just prior to it, or shortly afterwards). This is usually the most appropriate time also for the review of relatively minor elective procedures (such as herniorrhaphy). For those more persistent conditions in which optimal hospital management simply initiates therapy or inaugurates a rehabilitative program that will continue after discharge, an intermediate outcome assessment may be more appropriate. This may be arbitrarily defined anywhere from a month or two to a year or two after discharge. Examples might include a 6- to 12-month follow-up to determine the stability of control for hypertension, the induction and persistence of remission in lipoid nephrosis, or for assessing functional return after a serious leg fracture. Long-term outcome evaluation (2 years or more) may be more appropriate to the long-range assessment of the impact of restorative procedures such as coronary bypass operations, the impact of intervention in degenerative conditions such as joint replacements in rheumatoid arthritis, the cure rate in cancer chemotherapy, and so on. As Fig. 9-2 shows, the potential exists for outcome studies to reflect six different data bases relevant to the strategies used and their timing. The reader is therefore well-advised to bear this in mind in considering how and when it might be best to mount such studies or in evaluating and attempting to compare data from different outcome studies.

Care objectives

The natural history of a disease process must also be considered in determining whether a given clinical outcome is consistent with the objectives of care and therefore important to monitor. If, for example, the expected outcome of a disease entity is uniformly fatal, the clinical management objectives will be directed toward other aspects of care, and the occurrence of death in itself has little or no value as an indicator of inappropriate care. The reverse is true of course for a uniformly benign condition. Relevance exists only when the natural course of a disease process is potentially responsive to management or when any given outcome can be demonstrably related to the care process in a cause-effect relationship. An example of the latter would be typified by the restoration of motion in a limb after joint surgery and so on. Assuming these conditions are met, the objectives of the review program take on importance and will be discussed next.

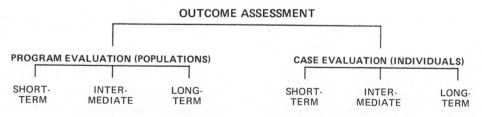

Fig. 9-2. Time frame for performing outcome assessments.

Review objectives

Again the objectives set for the review program determine what kind of care outcomes will come under surveillance. If, for example, the control of excessive costs is the chief concern and utilization review is the type of program employed, then the outcomes of interest are the number of unnecessary admissions denied, the number of hospital days saved (extensions denied), the number of unnecessary major procedures (such as operations) deferred, and the effectiveness of discharge planning (to arrange earlier discharges of patients or transfers to long-term care facilities).

If, on the other hand, the maintenance of high-quality care is the chief concern and quality review is the operational surveillance program,[19] then outcomes of general interest might include patient survival (in potentially lethal conditions), the prompt resolution of acute conditions, the regression (or arrest) of chronic ones, ambulation and mobility, and the patient's functional status (including one's ability to care for himself and to conduct his normal social activities such as employment). Outcomes of more specific relevance are those which directly relate to the disease process itself or its overt manifestations. If, for example, a diabetic was admitted to the hospital for the control of ketoacidosis, then his urine ketones should be under control at discharge. The same thing applies to the completion of planned procedures. If the patient was admitted to have a herniorrhaphy, the hernia should be promptly and satisfactorily repaired without complications, and so on.

COMBINED PROCESS AND OUTCOME REVIEW

Whether outcome assessment is more relevant or more important than process assessment seems to us to be a moot point at this moment in medical history. Until a great deal more is known about what kind of care is being delivered now (how good it is and whether costs can be contained without sacrificing quality), it is difficult to rationally defend one preference over the other. It is especially hazardous to argue for the exclusion of any program of peer review that can tell us anything we do not already know about what valid current care practices are and what their actual impact is on the health status of patients and on the cost equation. We therefore conclude this discussion with reflections on the merits of a measured incremental approach toward combining process and outcome measurements.[3]

First, there seems to be an evolutionary trend building that favors the development of fairly comprehensive review methodologies[20] meriting an endorsement of the concept by the staff of the Bureau of Quality Assurance.[21] There are several reasons for this, but the most persuasive is the need to overcome the disadvantages of incomplete or misleading feedback when only limited review programs are employed. Quality assurance programs that monitor only the efficacy of care may achieve their objective of fostering better care for the individual but at an unconscionable expense in manpower and resource utilization. Similarly cost control programs that monitor only the efficiency of care may be successful in containing costs and resource utilization but at the expense of an unconscionable degradation in the quality of personal care.[5] The best assurance that quality control programs do not promote reckless spending is to monitor their cost impact, and the best way to assure that utilization review programs do not degrade medical care is to monitor their clinical impact (outcomes). These functional interrelationships are illustrated in Table 9-2.

Thus it can be seen that natural evolutionary pressures do favor a convergence of purpose if not a complete synthesis of methodologies.

Second, if it is a safe assumption that evolutionary change will be directed toward comprehensiveness in review systems (as in care systems), then the actual

Table 9-2. Interrelationships of quality and utilization review

Review program	Review objective	Negative impact	Monitoring needs
Quality	Promote efficacy in care process	Excessive cost?	Resource consumption
Utilization	Promote efficiency in care process	Degraded care?	Clinical outcome

starting point (initial review methodology) is less relevant than the commitment to a flexibility in the review system that can change in this direction. What this means in terms of evaluating existing systems is to look for the abundance of linkage points where quality can be tied to utilization (and vice versa) and the degree of resilience in the supporting structures (for example, data systems) to effect this linkage logically and economically.

Third, if review systems do undergo significant evolutionary changes toward comprehensiveness, demands for greater efficiency will likely favor the eventual incorporation of progressively more technologic advances into the review process. In the meantime one should probably remain open-minded about what new capabilities can be brought to peer review through advances in both computer hardware and software.[22] Data-handling chores that are technically unfeasible or economically impractical by today's standards could become tomorrow's routine way of doing things. This would have the effect of expanding the scope of cost-effective peer review.

If a significantly greater amount of automation does become available to support review activities at the hospital level, then this is likely to stimulate evolutionary changes in review strategies. Already presented in Chapter 7 has been a technical explanation why the incorporation of more automation in review systems would favor a shift from a retrospective to a prospective strategy for conducting review operations. Explained in simpler terms, the rationale amounts to the ounce of prevention concept. It is far better to be sure

in advance that the patient will receive quality medical care (or that unnecessary costs will be avoided) than it is to attempt to do something about it after the fact. This we submit may be the strongest long-range determinant to shape the kind of peer review systems that exist a decade or two from now.

REFERENCES

1. McNeil, B. J., and Adelstein, S. J.: The value of case finding in hypertensive renovascular disease, N. Engl. J. Med. **293:**221-226, 1975.
2. McNeil, B. J., Keeler, E., and Adelstein, S. J.: Primer on certain elements of medical decision making, N. Engl. J. Med. **293:**211-215, 1975.
3. Thorner, R. M.: Health program evaluation in relation to health programming, Technical Rep. **86:**525-532, 1971.
4. Hospital review expansion seen, Am. Med. News, Feb 17, 1975, p. 6.
5. Welch, C. E.: PSRO—pros and cons, N. Engl. J. Med. **290:**1319-1324, 1974.
6. Williamson, J. W.: Evaluating quality of patient care, J.A.M.A. **218:**564-569, 1971.
7. Curtis, P.: Problems in primary care, Update Int., pp. 296-298, 1974.
8. Donabedian, A.: Promoting quality through evaluating the process of patient care, Med. Care **6:**181-202, 1968.
9. Harrington, E. D.: A major pitfall: inadequate assessment of the patient's needs resulting in inappropriate treatment, Pediatr. Clin. North Am. **12:**141-173, 1965.
10. Dukelow, D. A.: Health approval of school children, ed. 4, Washington, D.C., 1969, Joint Committee on Health Problems in Education, National Education Association and the American Medical Association.
11. Fried, C.: Rights and health care—beyond equity and efficiency, N. Engl. J. Med. **293:**241-245, 1975.
12. Vaughn, V. C., McKay, J. R., and Nelson, W. E.: Textbook of pediatrics, Philadelphia, 1975, W. B. Saunders Co., p. 971.
13. Norton, A.: The new dimensions of medicine, London, 1969, Hodder & Stoughton.

14. Abse, D.: Medicine on trial, New York, 1969, Crown Publishers.

15. Abelson, P. H.: Cost-effective health care, Science **192:**620, 1976.

16. Davidson, G. R.: Medicine through the ages, London, 1968, Methuen & Co.

17. Aldridge, M. C.: Self-care as an alternative future for community health systems, Denver, October 1976, Medical Futures Committee of Planned Parenthood, p. 14 (working paper).

18. Rushmer, R. F., and Huntsman, L. L.: Biomedical engineering, Science **167:**840-844, 1970.

19. Jessee, W. F., Munier, W. B., Fielding, J. E., and Goran, M. J.: PSRO an educational force for improving quality care, N. Engl. J. Med. **292:**668-676, 1975.

20. King, L. S.: The growth of medical thought, Chicago, 1963, University of Chicago Press.

21. Goran, M. J., Roberts, J. S., Kellogg, M. A., Fielding, J., and Jessee, W.: The PSRO hospital review system, Med. Care **13**(suppl.):1-32, 1975.

22. Barnett, G. O.: Medicine and computers, The New Physician, February 1970, pp. 119-120.

10

Management information systems and the costs of systematic peer review

JAMES E. SORENSEN
PAUL Y. ERTEL

Medical peer review starts with the management control system of the health service deliverer. A health care management control system enables health care managers

1. To make better plans that relate to organizational goals and objectives based on the relative benefits and cost of alternative courses of action
2. To have better control that assures efficient and effective action in pursuing the organization's objectives

But plans and controls require four generic types of information: *planning information,* which concerns what services the organization will render and to whom and what resources the organization will use to provide these services, and *performance information,* which concerns how effectively the organization is doing its job and how efficiently the organization is using its resources. Developing the capacity to provide planning and performance information requires a management information system (MIS). The MIS must be dominated by what information is needed in decision making. The MIS must produce information that

1. Defines how current resources are required and consumed (for exam-

ple, how professional staff are deployed)
2. Assesses the pattern of service delivery (for example, who receives what types and amounts of services)
3. Provides monitoring aids for various health care providers and managers (for example, report on whether particular admissions were inappropriate)
4. Develops data for multiple reporting requirements (for example, reporting to funding agencies or payment agents such as the Social Security Administration or PSRO review)
5. Creates a data base for planning (for example, identifying changing patterns of utilization)
6. Assesses outcomes of rendered services (for example, level of functioning of client, changes in symptoms)

As varying forms of medical peer review emerge (for example, PSRO, PSRO hospital-delegated review, hospital-based and self-initiated reviews), both service deliverers and service monitors will sense the vital role of and the demands placed on an MIS in their respective organizations. While this chapter focuses initially on the information system of a hospital deliverer, a service monitor (for example,

PSRO) can benefit from and use the same analysis, since they too must develop systems to develop planning and control information.

But information systems are not free. The balance between enough information to make adequate planning and control decisions and the cost of developing and maintaining an information system is a constant cost-benefit struggle. Whenever any organization expands its information system beyond the satisfaction of minimal legal requirements and routine problem solving, the continuing question becomes: Are the benefits worth the investment?

The themes of this chapter are simple:

1. Effective medical peer review starts with the development of a management information at the level of service delivery. The requirements and characteristics of management information vary by level of decision making and type of organizational function. The physician, the nurse, the skilled attendant, and their immediate managers collectively require considerably more detailed information to perform their tasks than higher level superiors or reviewers. Quality assessment and utilization review, for example, extract or aggregate specific key items for analysis and comparison by drawing information from patient records or clinical files and management records. Without an adequate information system, quality or use reviews are stymied and diminished in effectiveness. Organizations who may review deliverers of services are dependent on the service deliverer's information systems—input to the reviewer is the output of the deliverer.

2. An understanding of the content and underlying concepts of information systems is required to build and operate an effective yet efficient medical peer review system. Not all information that health care managers or reviewers receive, need, or use comes from the information system. A phone call from a close friend or a casual comment by a medical colleague in a group discussion may have a large impact and can change the whole course of an organization. This informal information system is acknowledged as important, but this chapter focuses on the formal, structured information system planned for managing the organization and the medical peer review.

3. Information is not free or even inexpensive. Information should be viewed as a valuable but expensive resource, should be used in improving and in managing the delivery of health care services, and should be evaluated for its own cost-effectiveness. A highly specific but timely look at emerging PSRO requirements highlights inadequate concern for the costs of information systems and medical peer review.

REQUIREMENTS AND CHARACTERISTICS OF MANAGEMENT INFORMATION
Level of managerial activity

The information needs of a health care manager vary by levels of managerial activity. Because the level of the management activity influences the characteristics of the information used, information systems must be designed to provide different types of information at different levels. Four general managerial levels may be identified within health care organizations:

1. Strategic planning
   a. Setting organizational goals
   b. Outlining policies and objectives
   c. Identifying general range of appropriate organizational activities
   d. Long-range planning
2. Tactical or managerial control
   a. Short-range activities for acquiring and allocating resources
   b. Identifying new services or locations or services
   c. Deciding on service location layout and personnel requirements
   d. Analysis of budgets and variances from budget
3. Operational control
   a. Ensuring specific tasks are imple-

mented in an effective and efficient manner

b. Accepting or rejecting specific clients

c. Ensuring quality of service at point of delivery

d. Allocating personnel to predetermined programmatic plans

e. Determining reasons for variations of expenditures from budgeted amounts

4. Clerical inputs

a. Completing data capture forms according to prescribed procedures

b. Performing assigned functional tasks

Clerical systems feed information into the decision-oriented information systems at higher levels of the organization. As management activity moves from the lower levels of the organization to higher levels, the decision emphasis turns from operations to control to planning and policy making,[1,p.12] while planning and control operate throughout the entire organization. The emphasis is decidedly different at the varying activity levels. Data are condensed and filtered until they become information for decision making.[1,p.10] Conceptualization of the data-to-information process through varying levels of managerial activity is presented in Fig. 10-1.

Medical peer review has its beginning in the clerical inputs, since the primary re-

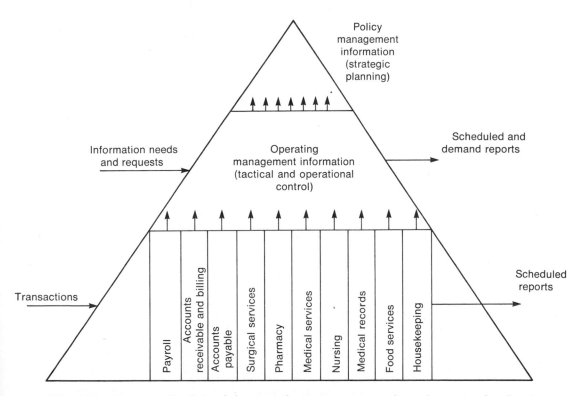

Fig. 10-1. Conceptualization of data-to-information process through varying levels of managerial activity. *Transactions* refer to interactions with the system in connection with its operation (patients using services, purchases from outside vendors, paying the medical and nursing staff, and so on). *Scheduled reports* refer to outputs from the processing system in a fixed format at a fixed time (census reports, drug inventory status, payroll summaries, budget variances, balance sheets, income statements, and so on). *Demand reports* refer to outputs based on special requests (explanation of admission, cost of a certain service, explanations why costs exceed budget, and so on). (Adapted from Head, R.: Datamation, May 1967.)

view team is focusing on the day-to-day operations such as surveying new patient admissions and assessing patient progress and readiness for new interventions. Often preestablished procedures and decision rules are used and specific data capture forms utilized to encourage consistent, efficient, and effective health services to clients.

Utilization review is basically another form of operational control. Only at a level 2 review–a peer review committee focused on utilization, medical audit, evaluation, continuing education–are higher levels of control activated. Level 2 review (and level 3 appeal) incorporates strategic planning through the setting and reviewing of objectives as well as managerial (or tactical) control by assessing deviations from objectives.

The characteristics of information needed for planning and management vary by level of managerial activity. Strategic decision making, especially long-range planning, requires greater amounts of external information, lower levels of accuracy, and higher levels of summarization. Tactical decisions require more accurate, precise, current, and more repetitive information. Operational decisions, however, require the most detailed information. Specific, accurate, frequent, and current data are required for health care deliverers and managers to evaluate the immediate response required for short-range changes in day-to-day operation. Table 10-1 summarizes the interaction of characteristics of information and level of decision making.

Organizational function

Another source of variation in the characteristics of information stems from organizational function such as the service delivery, personnel, and finance/accounting or evaluation function. Often each functional area of organization requires specific types of information, and this frequently leads to functional information subsystems that merge ideally as an integrated management information system. This federation of functional subsystems, while processing functionally specific informational needs, may often use a common data base (but maintaining some unique files) while sharing common computer programs. A matrix of functional subsystems and managerial activities is summarized in Fig. 10-2. The size of the subsystem is usually inverse to the level of the managerial activities and is pictorially represented by varying-sized rectangles, with more of the subsystem being devoted to lower level managerial activities and comparatively smaller portions being devoted to higher level activities.

Characteristics of information change as the managerial function changes. The service delivery function needs data, for example, on the population at risk, clients,

Table 10-1. Information characteristics by decision category*

Characteristics	Decision making	
	Operational ←——— Tactical ———→ Strategic	
Source	Largely internal	Largely external
Scope	Well-defined, narrow	Very wide
Level of aggregation	Detailed	Aggregate
Time horizon	Historical	Future
Currency	Highly current	Older
Required accuracy	Higher	Lower
Frequency of use	Very frequent	Infrequent

*Adapted from Gorry, G. A., and Morton, M. S. S.: Framework for management information systems, Sloan Management Rev., Fall 1971, p. 59.

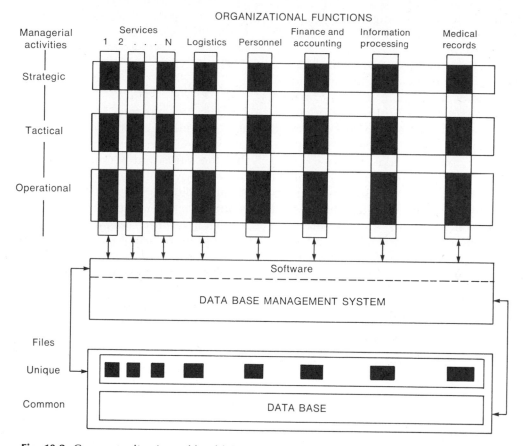

Fig. 10-2. Conceptualization of health care information systems. (Adapted from Sorensen, J. E., and Elpers, R.: Developing information systems for human service organizations. In Attkisson, C., et al., editors: Evaluation of human service programs, New York, 1977, Academic Press.)

historic and current utilization of services, and progress on treatment plans. The personnel management function, however, needs data on employees' professional training, experience, years of service, and pay grade. Some data will be associated with only one function, while other data will be used by several functions. Years of service may only be used by the personnel department, but hours of rendered service may be used by managers in service delivery function as well as by payroll, cost-finding, and billing in the accounting/finance function. Managers in the service delivery function could use hours of rendered service to evaluate the level of effort by various professional staff, while accounting/finance may use the same information for billing a specific client, insurance, agency, or reimbursing an agency for services received by the client.

Information characteristics[2] such as accuracy or precision (less to more accurate), age of data (younger to older), repetitiveness (less to more repetitive), summarization (less to more summarized), descriptive contents (less to more descriptive), and source (less to more outside) also seem to vary by the particular managerial function. The accounting function, for example, requires precise, older, repetitive, and summarized data at one extreme, where a service delivery function (for example, medical nursing station) requires accurate, up-to-date, detailed, and often descriptive data.

The characteristics of information vary both by level of decision making and by organizational function. The information system created as a health care organization grows must be correspondingly varied and complex. If it is created in an unsystematic, piecemeal fashion, as is often the case, it can be excessively redundant and ineffective. The MIS designer attempts to integrate existing and needed information functions to best serve the organization at its current size and stage of development. Now this discussion focuses on the content of the information system.

CONCEPTUAL CONTENT OF HEALTH CARE INFORMATION SYSTEMS

Within a health care organization, information is needed for a variety of purposes. Information is required for
1. Clinical monitoring
   a. Supervision and review of medical and surgical treatment interventions
   b. Communication of background and instructions to those who deal with the patient
2. Research
3. Management
   a. Planning and controlling the acquisition and use of the organization's resources
   b. Assessing the efficiency and effectiveness of the organization's performance

Weinstein[3,p.397] has commented on the changing role of information in health care organizations:

Traditionally in medicine, individual physicians and other therapists have assessed for themselves how well individual patients responded to particular treatment procedures. . . . Much of the information needed to evaluate the treatment of individual patients is the same information needed to treat these patients . . . and is [the] information . . . assembled for statistical analyses of groups of patients. . . . With imaginative use of modern information handling . . . a given piece of information [is] recorded only once and used any number of times for a variety of purposes.

Overlapping systems

Clinical monitoring, research, and management information requirements overlap, but an intensive examination reveals that the kinds and extent of data needed for each system vary considerably. The commonalities and differences are conceptualized in Fig. 10-3.

Clinical records systems. Clinical record data for monitoring a patient's treatment needs and progress must be explicit and as objective as possible. Historically these files were developed manually and often could not be manipulated statistically because of inconsistencies in recording and difficulties of retrieval from hand-prepared records. With the advent of peer and utilization review, specific elements of the clinical record system must be extracted, summarized, and compared to specific criteria for operational and managerial control. Length of stay (LOS), types of service, and admitting diagnosis, for example, are elements that serve both the clinical records and management information systems. While an inappropriate LOS for a given diagnosis may be flagged for possible review by a physician advisor or a peer review committee for inappropriate treatment, a hospital administrator may desire profiles of the LOS by diagnosis and service to assess the need for modifying the types of services offered or adding additional staff because of changing admission patterns.

Research information systems. Research on medical problems requires extensive, often expensive to obtain, information on samples of (or in some cases on total) patient populations. The distinction between complex research approaches and simpler managerially oriented program operations evaluation should be drawn clearly. A long-term prospective controlled study examining the clinical cost-effectiveness of

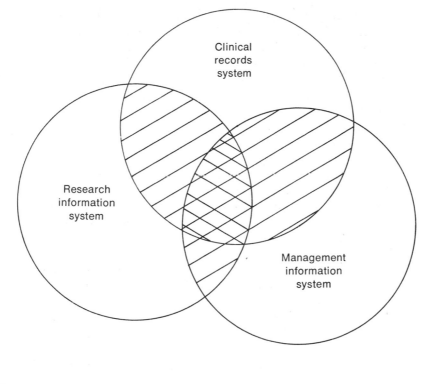

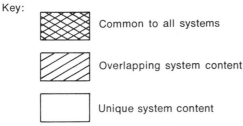

Key:

Common to all systems

Overlapping system content

Unique system content

Fig. 10-3. Commonality among clinical records, research information, and management information systems.

short-term hospitalization as an alternative to long-term hospitalization for schizophrenic patients (where either type of case is clinically feasible such as in the study by Glick et al.[5]) requires an elaborate design using classic evaluation procedures. On the other hand, less complicated approaches may be used in ascertaining that a given community mental health center (CMHC) target group received services that achieved a treatment plan objective and at what cost during the past 3 months or ascertaining which of two modalities used by a CMHC treating manic depressives was most effective for the costs incurred. The first example of evaluation is more clearly in a research area where

the second and third type have a greater management flavor.

There should be a clear-cut separation between studies designed to determine relationships between treatment modes and effects and evaluation studies. The former studies should be undertaken within a pure science content. . . . For evaluation purposes, it is necessary to monitor treatment programs to see that any given approach does not fall below some experimentally determined lower limit of production.[4]

Management information systems. As quality and utilization reviews develop, more elements of the clinical record systems will become part of the required inputs of the management information system. Initially the process may be done by manual extractions from manually prepared records done by humans. Eventually the overlaps will be automated, and computers (ranging from mini to midi to maxi) will perform routine processing and report preparation for key manager/decision makers within (and outside of) the delivering organization. Medical audit teams may want to be alerted to possible cases of poor health care, while administrators may be interested in the overall incidence and resolution of the same cases. The medical audit team may be expected to press for more detail, while hospital administrators are likely to press for greater summarization.

Management requires select data on all clientele (usually less detailed) and on the resources acquired and devoted to providing various services.[6,pp.10-11] Managers at varying levels usually require report information focused around five broad classes of questions:

1. Questions assessing patterns of patient or client care and services; illustrative reports would include
   a. Disposition of intakes by organizational service
   b. Ethnic/racial background by sex and type of service received
   c. Residence of patients admitted by organizational service
   d. Patients added by major presenting health problem
   e. Patients discharged by major and minor discharge diagnosis
   f. Number and proportion of admissions (apparently) eligible for third-party reimbursement
   g. Volume of services by type of service and organizational unit
   h. Patient load by individual staff or staffing units
2. Questions defining how various types of resources are acquired and consumed; typical reports include statistical and financial data:
   a. Statistical
      (1) Distribution of staff time by discipline and service
      (2) Volume of services provided by staff or staffing units
   b. Financial
      (1) Cost per unit of service
      (2) Comparison of program costs and fee revenue by type of service
      (3) Comparison of budgets and expenses by organization components
3. Questions that create monitoring aids for health care managers for medical peer review and utilization review; reports might include
   a. Statistical/medical
      (1) Concurrent review aids
         (a) Admissions not meeting admissions justification profile criteria by type of admitting diagnosis or problem
         (b) Listing of admissions exceeding average LOS criteria (local norms)
         (c) Extended length of stay by service and complications
      (2) Retrospective review aids
         (a) Admitting diagnoses not validated by physician
         (b) Admission justifications not confirmed
         (c) Case listings of diagnoses not accompanied by critical diagnostic or therapeutic services
         (d) Case listings of diagnoses accompanied by potentially harmful medical services
   b. Financial
      (1) Concurrent review aids
         (a) Admission without determination of third-party payment source
         (b) Cumulative charges in excess of Medicaid or medicine allowances
      (2) Retrospective review aids
         (a) Cases where cost per spell of illness exceeds average cost criteria (mean ± 1 standard deviation)

4. Questions identifying patient outcomes
   a. Discharge status by diagnosis and LOS
   b. Specific complications by diagnosis and LOS
   c. Specific complications by service and attending physician
5. Questions responding to external requirements; usually these reports should be completed from existing internally generated reports or by a search of an external source (for example, census data)

Areas of managerial overlap between clinical and, to a much lesser extent, research information systems should be clear. Whether these three kinds of data can be easily and economically integrated into a single data system is problematic because of the variations in the depth, nature, and manipulations of their respective system data bases. Information systems for each major system pose challenging but differing design and reporting requirements. Selected medical information about a patient's allergies, for example, must be immediately accessible for the physician prescribing medications, while the length of stay may need to be accessed only periodically. Readings on an experimental group may be analyzed long after the patient has been discharged, but the information may have to meet exacting measures of calibration and time of administration.

Distinction between these three systems adds clarity to the design (or redesign) of an information system to serve medical peer review. While drawing heavily on medical records systems, the medical peer review process is likely to cause more records to become part of the management information system. Medical peer review is a management control process that depends on two interlocking information systems for its success and adds another demand on the provider of care and the often inadequate and overburdened information system. To be economical yet effective requires an integrated approach to information system design—an approach seldom considered in most health care organizations.

INTEGRATING THE INFORMATION SYSTEM IN A HEALTH CARE ORGANIZATION*

Two overriding considerations of how the information system is integrated flow from top management's view of how they want to manage the organization and the level of diversity within the organization—the level of separateness or interdependencies within the functions and operating units.

Management comes in many forms and so do approaches to information systems. Information systems may be hierarchically oriented with either centralized data processing or decentralized data processing or systems oriented with either integrated processing or distributed processing. While these distinctions are not easy to differentiate, this rough classificatory scheme provides an organizing framework for probing optional approaches to designing organizational information systems. The hierarchical approach reflects what has been achieved historically, while the systems approach offers an alternative basis for conceptualizing logical rather than practical issues.

Hierarchical approach

Superordinate and subordinate relationships channel the flow and processing of information. Hierarchical organizational units (functional, departmental, or divisional) provide the lines through which information flows upward or downward. The data bases are segregated along functional or other specialized lines. For example, the service delivery function may be separate from personnel, which may be separate from the accounting or finance function. Often communications

---

*This section of the chapter draws on discussion developed in Sorensen, J. E., and Elpers, J. R.: Developing information systems for human service organizations. In Attkisson, C., et al., editors: Evaluation of human service programs, New York, 1977, Academic Press.

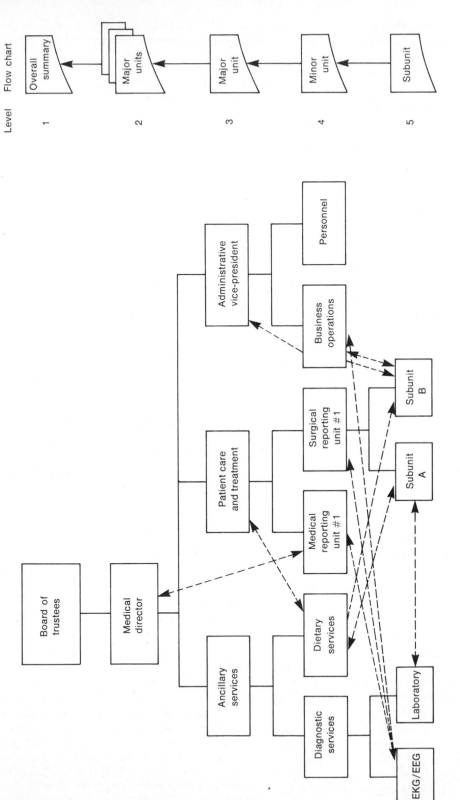

Fig. 10-4. Simplified sample of organizational chart and reporting level.

between the functions are problematic, since the data-processing activities of each function or organizational units are unrelated to each other. The solid line relationships in Fig. 10-4 reveal this approach.

Actual data processing may be done with centralized or decentralized facilities. Centralized processing may be done by a separate electronic data-processing department, service bureaus, time-sharing computer facilities, or facilities under contract. The general condition is that the separate data bases of different functions, for example, are processed by a common unit such as an electronic data-processing (EDP) department. Decentralized data processing still retains vertical (for example, hierarchical) information processing, but the EDP department is separated from the other areas. The essential characteristic of the hierarchical approach is that the data processing is geared to specialized interests (that is, functions, departments, services), which results in separate data bases for each of the functions, departments, or divisions, and is controlled by the area to whom the information is reported.

Systems approach

An alternative approach focuses on the systems perspective—one which makes available a broad base of comprehensive information on a timely basis to internal and external users for observations, reaction, and decision making. Strategic, tactical, and operational levels of decision making are incorporated, as well as planning and controlling activities, into an interlocking network of subsystems (rather than a vertical organizational hierarchy). *Information flows directly to users who need and are supposed to receive it.* The superordinate-subordinate reprocessing of data is reduced, thus permitting lateral and vertical flows of information. The dotted lines in Fig. 10-4 illustrate this perspective. Two general systems approaches exist: (1) integrated (analogous to the centralized data processing used in the

hierarchical approach) and (2) distributed (analogous to the decentralized data-processing method in the hierarchical approach).

Integrated system. The integrated system channels all organizational data into a common data base and services all data processing and information functions for the entire organization. Traditional methods of handling data and information are changed, since data collection, data processing, production of information (for example, reports), and communication of information are integrated. Client records systems (for example, medical and demographic data), financial data (for example, accounting, cost-finding, budgeting), and managerial data (for example, personnel, outpatient services, patient days, intakes) are largely consolidated. When a service is rendered, patient and professional staff data are captured and used to update patient and professional personnel files for purposes of summarizing services (1) received by specific client, including billing of client or third-party; (2) rendered by type of service and specific individual professional, as well as by classes of varied professionals; (3) accumulated by delivered units of service by program and geographic location; and (4) compared against time, size, or appropriateness criteria (for example, when last medication was given, dosage, inappropriateness because of allergic reactions).

Fig. 10-5 reveals major components of an integrated information system with a common data base. Characteristics of this system are[7-9]

1. Instantaneous and simultaneous updating of files
2. High-speed response to inquiries via remote terminals
3. Massive on-line storage
4. Both centralized batch data processing and on-line processing (although on-line processing is not always necessary)

The advantages of the integrated system include[7-9]

1. Reduction of duplication and redundancy of files and programming
2. Increased standardization
3. Reduction of clerical work and involvement in input, processing, and output, thereby reducing errors
4. Instantaneous and simultaneous updating of files
5. Concurrent retrieval, update, or deletion of data from the common data base by multiple users
6. Greater security, controls, and pro-

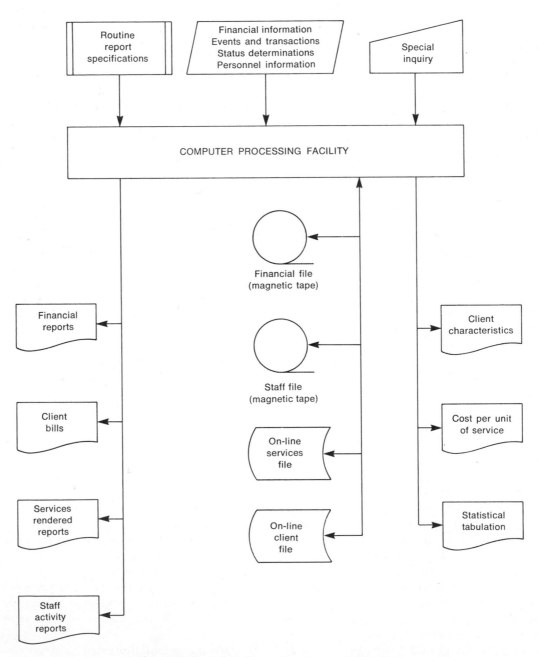

Fig. 10-5. Partial outline of an integrated system.

tection of common data base against unauthorized users

7. Retrieval of data on an economical basis, since economics of scale can lead to lower overall costs, fewer errors, and more timely reports

On the other hand, integrated systems have the following possible disadvantages:[7-9]

1. A high level of financial and personnel resource and management commitment are required to make the system successful; cost of development is high.
2. Withheld cooperation at any level of management can destroy the potential benefits of the system.
3. Downtime can be catastrophic; if the central processing unit (for example, computer) is down, the system is completely degraded, and backup facilities can be costly and redundant.
4. Modifications are difficult because of the interdependencies within the programs.
5. Threats to client confidentiality may be increased.

Distributed system. The distributed system, recognizing the disadvantages of the integrated system, uses a group of relatively independent information subsystems that are tied together via varying communication interfaces. Large files are broken down into several files with "need

to know" access criteria. An example of a distributed system is presented in Fig. 10-6.

Advantages accruing from the use of the distributed information system include[7-9]

1. Cost-effectiveness of distributed systems and their interaction with individual data bases are greater by using minicomputers and telecommunications.
2. Central facility costs are reduced (but may be offset by costs of interaction between data bases).
3. Modification is easier to meet user requirements.
4. The level of resources (personnel and financial) and level of coordination among levels of management is not as great (when compared to an integrated system).
5. Less sophisticated and less expensive technology is required with lower costs.
6. Organizational demands for volume, timing, complexity, and processing may be easier to meet.
7. Breakdown of one subsystem does not degrade the entire system.
8. New subsystems can be added more easily and without upsetting other subsystems.

The distributed system, however, is not without its disadvantages. Some of these include[7-9]

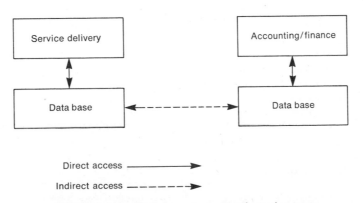

Direct access ⟶

Indirect access ⤍

Fig. 10-6. Two functions in a distributed system.

1. Difficulty in extracting corresponding data from different files or in making inquiries into different files
2. Increased possibility of inconsistencies in different systems leading to errors (for example, mismatches of data files on the same client)
3. Duplication of data capture and storage
4. Difficulty in maintaining coordination and communications

Summary

Distributed systems possess some integration, while integrated systems possess some distribution. In brief, the varieties of combinations are endless. *The basic decision is whether to favor a highly integrated system or a distributed system with some integration.* Conditions such as the following flavor the choice:

1. Type of activity of the organization (How diverse are the activities of the organization?)
2. Type of management style (Does management want to operate as an integrated unit or to decentralize so that each unit makes important decisions about its own activities?)
3. Extent of geographic dispersion (Are the organizational units geographically dispersed?)

Commercial airlines, for example, favor integrated systems because of their similarity in operations and the central role of reservations in determining requirements for personnel (for example, pilots, stewardesses, maintenance) and other resources (for example, airplanes). Large manufacturing operations, where the diversity among functional areas is great, lean toward distributed systems. Health care information systems can be successfully developed with both approaches but should lean toward integrated systems. The degree of integration occurs by integrating data into a data base (for example, eliminating numbers of files and provide for planned retrievals), data-processing functions (for example, single and general programs process data at common facilities regardless or sources), data flows (for example, developing flow around natural mainstream and collecting all information needed downstream at appropriate sources), and the outputs (by integrating networks, copying individual files, or using general retrieval programs, the report response capability can be similar to an integrated system).

INFORMATION SYSTEMS FOR MEDICAL PEER REVIEW

Integration of health care information systems begins with the design process by asking questions about how could the sys-

Table 10-2. Standard task list of the work breakdown structure for project control*

I. Study phase	
Task 1	Study organization goals and problems.
Subtask	1.1 Interview managers and study internal documents.
Subtask	1.2 Survey operating problems.
Subtask	1.3 Study informational problems.
Task 2	Study hospital resources and opportunities.
Subtask	2.1 Evaluate hospital resources.
Subtask	2.2 Study needs of care system and environmental trends.
Subtask	2.3 Evaluate competitive position.
Task 3	Study computer capabilities—equipment and manpower skills.
Task 4	Prepare proposal for MIS design study.
II. Gross design phase	
Task 1	Identify required subsystems.

*From Murdick, R. G., and Ross, J. E.: Information systems for modern management, ed. 2, Englewood Cliffs, N.J., 1975, Prentice-Hall, pp. 260-261.

Table 10-2. Standard task list of the work breakdown structure for project control—cont'd

Subtask	1.1	Study work flow and natural boundaries of skill groupings and information needs.
Subtask	1.2	Develop alternative lists of subsystems.
Subtask	1.3	Develop conceptual total-system alternatives based on the lists of sub-systems.
Subtask	1.4	Develop scope of work to be undertaken based on need of the hospital and estimated resources to be allocated to the MIS.
Subtask	1.5	Prepare a reference design showing key aspects of the system, organizational changes, and computer equipment and software required.

III. Detailed design phase

Task 1	Disseminate to the organization the nature of the prospective project.
Task 2	Identify dominant and principal trade-off criteria for the MIS.
Task 3	Redefine the subsystems in greater detail.
Subtask 3.1	Flowchart the operating systems.
Subtask 3.2	Interview managers and key operating personnel.
Subtask 3.3	Flowchart the information flows.
Task 4	Determine the degree of automation possible for each activity or transaction.
Task 5	Design the data base or master file.
Subtask 5.1	Determine routine decisions and the nature of nonroutine decisions.
Subtask 5.2	Determine internal and external data required.
Subtask 5.3	Determine optimum data to be stored in terms of cost, time, cross-functional needs, and storage capacity.
Task 6	Model the system quantitatively.
Task 7	Develop computer support.
Subtask 7.1	Develop computer hardware requirements.
Subtask 7.2	Develop software requirements.
Task 8	Establish input and output formats.
Subtask 8.1	Develop input formats (design forms).
Subtask 8.2	Develop output formats for decision makers.
Task 9	Test the system.
Subtask 9.1	Test the system by using the model previously developed.
Subtask 9.2	Test the system by simulation, using extreme value inputs.
Task 10	Propose the formal organization structure to operate the system.
Task 11	Document the detailed design.

IV. Implementation phase

Task 1	Plan the implementation sequence.
Subtask 1.1	Identify implementation tasks.
Subtask 1.2	Establish interrelationships among tasks and subtasks.
Subtask 1.3	Establish the performance/cost/time program.
Task 2	Organize for implementation.
Task 3	Develop procedures for the installation process.
Task 4	Train operating personnel.
Task 5	Obtain hardware.
Task 6	Develop the software.
Task 7	Obtain forms specified in detail design or develop forms as necessary.
Task 8	Obtain data and construct the master files.
Task 9	Test the system by parts.
Task 10	Test the complete system.
Task 11	Cut over to the new MIS.
Task 12	Debug the system.
Task 13	Document the operational MIS.
Task 14	Evaluate the system in operation.

tem be designed. While systems analysis focuses on what a system is doing or what it should be doing to meet user needs, systems design seeks answers to how could the system best meet user requirements. Systems implementation focuses on the installation, development, testing, and evaluation of a detailed system design. In Table 10-2 Murdick and Ross,[8] through a suggested standard task list for project control, provide a convenient but highly condensed overview of the entire systems development process. (While the table suggests the use of a computer, manual or keysort or other data-processing approaches may be appropriate.)

Study and gross design phase. During the study phase varying organizational constraints and requirements will be weighted differently by different health care organizations. For example, weighting on cost of acquisition, cost of maintenance, reliability, life expectancy, level of performance, flexibility, potential for growth, ease of installation, and accuracy will vary widely among health care organizations, but each variable must be considered in arriving at a preliminary design.

The sequence of events in these two phases is also crucial:

1. Formulation of organizational goals and objectives
2. Determination of questions (or hypotheses) to be addressed by information systems for assessing achievement of goals/objectives in step 1
3. Formulation of reports that address the question in step 2
4. Determination of data elements to be used in formulating reports in step 3
5. Creation of data capture instruments to accumulate data for report in step 4
6. Identification of most cost-effective approaches to error control
7. Estimation of volumes of data-processing and storage requirements

8. Simplification of report requirements, document requirements, and error control mechanisms
9. Derivation of data-processing recommendation
10. Review of design by management and staff for decision to move to detailed design, modify design (for example, use a manual system by reducing reporting requirements), or abandon the project entirely

A common fault is to plunge into the creation of data capture instruments (step 5) with little regard for the crucial role of the first four steps. Inefficient and ineffective systems often result and create frustrated and disappointed users. Add-on or redesigned information requirements to accommodate medical audit review and utilization review are not exempt from the requirement to be developed using sound systems design methodology. The temptation to pass off the requirements as too time consuming or too rigorous is great. Only good system design can produce good clinical and managerial information.

Detailed system design. This phase of system design (or redesign) usually involves[10,pp.4-1 to 4-52]

1. Design of improved record flow that integrates required MIS documents with existing forms. Most systems grow like Topsy, medical peer review is added, old forms are patched, and new ones added. Data gathering becomes inefficient, accuracy drops, and staff resistance grows. An easy way to counteract opposition is to simplify through record-keeping integration (the sequential step of charting current record flows), integrating MIS documents with current flow, and simplification of record flow.
2. Design of input documents or forms design. Use of demonstrated techniques on item coding, item format, and form layout reduces the burden of recording data (written document or

CRT input) and enhances accuracy and completeness.

3. Preparation of data-processing specifications including
   a. Criteria for editing data inputs for documents and internal processing (for example, merge edits)
   b. Procedures for selected computations (for example, age, units of services, indices, exception listings)
   c. Formats and guides for reports
   d. Performance criteria for data processing including programming deadlines, confidentiality, and financial arrangements.

4. Determination of firm cost estimates.

5. Design review that leads to final approval for implementing the information system.

Implementation of the design. Installing the information system requires[10,pp.5-1 to 5-18]

1. Prepare detailed plan of implements (using program evaluation and review techniques [PERT]).
2. Pretest forms.
3. Prepare procedures manuals and conduct orientation and training sessions.
4. Decide about inclusion of current case load and historical data in data base. (A good way to start is with current case load and to be sure that all of the data loaded into the base have been thoroughly edited.) This approach ignores most historical data captured under different systems, since the accuracy and completeness are nearly always seriously deficient.
5. Develop and test computer programs (if used).
6. Initiate collection of essential data for data base for existing case load.
7. Initiate collection of current data and delivery system operation.

Guidelines for design

The level of integration of conceptual content in managerial decision levels and functions hinges on the approach outlined in the discussion in the systems approach, that is, integrated or distributed. While adhering in varying degrees, health care information systems should observe some of the key guidelines of good systems design:[7-9]

1. Source data should be collected only once, even if used several times by the system (to reduce redundancy and error).
2. The number of steps in data capture should be at a minimum (to increase accuracy).
3. Subsystems should produce data compatible with other subsystems; one subsystem should not have to re-enter data received from another subsystem.
4. Timing of reports should be geared to timing and processing of supporting data; data should not be captured any sooner than required for reports.
5. Changes of innovations be cost-effective from an overall system perspective (for example, cost of capturing data, correcting errors).
6. Source data should be thoroughly edited so only valid data will be input into the information system.
7. Audit trails and record reproduction should be available on demand.
8. Back-up and security procedures should be maintained for all files.

In summarizing a technical approach to system design and the context in which the approach can be used, Chapman[10] observes that a MIS for any organization

1. Can be helpful only to the extent that a climate prevails that welcomes the assistance that can be provided by a management tool
2. Must provide information about resource expenditures that can be compared to objectives, intuitive or structured, that can influence decisions about future resource allocations
3. Must determine information collection requirements primarily in terms

of the structuring of data for decisions

4. Must be designed by an iterative process in which the broad outlines of organizational structure, as it implies feedback needs, report requirements, data collection needs, and of maintaining data integrity, are determined in sequence

5. Must determine the details of record-keeping integration, data-processing specifications, and input document contents and format only after a total system concept has been conceived, so that implications of cost-effectiveness trade-offs can be traced throughout the system

6. Must be implemented according to the carefully prepared plan that minimizes the consternation of organizational change and gets the system operational without delay and loss of credibility in the eyes of the agency staff

ECONOMICS OF INFORMATION SYSTEMS FOR QUALITY ASSESSMENT AND UTILIZATION REVIEW

Developing integrated information systems for medical peer and utilization review consumes resources. The outlays should be cost effective. Another way to state the question is, What costs and in what amounts will be different because of medical peer review information requirements? Many people, often well-intended observers, make the mistake of thinking that incremental information requirements can be added to an existing system with little or no inconvenience or expense. Wrong! Others misguidedly believe that the major cost of a system is the computer configuration. Wrong again! Costs of information systems are extensive and pervasive. A partial list follows:

1. Computer configuration
2. Renovation (for example, facilities, air conditioning)
3. Training (for example, including users and preparers of input)
4. Programs and program testing
5. Conversion (for example, preparing and editing records for completeness and accuracy, setting up file library procedures, preparing and running parallel operations)
6. Operations (for example, staff, supplies, maintenance, insurance, light and power, computer rental [or amortization])
7. Professional staff and support personnel time complying with data capture requirements
8. Error detection and correction process; tracking specific cases emerging in various appeal processes
9. Information system changes or modifications excited by changing external reporting requirements or controls
10. Preparation of new materials to accommodate changing external requirements

The growth of information systems costs start with project planning and grow into an operational state. Fig. 10-7 is an integrated performance/cost/time (PCT) chart used for controlling the three key variables in a system development and clearly reveals the pattern of growth of costs over time.

The information economics of PSROs*

To explore the financial impact of peer review information systems within a contemporary frame of reference, we must examine the current and announced PSRO information requirements for their impact on direct and indirect care provider costs. Unless this discussion is so circumscribed, an inclusive catalog of all costs and related economic determinants associated with all conceivable forms of peer review could consume this entire book.

---

*This section of this chapter draws on source materials published by the U.S. Department of Health, Education, and Welfare, Bureau of Quality Assurance (BQA).

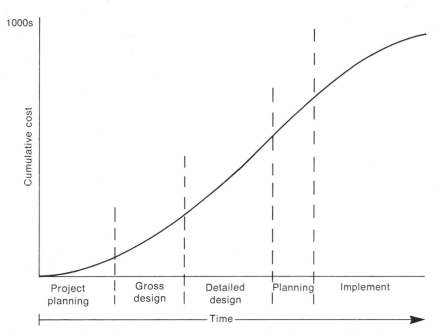

Fig. 10-7. Integrated performance/cost/time (PCT) chart for controlling three key variables (labor, materials, and computer charges) in system development. (Adapted from Murdick, R. G., and Ross, J. E.: Information systems for modern management, ed. 2, Englewood Cliffs, N.J., 1975, Prentice-Hall, p. 264.)

This discussion also provides a clearer look at the impact of PSRO directives on hospital information systems.

A prime concern of hospitals is the urgent need to implement (and to pay for) the unfolding data-handling requirements of the PSRO program. If PSRO is either to succeed or fail at the local hospital level, then the economic impact of its information-handling requirements on hospitals could become a major determinant in the survival of either the PSRO program or the hospital or both. The overall economic impact of any program on a hospital can be roughly divided into those factors that affect total revenues (hospital income) and those that divert portions of the hospital's income to nonreimbursable expenses. An effective PSRO program will be expected to reduce hospital admissions, shorten patient stays, and curtail unnecessary services (all of which happens to be the expressed hope of Congress and the federal establishment). The resultant reduction of income could pose a potential long-range threat to the survival of many hospitals. But participation in the PSRO program as a delegated hospital could also have more immediate economic consequences. Stated simply, the issue concerns what it costs hospitals to comply with information requirements as compared to what reimbursement they will receive in return. The sources of costs that are likely to be encountered can now be fairly well identified for PSRO-delegated hospitals irrespective of the specific type of information system they employ.

Catalog of PSRO requirements. The first step in addressing the cost impact question is to enumerate all of the various PSRO informational requirements that have been officially promulgated or formally announced to be in the planning stage. These requirements are scattered among a number of BQA transmittals and other HEW documents. Table 10-3 contrasts the sources of information-handling costs that are directly involved in meeting specified PSRO reporting requirements and are

Table 10-3. Sources of PSRO data requirement costs

Recognized costs	Unrecognized costs
Concurrent review activity summary	PSRO document control system
Medical care evaluation (MCE) abstract	Coding of diagnoses, procedures
MCE restudy report	Collection/reporting of PSRO optional data
MCE study status report	Patient/provider file access records
PSRO hospital discharge data set	File access notification system
Quarterly PSRO function cost summary	Accuracy verification procedures (files)
Quarterly delegated hospital function cost summary	Compartmentalized file access
	System for purging files of identifications
Patient profile generation	Personnel training re: privileged information
Practitioner profile generation	File data removal records
Provider (hospital) profile generation	Claims appeal disclosures
Diagnosis profile generation	Sanction report disclosures
Procedures profile generation	Conversion to prescribed data abstract forms
Deficiency analysis (PMIS)	Transmission of data to processor/PSRO
Corrective action reporting	Reporting PSRO decisions to payors
	Data-base layout/logistics for data interchange
	Changes in data requirements/instructions

therefore readily recognized in contrast to those costs that are indirect (supporting activities that are necessary to comply with requirements). The latter are not nearly so obvious and have therefore been termed "unrecognized." Only by examining the sum total of all information-handling activities related to PSRO can we fully appreciate their overall demand on hospital resources. A precise calculation of the actual costs of PSRO data handling at the hospital level could only be ascertained by examining in a given institution all those functions likely to generate some kind of expense to the hospital in the context of how those functions are performed. Seen in the aggregate, one can better appreciate the magnitude of present and anticipated demands required by PSRO participation and relate these to expenses for which hospitals must budget and fund from one source to another. Indirect data-handling activities are dictated by the specified requirements of a data system with this kind of mission and therefore will be discussed later.

SPECIFIED (RECOGNIZED) PSRO INFORMATION REQUIREMENTS

The official HEW requirements are summarized through extracts cited by item or page number from communications prepared by the Bureau of Quality Assurance (BQA) of the Health Services Administration. In the first of these, the *Federal Reports Manual: PSRO Management Information System* (PMIS),[11] section I (1.1) states that "This manual describes the requirements for routine reporting from the Professional Standards Review Organizations (PSROs) to the Federal Government. The reports specified in this manual request data on hospital review activities, PSRO and delegated hospital costs, and on hospital utilization by Federally covered patients" (PI-1). It is further stated that: "The intent . . . was to provide guidance to local PSROs for developing the management feedback necessary for sound operation as well as to meet the routine information requirement of DHEW and the National Professional Standards Review Council" (PI-2).

The types of information collected, used, and generated by the PSRO program were determined by the functions to be performed and the level of aggregation of data required. These requirements have been categorized as follows (p. 1, PI-1):

    I. Concurrent review activity summary

II. Medical care evaluation study reporting

III. PSRO hospital discharge data set

IV. Cost reporting

Reports in all four areas are to be sent to the BQA on various due dates, and a hospital's concurrent review is to be reported quarterly. "Data for delegated and non-delegated concurrent review are to be reported separately" (PII-1). The content of each of these reports is briefly summarized below.

I. Concurrent review activity summary

The reporting PSRO and the hospital itself must be identified along with the identity of federal payment programs of which reported patients are beneficiaries, and then counts are requested of how many cases were reviewed concurrently or by preadmission procedures, the number referred to physician advisors, those granted or denied admission certification or continued stays, and for how long, and so on.

II. Medical care evaluation study reporting

Three routine, formatted PSRO reports are related to this review activity, and the purposes they are expected to serve are described as follows (p. 2, PIII-1):

1. To fulfill the intent of section 1155(f)(1) of Public Law 92-603, the 1972 amendments to the Social Security Act, which authorized HEW to establish federal reporting requirements for PSROs

2. To define that set of information which will both assist each PSRO to monitor and assess its activities at the local level and allow the federal government to meet its monitoring responsibilities

3. To build a data base for preparing reports allowing PSROs to compare the extent and type of their activities and expenditures with the pattern for similar PSROs and providing technical assistance to PSROs.

4. To allow the federal government to obtain summary information on PSRO activities and costs to contribute to contract renewal decisions.

The contents of these reports are summarized as follows:

Medical care evaluation study abstract (BQA 131). This report describes the problem under study with respect to diagnostic or treatment aspects. The perceived need for the study and the method for selecting it are requested along with the review and analysis methodology; characteristics of the study topic such as its prevalence, morbidity, cost, and so on; the responsible review authority; personnel participation; derivation of criteria used; the study site; review strategy; sample characteristics; type of data instruments (forms) used; data quality controls; how data were processed; what compliance with standards was found; whether deficiencies were justified, and if not, what was their primary cause and who (or what) caused them; what types of corrective actions were taken and by whom; what recommendations grew out of the study; and finally the person hours utilized in all major phases of each study from its design to the analysis of its results (pp. III-3 to III-11). The cost of preparing this particular report is not so much in filling out the report form as it is in setting up and using de novo data-capturing instruments to record the required wide-ranging descriptive data and especially in documenting the personnel activities, both of which may vary enormously from study to study.

Restudy report (BQA 133). This report form differs more in purpose and format from BQA 131 than it does in what basic kinds of source data must be collected. Its purpose is to "assess the effectiveness of corrective action(s) taken in MCE studies" (PIII-13). It therefore covers much of the same investigative ground conceptually.

Medical care evaluation study status report (BQA 135). This report differs from the other two in that it examines the activity status (or progress) of conducting MCE studies within the individual hospital. After identifying the institution and study topics, this report examines the number of studies conducted, their characteristics (technical rating), planned and actual duration, restudy plans, and impact rating.

III. PSRO hospital discharge data set (PHDDS)

The provisional policies for PSRO data routing and processing published in PSRO transmittal no. 20[12] defined the PHDDS as being comprised of two subsets of data items (p. 2). Part A, the uniform hospital discharge data set (UHDDS), was developed in 1971 "to be a minimum set of data, uniformly defined, capable of providing to all users basic and comparable information on all hospital discharges" (p. 1). This is supplemented by Part B, which is described as "a limited number of PSRO-specific data which has evolved from PSRO policy development" (p. 2). Its content was essentially described in the Concurrent Review Activity Summary.

As defined in the *Federal Reports Manual* (PMIS), Part A calls for reporting the following data items on a case-specific basis: patient identification, date of birth, sex, race, residence, hospital identification, admission date and hour, discharge date, attending physician, operating physician, diagnosis (principal and others), procedures (principal and others), disposition of patient, and the expected principal source of payment (pp. IV-1 to V-5).

IV. Cost reporting

Two quarterly reports are required under this data category and are intended to provide HEW "with necessary management information" (p. V-1).

Quarterly PSRO function cost summary (BQA 151). The cost components to be reported by the PSRO include that of review personnel salaries, fringe benefits, premium pay, and the use of various consultants. These costs are to be broken out with regard to how much of the expenditures went into concurrent review, MCEs, profile and norm determinations, hospital versus long-term or ambulatory care review, and administrative costs. The PSRO

must also report on its furniture and equipment, supportive office costs, travel, indirect costs, and so on.

Quarterly delegated hospital function cost summary (BQA 153). Cost components to be reported by a delegated hospital are essentially a subset of the PSRO cost summary. Required data items include personnel costs broken out by functional areas and other direct costs such as telephone, data processing, and so on.

Once again, the effort to obtain a reliable accounting for the fraction of time and effort spent among these various functional areas requires the recording and collating of data by review personnel, which is in addition to (that is, outside) their peer review activities and which therefore adds to the cost of review.

Statement 2.2 in transmittal no. 20 fixes responsibility for who is responsible to deliver what in complying with the above-listed data requirements:

The conditional PSRO shall at a minimum obtain from the data processing contractor, patient, practitioner, and institutional profiles and management reports of concurrent review activities on a regular basis with the format and frequency of these reports to be mutually agreed to by the PSRO and the PSRO-delegated hospital.

This statement carries with it the implication that both the PSRO and the hospital should understand what is involved in meeting these requirements and rationally contract for handling the flow of required data elements at a rate of compensation that neither takes advantage of the PSRO nor penalizes the hospital economically. For this reason we will now examine some of the less easily recognized (or hidden) costs a hospital would likely encounter in complying with data requirements of the type and quantity required by the PSRO program.

UNSPECIFIED (UNRECOGNIZED) PSRO INFORMATION REQUIREMENTS

A broad range of implicit data handling and storage chores are described under several PSRO transmittals. In the main these are obligatory in the sense that they are typically necessary to support the prescribed activities essential to comply with (recognized) operational information requirements. Each item cited below will be identified by the page number of the transmittal from which it is derived.

Table 10-4 presents and comments on representative elements of indirect costs that are incremental to the immediate costs of processing the currently specified PSRO information or data requirements.

Among the major determinants of the hospital impact of costs relating to the requirements cited in Table 10-4 are (1) whether the costs are to be borne by the hospital or by the data processor, (2) whether data may be transmitted by the hospital in clusters or on a case-by-case basis, and (3) the nature of security and audit trail functions required in the name of preserving confidentiality. The latter merit some discussion here.

The information access safeguards imposed by administrative requirements are clearly timely and prudent considering the sensitivity of the information involved and the risk exposure for millions of patients and thousands of physicians. So long as peer review processes remained entirely internal (confined within the hospital) there was far less exposure risk and thus less justification for extensive requirements for audit trails, compartmentalized file access, selective external reporting, appeals

mechanisms, and so on. New access control systems become necessary precisely because of external data-sharing and reporting requirements.

Before contracting to conduct the delegated review, a hospital is well advised to ascertain the full range of legitimate costs involved in complying with all PSRO data requirements at the hospital level and whether all of these costs can or will be reimbursed by the PSRO program.

From a hospital's viewpoint then the pertinent economic questions are, How much of the institution's personnel time and other resources will be consumed in complying with PSRO data requirements and information handling policies? and How much will the hospital be compensated for doing so? Transmittal no. 20, policy statement 3.3.6 (p. 13) says:

The PSRO will be funded a maximum of seventy-five (75) cents per Federal discharge reviewed which will cover:

a. Incremental costs of forms, handling, editing, and keying additional PSRO-specific data elements into machine reproducible language.

b. Full costs of preparing and furnishing a magnetic tape to the PSRO or its processing agent where applicable (routing).

It is probably too early to know whether a predetermined and fixed figure for reimbursement to PSROs will enable them to let contracts that constitute a fiscally sound risk for each hospital. Such a determina-

Table 10-4. Data-handling and storage chores representing indirect costs of PSRO information requirements

Quote	Source	Comment
1. "The PSRO, data processing organization and delegated hospitals must agree to the establishment of in-house procedures for controlling the quality of data. Suggested procedures for data collection will be furnished by BQA."	PSRO transmittal no. 20,[12] policy statement no. 3.1.4	Quality control and error surveillance of data is important and makes sense. But this is virtually an open-ended activity with regard to how much time and resources might be dedicated to it. In other words, what it will cost a hospital to comply will be defined by whatever those "suggested procedures" turn out to be.

Continued.

Table 10-4. Data-handling and storage chores representing indirect costs
of PSRO information requirements—cont'd

Quote	Source	Comment
2. "The PSRO will require the use of the ICDA-8 for coding diagnosis and surgical procedures to the fullest extent possible."	PSRO transmittal no. 20, policy statement no. 3.1.5	It is not clear at this writing as to who will be required to code diagnoses and procedures. Coding uniformity and accuracy could be better controlled if centralized data processors (brokers) performed this task. Obviously, if hospitals must assume it, this will add to their cost of supplying PSRO data. Another unknown is whether there will be a maximal limit to the number of diagnoses or procedures that must be supplied for each patient. (Some patients may have a considerable number of each over a long hospitalization.) Involved here is a trade-off between the value of completeness in reporting as opposed to the cost of coding minutia.
3. "The third category of data, optional data elements to be determined by local PSROs, is variable and periodic. These data are to be selected locally to respond to specific needs within a PSRO area."	PSRO transmittal no. 20, policy statement no. 1.3.2	This represents another open-ended data-handling requirement. Whatever data items the local PSRO opts to require local hospitals to collect will, once again, be additional to the federal requirements.
4. Patients and providers "must be allowed access, upon request, to their individual PSRO data."	PSRO transmittal no. 16,[13] policy statement no. 3	Verifiably controlled case-specific data retrieval (on unpredictable requests) can add a significant security dimension and cost to file access techniques whether automated or manual.
5. "Physicians of record must be notified in writing at least ten working days prior to patient access."	PSRO transmittal no. 16, policy statement no. 4	Such a requirement necessitates that a tickler file and access record be kept plus a reporting structure either within or external to the monitoring system. Specifications on timeliness of notification could increase system costs considerably.
6. "The PSRO must establish and implement procedures to verify the accuracy of the data and information accessed."	PSRO transmittal no. 16, policy statement no. 3	Verification of data already stored in files requires not only look-up and confirmation functions but also concomitant security measures including audit trails (permanent records of personnel authorization and their access to data) to prevent unauthorized data alterations.
7. "Each component of the PSRO review system will have access only to that PSRO information and	PSRO transmittal no. 16, policy statement no. 6	File compartmentalization must occur at several layers or levels within file structures, and each separate level must possess concomitant access security, authority checks, and audit

Table 10-4. Data-handling and storage chores representing indirect costs
of PSRO information requirements—cont'd

Quote	Source	Comment
data necessary to carry out its functions within the system."		trails. This requirement both complicates and enlarges automated or manual systems while requiring some form of keyed (secure) access, both of which are costly.
8. "Each PSRO must purge such files of all personal identifiers as soon as such identifiers are no longer necessary . . . for purposes of review appeals, program monitoring and program evaluation."	PSRO transmittal no. 16, policy statement no. 9	File purging may be required at times convenient or inconvenient to the data system. Since care episodes (hospital stays) can vary from hours to more than a year, there must be a systematic method for recognizing and protecting active cases from purge routines. This is another requirement that can add complex sort routines, increase file space requirements, and thus add costs to the information system.
9. "It is the responsibility of the PSRO to provide an ongoing program of training in the handling of PSRO privileged information. . . "	PSRO transmittal no. 16, policy statement no. 14	Full integrity of the information system requires that only trained personnel have access to files and programs. Verification of which personnel have this competency requires information exchange between the training program and the data system.
10. "Each access to privileged data and information which requires removal of the data or information outside of a PSRO review system component, must be recorded in such a manner as to indicate what material was accessed, for what purpose, when, by whom, when the material was taken, and when returned."	PSRO transmittal no. 16, policy statement no. 15	Ongoing access logs require dedicated file space and summarization. If the review process captures data of value, then it is likely to stimulate user access to these data, and the BQA requires that the traffic of this access be monitored. Required monitoring leads to more data security and audit trail functions, which must be instituted at the point of data origin—the local hospital. Such layers of add-on control system requirements may spawn relatively small or relatively large cost increments for the hospital, depending on the type and capabilities of its existing information system.
11. "In claims appeals disclosure of privileged data or information to other than the claimant or his representative must be limited to those parties involved in the appeals process."	PSRO transmittal no. 16, policy statement no. 18	This requirement would appear to enlarge the audit trail function called for under step 13.
12. "Copies of sanction reports forwarded to the	PSRO transmittal no. 16,	A tickler file would likely be needed to monitor and assure the timely notification of providers.

Continued.

Table 10-4. Data-handling and storage chores representing indirect costs of PSRO information requirements—cont'd

Quote	Source	Comment
Secretary of DHEW . . . may at the same time be forwarded to state licensing boards. However, the practitioner or facility must be notified in writing at least 15 working days prior to disclosure to permit the submission of a statement to accompany the disclosed sanction report."	policy statement no. 16	This function may be suited to properly designed automated systems, but, as with the other add-on requirements, contributes both the size and complexities of the information system.
13. "If sanctions are levied on health care practitioners or health care providers . . . the name of the sanctioned party, the action taken and the nature of the sanction must be made a matter of public record by both the Secretary and the PSRO."	PSRO transmittal no. 16, policy statement no. 21	While the responsibility for reporting is clearly fixed at the PSRO level, the source information can only originate at the institutional (hospital) level. Pass-through requirements such as this one require structured data capture and reporting by hospitals of confirmed corrective actions and remedial processes instituted in response to sanction proceedings. This constitutes a wholly separate data-handling function.
14. "NOTE: BQA is working with other HEW agencies to finalize a departmental UHDA (Uniform Hospital Discharge Abstract) and instructions for recording elements of the UHDDS."	PSRO transmittal no. 26[14,pp.1-3]	Some forms are easier and less expensive to use than others. The instructions for recording and operationally defining individual data elements also influences the cost of data acquisition, and the impact of neither of these factors can be assessed until the announced instructions are issued.
15. "Attached to this transmittal are changes to be made in the Provisional Policies for PSRO Data Routing and Processing and the Federal Reports Manual of the PSRO Management Information System (PMIS) forwarded as enclosures [in previous Transmittals]."	PSRO transmittal no. 26, p. 1.	Every time there is a change made in any aspect of data handling, all personnel involved in operationalizing these changes must be notified and properly instructed as to how to proceed. The making of changes in data collection forms themselves requires designing new forms and discarding the old. Changes in specific data items requires the issuance of new instructions to data collectors and changes in file structures and in the procedures to process, route, and store data. The magnitude of the changes determines the magnitude of their cost. The point is that if the changes to be made are of any consequence or occur with any frequency, they will add significantly to the total costs that must be borne by a hospital in complying with PSRO requirements.

tion will depend first on whether the total PSRO information requirement and data-handling activity were fully specified as to content and format, so that cost projections could be calculated and found to be within a reasonable range. Apparently not all the relevant parameters are yet known. Therefore it cannot at this time be determined whether a reimbursement of 75 cents per case will be insufficient and thus compromise the solvency of a hospital or not. However, three messages are unmistakably clear from analyzing what has been established.

First, a hospital must take considerable care to be certain that it knows what the true cost of its participation in the PRSO program is. Second, a hospital is well advised to carefully document all of the actual expenses that contribute to the final figure it must charge the PSRO. Third, any (all) health care dollars spent on reporting requirements cannot also be spent on the delivery of health services.

Taking a broad view of these still-proliferating PSRO informational requirements, one may wonder at what point the diversion of a finite number of health care dollars into any form of health care evaluation ceases to have a favorable cost-benefit margin. But it must be remembered that the best break on the cost side of that equation may come from an integrated rather than a distributed data system. However this aspect works out for the individual hospital, it should make every effort to utilize all collected data to serve its own decision-making and internal management needs as well as to comply with externally imposed data requirements. It is ultimately in collecting whatever data it must in a way that eliminates duplication and in utilizing all data in a way that contributes to internal efficiencies that the economics of data handling tip in the hospital's favor. In short the hospital should be far more than just a passive conduit for channeling data elsewhere.

From a still broader point of view, the acquisition of health care evaluation data is an asset only so long as it serves to improve the health of people. When that is at the bottom line of a data system, very likely it makes good economic sense, too.

REFERENCES

1. Hoffman, T. R., Chervany, N. L., Dickson, G. W., and Schroeder, R. G.: Health maintenance organizations: management and information systems, monograph no. 4, Minneapolis, 1973, University of Minnesota, MIS Research Center, College of Business Administration.
2. Adams, C., and Schroeder, R.: Current and desired characteristics of information used by middle managers: a survey, no. 72-01, Minneapolis, 1972, University of Minnesota, MIS Research Center (working paper).
3. Weinstein, A. S.: Evaluation through medical records and related information systems. In Streuening, E. L., and Guttentag, M., editors: Handbook of evaluation research, Beverly Hills, Calif., 1975, Sage Publications, vol. 1, pp. 397-481.
4. Levine, A., and Levine, M.: Evaluation research in mental health: lessons from history. In Zusman, J., and Wurster, C. R., editors: Program evaluation: alcohol, drug abuse and mental health services, 1975, Lexington Books, pp. 79-91.
5. Glick, I. D., Hargreaves, W. A., and Goldfield, M. D.: Short vs. long hospitalization, Arch. Gen. Psychiatry **30:**363-369, 1974.
6. Cooper, E. M.: Guidelines for a minimal statistical and accounting system for community mental health centers, publ. no. ADM-74-14, Washington, D.C., 1973, U.S. Dept. of Health, Education, and Welfare.
7. Burch, J. G., and Strater, F. R.: Information systems: theory and practice, Santa Barbara, Calif., 1974, Hamilton Publishing Co.
8. Murdick, R. G., and Ross, J. E.: Information systems for modern management, ed. 2, New York, 1975, Prentice-Hall.
9. Davis, G. B.: Management information systems: conceptual foundation, structure, and development, New York, 1974, McGraw-Hill Book Co.
10. Chapman, R.: The design of management information systems for mental health organization—a primer, Rockville, Md., 1976, National Institute of Mental Health.
11. Federal reports manual: PSRO management information systems, Washington, D.C., September 1975, U.S. Dept. of Health, Education, and Welfare, Bureau of Quality Assurance.
12. PSRO data routing and processing policies and the federal reports manual of the PSRO management information system (PMIS), PSRO transmittal no. 20, Rockville, Md., May 30, 1975,

U.S. Dept. of Health, Education, and Welfare, Bureau of Quality Assurance.

13. Specifications for confidentiality policy on PSRO data and information, PSRO transmittal no. 16, Rockville, Md., February 14, 1975, U.S. Dept. of Health, Education, and Welfare, Bureau of Quality Assurance.

14. Revisions to transmittal 20, PSRO transmittal no. 26, Rockville, Md., September 12, 1975, U.S. Dept. of Health, Education, and Welfare, Bureau of Quality Assurance.

PART TWO

PRACTICE

Earlier chapters were intended to make explicit some fundamental assumptions about peer review. If successful in doing so, the conceptual base laid down in the Theory Part would direct thinking toward a realization that evaluation technology per se is becoming almost as broad-ranging in its scope as is medicine. That notion carries three important implications for peer review:

1. No one methodologic approach can be proposed as the answer to all the technical problems in peer review (any more than one treatment can be expected to cure all diseases).

2. Evaluation technologies already available probably exceed by a considerable margin realistic funding possibilities or the organizational capabilities of hospitals to make full use of them (therefore careful selection is indicated).

3. The most rational approach to selecting or designing an effective peer review program begins with an accurate diagnosis of (that is, by defining) the problem(s) that needs correcting in care delivery at a given hospital, just as the most rational approach to medical problems begins with an accurate diagnosis in a given patient.

Thus the hospital must first specify the problems to be addressed and thereby determine the review functions it needs or wishes to undertake. Only then can the hospital rationally select from among available techniques and methods those particular peer review programs and strategies most appropriate to the environment of that particular hospital.

With these thoughts in mind, a number of illustrative examples of the tools and operating systems of peer review are presented in the chapters that follow. They were not selected for any reasons of endorsement nor is it intended that they represent in aggregate a complete compendium of all the tools and systems of merit and achievement. The chapters in the Practice Part were chosen because they illustrate major design considerations, reflect on important issues raised in the Theory Part, and because they represent the most mature and established review systems of their type with the longest operational experience, because they translate some aspect of review technology into everyday practical solutions to current problems, or because they reflect trends in the likely evolution of peer review.

While a number of these chapters will again focus on the hospital as the setting for peer review activities, ambulatory care is also explored, and general principles that apply to the review of health care wherever it is delivered will be emphasized.

Paul Y. Ertel

Basic instruments for peer review

11

The AMA model screening criteria

CLAUDE E. WELCH
ALBERT C. STOLPER

HISTORY

The AMA has been a strong advocate of local review of professional activities by professional equals for many years. Peer review in this context means review by equals. Approximately 5 years ago a peer review manual was published that included descriptions of model systems in operation at that time. The period since then has seen a rapid development of such methods, especially by foundations and EMCROs, and the formulation by Senator Bennett of his amendment that later was incorporated in Public Law 92-603 establishing the PSRO system. Subsequently this has led the Interspecialty Council of the AMA to institute preparations for the development of a more formal system of peer review that could be applied by the profession throughout the country.

The past 3 years have witnessed many changes in the attitudes of the profession and of government. In this dynamic environment it is not surprising that the underlying principle of the PSRO law—professional review by professionals—may have been lost in volumes of regulations, faltering financial support, and a profession reluctant to accept its responsibilities.

Nevertheless there has been a great deal of progress toward the goal that visualizes universal application of a peer review system. A major step to secure the cooperation of physicians throughout the country has proved to be far more difficult than to secure the approval of national specialty societies. Needless to say there still are strong groups scattered in many states who are opposed to the concept of PSROs.

However, after the House of Delegates of the AMA finally voted to support PSRO activities in June 1974, task forces that already had been at work accelerated their activities. Immediately thereafter the AMA signed a contract with HEW to develop and publish a manual containing model screening criteria that could be adapted by each individual PSRO and used as an aid to monitor the utilization of services and the quality of care delivered in their areas in short stay, acute care hospitals.

The history and decisions of the AMA Task Force on Guidelines of Care since its inception in 1973 have been recounted in two previous publications[1,2] and will not be considered in detail here. Suffice it to say that numerous alternatives have been considered and that at the present moment it appears to the various committees involved that an acceptable, functional format and methodology is described in *Model Screening Criteria to Assist Professional Standards Review Organizations.*[3]

The final development of a model format and screening criteria was the joint effort of a 34-member Project Policy Committee (that included representation from all major specialty organizations), a 7-member Project Steering Committee, a 6-member Technical Advisory Committee (all of whom had practical experience in peer review projects), and staff support from the AMA and HEW.

The criteria have been approved by the National Professional Standards Review Council and by the Office of Professional Standards Review (OPSR) in HEW. Consequently when the applicable, necessary local modifications are added, each PSRO would be reasonably assured of its acceptability by these agencies—a legal necessity before any PSRO criteria can be employed.

At this writing there has not yet been set into motion a review mechanism whereby local PSROs can receive this formal approval of whatever modifications or adaptations they feel constrained to make in the model criteria. Thus there has been no opportunity to learn whether the National PSRO Council will be liberal or strict in its interpretation of the norms, criteria, and standards set up by each PSRO. It was the experience of the AMA Task Force that the Council tended to be cautious in their approbation of the AMA material. It remains to be seen, however, whether time constraints and political pressures to speed program implementation may favor a more liberal approach in dealing with local PSRO criteria.

Before the system is described, several other introductory remarks should be made. In the past, several approaches to criteria format have been put forth. These approaches reflect a fundamental difference in philosophy regarding the scope of criteria necessary for an effective review system. Some review systems utilize criteria that are all-inclusive; thus they may include lengthy lists of "required," "usual," "optional," or "consistent with" diagnostic or therapeutic procedures. A format such as this would obviously be long and detailed; however, it could serve as a resource for in-depth quality review by retrospective audit such as in MCEs. It also would be appropriate for claims review regarding payment for services performed. Needless to say, however, such a detailed approach is not the most efficient method of reviewing the large number of cases that would be involved in PSRO review. In addition the legal ramifications and inflationary pressure caused by such an approach are causes of concern.

It was the opinion of our committee that an alternative course should be chosen. On the basis that the primary objective of PSROs is quality control, it should be possible to cull from a large number of applicable items a relatively small number of key questions that when answered either in the positive or negative, would effectively screen out only those cases for physician review where there is a higher probability that a problem exists in terms of substandard quality. The result is that the present format is comparatively brief and as such is simpler to use, more flexible, and less likely to be inflationary by limiting the listing of procedures to only those critical to good patient care.

THE MODEL FORMAT AND SCREENING CRITERIA

Our committee discussed in detail several methods to achieve the objectives of Public Law 92-603. Theoretically one way should be to specify a model format and then have each PSRO develop its own criteria using that format for each problem or diagnosis it would encounter. Such a course would have been relatively simple. If it had been followed, the educational impact on local groups might have been enhanced, but in addition to frustration and delay either the wheel would

---

MODEL FORMAT
(code number)

Title (diagnosis or problem)
 I. Justification for admission (5 or fewer entries)
 II. Length of stay
  A. Initial length of stay assignment for primary diagnosis or problem (numerical determinations to be established locally based on statistical norms)
  B. Extended length of stay assignment (numerical determination to be established based on individual patient's condition at end of initial length-of-stay period)
   1. Reasons for extending the initial length of stay
 III. Validation of (5 or fewer entries in A or B)
  A. Diagnosis
  B. Reasons for admission
 IV. Critical diagnostic and therapeutic services (5 or fewer entries)
 V. Discharge status (5 or fewer entries)
 VI. Complications (5 or fewer entries in A or B)
  A. Primary disease and treatment—specific complications
  B. Nonspecific indicators

---

have to be reinvented time and again or many individual criteria sets would have been rejected by central review authorities.

The decision of the committee therefore was to first prepare an acceptable format. Thereafter criteria would be developed for screening by individual diagnoses and admitting problems and then used as models for local review and adaptation by PSROs. To achieve this objective some limit had to be set on the number of criteria sets that should be prepared. It was decided that each major specialty society concerned directly with patient care should develop criteria for those diagnoses and medical problems that account for 75% of their admissions to short-term, general hospitals. Criteria sets for additional diagnoses could be developed, if deemed appropriate, by a specialty. Thereby the major needs of nearly all hospitals could be filled. It was considered to be inappropriate for any hospital to require criteria for any given diagnosis made on less than 30 patients admitted in a year. This arbitrary cut-off point was based on the consideration that the individual review of such a manageable number of records would be simpler and more economical than developing criteria sets for use with a screening device. Data concerning frequency of admission to hospitals by diagnosis or problem was obtained from the Professional Activities Study (PAS) of the Commission on Profession and Hospital Activities through the cooperation of Dr. Vergil Slee.

The first publication—a draft issue of *Model Screening Criteria to Assist Professional Standards Review Organizations*—is an 800-page volume containing more than 300 criteria sets covering over 760 diagnoses or problems. At the present the first printing of 15,000 volumes has been exhausted.

THE SIX MAJOR CRITERIA ELEMENTS

The model format followed for each diagnosis or problem includes six major elements (see boxed material). The applications of this format can be shown by a specific example (see p. 278).

USE OF MODEL CRITERIA

It is important that anyone who uses these criteria should understand the reasoning behind their formation. As a detailed explanation has already been made in the AMA manual (pp. 8 to 12), only a few comments will be made here on each of these items.

Code number. For any analysis some established system of diagnostic classification is necessary. To date, none has been entirely satisfactory. Broad, often muddy groupings exist, and terminology is vari-

EXAMPLE FROM MODEL FORMAT*

H-ICDA
560

Intestinal obstruction, small intestine
  I. Justification for admission
     A. Suspicion of or diagnosis of intestinal obstruction
 II. Length of stay
     A. Initial length of stay assignment for primary diagnosis or problem (numerical determinations to be established locally based on statistical norms)
     B. Extended length of stay assignment (numerical determinations to be established based on individual patient's condition at end of initial length of stay period)
        1. Reasons for extending initial length of stay
           a. Unresolved obstruction and/or ileus
           b. Wound complications including hematoma, dehiscence, infection, fistula
           c. Persistent fever (peritonitis, intra-abdominal abscess)
           d. Prematurity (weight less than 2500 grams)
           e. Weight gain of less than 20 grams per day on oral intake (infants)
III. Validation of
     A. Diagnosis
        1. Abdominal pain, abdominal distention, vomiting, obstipation
        2. X-ray evidence of obstruction
        3. Operative findings of obstruction
        4. Pathology report of excised tissue
     B. Reasons for admission
        No entry necessary
 IV. Critical diagnostic and therapeutic services

	Screening benchmark
A. X-rays of abdomen and chest	100%
B. Serum electrolytes	100%
C. Fluid and electrolyte replacement	100%
D. Nasogastric intubation and/or operation	100%
E. EKG (over 40 years of age)	100%

  V. Discharge status
     A. Alive
     B. Tolerating diet
     C. Afebrile (temperature less than 100° F for more than 24 hours)
     D. Wound healing satisfactorily
 VI. Complications
     A. Primary disease and treatment-specific complications
        1. Persistent obstruction or anastomotic leak
        2. Electrolyte imbalance
        3. Sepsis
        4. Wound complications including hematoma, dehiscence, infection, fistula
     B. Nonspecific indicators
        1. Any extension of initial length-of-stay assignment
        2. Prolonged (over 10 days) nasogastric intubation
        3. Second operation
        4. Persistent fever

*Developed by the American Pediatric Surgical Association and the American College of Surgeons.

able. ICDA-8* and H-ICDA-2† have been used most commonly. Conversion tables are available for translating from H-ICDA-2 to ICDA-8.

Title. Preferably the title (diagnosis or problem) should correspond to a code number. However, uncoded broad titles may be necessary for criteria sets applicable to more than one coded diagnosis or problem. Such grouping allows for more efficient review by permitting related cases to be reviewed together. In some instances the title should be sharpened; for example, peptic ulcer could be divided into "gastric" and "duodenal" ulcer.

Provision needs to be made for the inclusion of problems that are frequently present on admission (for example, headache, chest pain, abdominal pain) as well as definite diagnoses. This classification allows the review and analysis of those cases where a physician cannot establish a diagnosis prior to admission. During a period of hospitalization nearly all problems will be replaced by definitive diagnoses, so that a limited length of hospital stay should be allowed for a problem to be replaced by a diagnosis of a specific disease.

Justification for admission. Some diagnoses by their very nature require the patient to be hospitalized. For example, merely the diagnosis or suspicion of an acute myocardial infarction is sufficient to justify admission. However, in most cases merely the presence of suspicion of a specific diagnosis is not the sole indication that hospitalization is required. Other factors, which we shall refer to as modifiers, must be present. These modifiers include

1. Symptoms present at a stage of the disease that necessitate hospitalization for acute care: for example, this

type of modifier for bronchial asthma could include respiratory distress or cyanosis.
2. Complications of the admitting diagnosis or its treatment that require hospitalization for acute care: for example, a complication of bronchial asthma could be atelectasis.
3. Diagnostic or therapeutic procedures to be performed requiring hospitalization: examples of such procedures include surgery, radiotherapy, radiography, and chemotherapy.

Length of stay (LOS). These figures must be inserted by each local group. Statistical studies such as those made by PAS may be used as sources. The length of stay usually will be reviewed at the fiftieth percentile; thereafter any reasons for extension of hospital stay must be listed.

Validation of diagnosis. A few items should be identified. Laboratory test results, physical examination findings, and history items are important in that order, as explained below.

Validation of reasons for admission. The purpose of this format element is to validate, where appropriate and where medical consensus exists, each reason for admission listed under Justification for Admission. Laboratory test results are considered to be the most important in the sense of objective documentation, physical examination findings are less so, and history items are considered the least objective validation for admission. There is little reason to question an admission for back pain which a positive myelogram reveals is due to a lumbar disc problem. Of course it is also possible that the physical examination could be positive even though the myelogram was negative. Finally, some patients may be admitted with such a diagnosis on the basis of a suspicious history alone in the absence of either a positive myelogram or positive physical finding. Irrespective of the ultimate medical necessity of such admissions, these examples illustrate progressively less objectivity in justifying hospitalizations:

International Classification of Disease (World Health Organization, 1965), 8th ed. rev., adapted for use in the United States, Public Health Service publ. no. 1693.
†Commission on Professional and Hospital Activities, *Hospital Adaptation of ICDA*, ed. 2, Ann Arbor, Mich., 1968, The Commission.

1. When the reasons for admission are complications or symptoms, the question becomes, What lab, physical, or history findings would provide the best evidence retrospectively that these complications or symptoms were present on admission? For example, if a reason for admission for bacterial pneumonia is respiratory distress, then the validation of respiratory distress would be a respiration rate greater than 30 per minute.

2. When the reasons for admission are to perform diagnostic and therapeutic procedures, the question becomes, What would constitute adequate objective evidence in terms of the patient's condition that can be verified by other laboratory data or by physical or history findings which would indicate that the specific type of planned diagnostic or therapeutic procedure is necessary?

It is recognized that for certain listed reasons for admission, no objective data are possible or appropriate. For example, no validation is required when the reasons for admission are projectile vomiting or severe pain.

Critical diagnostic and therapeutic services. The entries listed here are only those services having a critical relationship to outcome. The benchmark of 100% is only a screening aid to indicate those services that, if not provided in a given case, should be referred for physician review. The benchmark of 0 is only a screening aid to indicate those services that, if *not* provided in a given case, should be referred for physician review. The benchmark of 0 is also only a screening aid to indicate those services that, if provided in a given case, should be referred for physician review. The screening benchmarks (0 and 100%) are only screening devices and are not intended to suggest the frequency with which such services should be provided. Clearly a few instances will exist where valid reasons exist for rendering or not rendering these services, depending on the needs of the individual patient.

Discharge status. These entries should reflect the goals of hospitalization to be achieved or the points at which the patient has gained maximum benefit from hospitalization. The clinical goals for all patients even with the same diagnosis obviously cannot be identical. For example, some patients with lower-leg amputations may be expected to be fully ambulatory, receiving physiotherapy in preparation for walking out of the hospital. For others who will remain bedridden the amputation may have been performed for the limited objective of relief of pain.

Complications. The most common complications either of the disease itself or the treatment can be listed. They should be potentially preventable and have a significant effect on morbidity and mortality. In other instances some nonspecific indicators that the patient's course has not been as smooth as desirable may be cited (such as long-continued fever without definite cause).

It will be observed that the maximum number of entries for each patient is 40. This is far from the encyclopedic list engendered for nearly every hospitalized patient. Rather it represents another practical cut-off point that in the opinion of the Task Force seemed to be a reasonable number of criteria items. The committee felt strongly that if the list was permitted to become too detailed, the program would become difficult to carry out. This emphasizes again that entries already required by other organizations need not be specified in PSRO review. Thus since such routine items as histories, physical examinations, and key laboratory items (admission urine, blood examination, and so on) are specified by the JCAH, they need not be repeated. On the other hand, if particular services need emphasis, they may be included; for example, preoperative white counts prior to appendectomy are important.

It also must be emphasized that these criteria have been developed primarily for screening purposes. In themselves they identify only those records that are to be submitted to physicians for further review.

Type of review. Review responsibilities of a PSRO include concurrent admission certification, concurrent continued-stay review, and retrospective medical care evaluation studies. By way of further definition, it should be emphasized that if the length of stay has already been extended, then the review should be conducted concurrently rather than retrospectively. The format shown on p. 277 can be adapted to each of these as follows:

1. Admission certification and concurrent continued-stay review. Elements I (Justification of Admission) and II (Length of Stay) are applicable for individual charts. Concurrent review may also include the use of elements III (Validation of Diagnosis and Reasons for Admission) and IV (Critical Diagnostic and Therapeutic Services), but are primarily designed for a retrospective analysis of a group of charts. Incorporation of items III and IV in a concurrent review process would require a very active review process carried out daily and would be beyond the present capability of many PSROs or hospital utilization review or quality audit committees.

2. Retrospective review. Elements V (Discharge Status) and VI (Complications) are intended for use in retrospective reviews only. Elements III (Validation of Diagnosis and Reasons for Admission) and IV (Critical Diagnostic and Therapeutic Services) also should be used in retrospective review but similarly may be used in concurrent review as previously mentioned.

Practical use of the screening criteria. Since the system has been introduced recently, no opportunity yet has arisen to assess the best method of implementation. Two methods could be suggested. In the first a certifying agent could inspect the chart within 24 hours of entry. A single-page form applicable to all diagnoses or problems would be inserted in the chart. Initial LOS assignment and reasons for admission and extension of stay could be listed by the physician on the same form. This sheet could serve for concurrent admission certification and concurrent continued stay review. Retrospective review would be carried out after discharge through analysis of the actual hospital chart rather than from an abstract form.

Another method would be to have the reviewer insert into the chart a duplicate sheet of the criteria applicable for the given diagnosis with appropriate boxes for checking entries as they are completed. Concurrent review would be facilitated, and retrospective review of such a record would be relatively easy. However, it would have the disadvantage that a physician might consider he had accomplished all of his tests as soon as all appropriate boxes were checked. Innovation could be stifled.

A chart demonstrating the possible action of the review coordinator would suggest that a large number of cases could possibly be referred for physician review (Table 11-1). In practice that number ideally should include less than 5% and probably should not exceed 10% of the hospital admissions to be practicable.

STRENGTHS AND LIMITATIONS OF THE CRITERIA (FORMAT AND METHODOLOGY OF USE)
Strengths

The advantages of the criteria may be listed briefly as follows: It is a comparatively simple method, and with the exceptions noted above, suitable for all types of review. Routine work may be performed by a nonphysician coordinator permitting 90% to 95% of all records to pass without further investigation. Data can be computerized easily. Physicians who will review

Table 11-1. Possible action of review coordinator to implement review system

Time	Coordinator	Physician review
Within 24 hours after entry (elements I and II)	Notes on diagnosis or problem	
	Criteria set is available	No
	No criteria set is available	Yes
	I. Justification for admission	
	One or more entries are present	No
	There is no entry under this element	Yes
Concurrent review—50th percentile of initial LOS (element II)	II. LOS	
	Assign initial LOS	No
	Extend LOS if new diagnosis appears	No
	If LOS is exceeded	Yes
Continued concurrent review—50th to 90th percentile of initial LOS (elements III and IV)	III. Validation of	
	Diagnosis	
	One or more entries present	No
	No entry present	Yes
	Reason for admission	
	One or more entries present	No
	No entry present	Yes
	IV. Critical diagnostic and therapeutic services	
	All 100% services done and no 0	No
	One or more 100% not done or one or more 0 done	Yes
Retrospective review (elements III, IV, V, and VI)	V. Discharge status	
	All entries present	No
	One or more entries lacking	Yes
	VI. Complications	
	Primary disease and treatment-specific complications	
	No entry present	No
	Any entry present	Yes
	Nonspecific indicators	
	No entry present	No
	Any entry present	Yes

the remaining 5% to 10% of records may at their option reduce or tighten the standards or insert other criteria if too few or too many records are sent for review. It should be expected that any significant variation from established practice would require approval by the National PSR Council. In regard to the present edition of the model criteria, the format is flexible and changes are foreseen and will be incorporated in the next publication.

These model criteria have been developed as a result of many hours of work by many special committees. Though in some cases the protocols may seem to be astonishingly brief, they represent the concurrence of specialists drawn from the entire country. The criteria mentioned before have been approved by the National PSR Council and the Office of Professional Standards Review.

Limitations

There are inherent weaknesses in any peer review system, and there is some question that any of them actually work very well. Furthermore it is difficult to prove that they improve patient care. This objection is particularly applicable to PSROs, since they will be involved in cross comparisons of health care data from various hospitals, something that has never been attempted before on such a large scale. The difficulty of acquisition of significant data should be stressed; even if LOS is reduced in the future, it may not be due to PSRO efforts but to increased availability of discharge facilities, for example.

Some critics would regard this system described herein as limited and inadequate. They would prefer to see a single, finely detailed system that covers all medical care in a comprehensive fashion. Our method does not do this; it builds on the strength of efforts previously accomplished by other organizations yet carves out a special mission that strives not to duplicate the activities of other organizations such as the JCAH and AHA. It is aimed precisely to adapt to the provisions of Public Law 92-603 for the purposes of PSROs and hospital utilization committees. This we believe is a major advantage rather than the opposite.

The major limitation of the criteria in terms of format and methodology of use is that only a portion—albeit a major part—of any peer review system is addressed. As prime examples, they do not approach the question of how norms or standards can be integrated. They probably are not adequate for most MCEs. The role of individual profiles of providers or recipients of medical care is not considered. Further discussions of these items follow.

FUTURE ACTIONS IN THE CRITERIA DEVELOPMENT PROJECT

After obtaining feedback from field-testing the criteria, revisions will be required. In the meantime, however, certain actions are already indicated to improve the first edition of the criteria document:

1. Titles (diagnoses and problems) require sharper definition and correlation with coding systems.

2. Despite many long hours of work already invested, there still are many diagnostic entities that should be included in the protocols or modified in some fashion. The specialty societies have been asked to review again the diagnoses for which they have written guidelines in the first edition to see if there are other diagnoses or problems they wish to include at their option in the revised edition. There is also to be a full review of all criteria by the involved specialty societies; this will include comments sent in from all sources including PSROs and hospitals using the guidelines from other specialty societies, from the American College of Pathologists, the American College of Radiology, the American Academy of Family Physicians, and from the American Osteopathic Association. The societies will then collectively decide which guidelines should be changed and proceed to do so for the next edition.

3. Further consultation between specialty organizations will be necessary. At present, medical specialties have been coordinated by the American College of Physicians and the American Society of Internal Medicine, and surgical specialties by the American College of Surgeons. Consultation between such coordinating groups and others (American Academy of Family Physicians, American College of Radiology, and College of American Pathologists) will be necessary.

4. In the present volume, at times two sets of criteria have appeared from different organizations for the same diagnosis. They may need to be combined.

Though these specific weaknesses can be corrected in the next edition, it is obvious that continued revision will be necessary to incorporate future advances in medical care.

Though the manual is a product of a great deal of work, much more is required. A prime objective will be the analysis of the strengths and weaknesses of the program, together with suggestions for change that will arise from careful study of the use of the manual by PSROs and hospital committees.

A consulting firm already has been procured to make an extensive study, and the program has been outlined. Reports should be available by the end of this year. At that time the findings and recommendations will be transmitted to the participating societies for their further considerations.

The second and final volume specified in the AMA-HEW contract included these changes and was published in June 1976. Most of the defects listed above were corrected.

THE INTERRELATIONSHIP OF SCREENING CRITERIA WITH NORMS, STANDARDS, AND CRITERIA

Section 1156 of Public Law 92-603 requires each PSRO to apply professionally developed norms of care and treatment, based on patterns of practice in its region, as principle points of review and evaluation. To clarify this statement, further definitions appear in section 709 of the *PSRO Program Manual:*[4]

norms numerical or statistical measures of usual observed performance of medical care.
standards professionally developed expressions of the range of acceptable variations from a norm or criterion.
criteria predetermined elements against which aspects of the quality of a medical service may be compared and that are developed by professionals relying on professional expertise and on the professional literature.

The relationship of criteria for screening, as prepared in the AMA manual, to norms, standards, and criteria requires examination.

Norms, as defined above, must be based on patterns of performance. Data have already been accumulated by PAS and other agencies that can provide the usual observed performance. As data banks are built from information provided by PSROs, these figures should become more refined and more readily available.

Standards likewise must be based on patterns of care. For example, if a death rate of 20% is the norm for a certain serious disease, a range of 15% to 30% might be accepted as a standard.

Criteria, as defined in the *PSRO Manual,* can be regarded as identical with criteria for screening developed in the AMA manual. However, screening criteria are only one type of criteria. The scope and content of criteria are dependent on the use to which they are put. MCEs and claims review require more comprehensive criteria.

After criteria have been established, norms identified, and standards set, retrospective review can be carried out either on individual charts or groups of cases. The chief task of the PSRO is to identify poor care and take action to improve it based on the results of this review. It was the considered judgment of the Task Force that if physicians find they are reviewing less than 5% of all records, then either patient care is superb or the criteria are drawn too loosely. Similarly if physicians are reviewing more than 10% of records, it was considered likely that either patient care is poor or the criteria are too strict.

Such systems, if they are to be acceptable to the profession, must be based on review by physicians. If such power should rest solely in the hands of bureaucrats, the needs of the public could be underestimated, and physicians would be certain to feel that they could not cooperate with such a system.

SCREENING CRITERIA AND CLAIMS REVIEW

The AMA screening criteria are not intended to be used for claims review by third party payors to determine whether payment for particular services should be made simply because there was no attempt to list all "consistent with" procedures. Most observers have regarded this feature as an advantage rather than a disadvantage. However, the need for claims review criteria still exists. Providers of care need to be involved in the development of criteria that will be used by third party payors for claims review, particularly where the appropriateness and level of payment for a particular service is involved.

THE USE OF SCREENING CRITERIA IN MCE STUDIES

Medical care evaluation (MCE) studies have been specified in the *PSRO Manual* and have been developed in detail by the Joint Commission on Accreditation of Hospitals (JCAH). A method of linking the AMA criteria with the Performance Evaluation Program (PEP) of the JCAH has already been developed by Mr. Charles Jacobs and examples have been published in their *Quality Review Bulletin.*

Without question MCEs are valuable both for patient care and physician education. However, we must quibble with the number of such studies that have been specified as desirable. Speaking from a background of many such clinical investigations that often took all of one's spare time for a period of many months, it is our impression that if many studies are required, all will become superficial and therefore be of little value. Hopefully PSROs will pay more attention to a few oaks rather than a lot of pumpkins.

Data acquired using only the AMA screening criteria sets may be satisfactory for those MCEs requiring minimal data. However, if an MCE study is to be of any depth, more observations will be necessary and more detailed criteria will need to be developed that are useful in accomplishing the objective of the MCE study. In such cases screening criteria nicely serve as the initial step in launching an in-depth MCE study. For example, when performing an MCE study to determine the cause of an unacceptable complication rate for a specific diagnosis, it would be necessary to establish detailed process criteria that relate appropriate preventive measures. Screening criteria would merely serve as the initial step by identifying those cases where the complication occurred.

The findings of MCEs can serve later as important sources to suggest changes to improve the quality of patient care as well as indicate that change may be required in criteria and standards. Again, relating back to the above example, an MCE study of an unacceptable complication rate may reveal that a critical preventive procedure is not being performed. Definitive steps can then be taken to improve the quality of care. On the other hand, an MCE study into a complication rate that has been unacceptable (not meeting the established standard) over a period of time may indicate that the established standard was too high rather than the care deficient. An analysis of the complication cases in this instance may show that given the current state of the art of medicine, all reasonable preventable resources were actually taken. Finally, MCE study results may indicate the need to add or delete specific entries under certain format elements for a criteria set covering a specific diagnosis. A study into a complication rate may indicate the need to add new nonspecific indicators to the future screens for that complication.

LOCAL PSRO ACTIONS REGARDING THE SCREENING CRITERIA

Local PSROs or hospitals that have received delegated review should review the AMA model screening criteria and take the following actions:

1. Determine an LOS for each diagnosis and problem. Lengths of stay are conspicuously absent from the protocols. They must be formulated by local PSROs on the basis of experience with similar cases. LOS data furnished by PAS or other data sources will be available for use initially but may require modification after local data are accumulated.

2. Determine whether or not additional criteria sets must be written. Many diagnoses and problems are not considered in this volume. Approximately 300 titles cover 75% of all short-term hospital admissions; if the other 25% had been included, an additional 4000 protocols would have been necessary. While new titles will be added in the coming volume, local PSROs may need to develop additional criteria sets if certain local medical problems occur more frequently or if

the local health status could be improved by the appropriate identification and treatment of certain local medical problems.

3. Determine whether or not psychosocial needs of patients need to be included in screening criteria. While such considerations are important in the individual care of patients, screening criteria are difficult to establish in this area and have not been approached in the AMA document.

4. Obtain approval of adapted criteria by the National PSR Council and OPSR.

THE FUTURE OF PEER REVIEW

There is no doubt about the fact that peer review will escalate in the future. Almost surely every third-party payor will need to develop some such system. Blue Shield, other insurance plans, foundations, health maintenance organizations, and prepaid health plans already have outstripped the peer review efforts of all but a few medical societies. It has been seriously contended that the secretary of HEW, through other provisions in Public Law 92-603, already has used a method to attempt to sidestep peer review by the profession; undoubtedly other federal or state governments will maintain steady pressure to contain the cost of medical care. If quality is to continue in the practice of medicine, only physicians can recognize it and support it. In this way peer review can remain as it should be—peer review by equals.

SUMMARY

The AMA has served to correlate guidelines for the development of screening criteria to be used by local PSROs. This has been accomplished through the agency of the National Specialty Societies combined with committee members appointed by the AMA and by HEW. A model format has been produced that can serve as a skeleton for the important diagnoses or problems that will be encountered by each PSRO. Over 300 model criteria sets have been produced for various diagnoses or problems; these also can serve as models for the local PSROs. The history of the development of the project is given, the method of use of the model criteria sets is listed, and comments are made about the strengths and weaknesses of the criteria. An initial publication, *Model Screening Criteria to Assist Professional Standards Review Organizations,* was published in 1975 and a revised final issue in 1976. Methods of validating the criteria are presented.

REFERENCES

1. American Medical Association Task Force on Guidelines of Care: PSROs and norms of care, J.A.M.A. **229:**166, 1974.
2. Welch, C. E.: PSRO guidelines for criteria of care, J.A.M.A. **232:**47, 1975.
3. American Medical Association: Sample criteria for short-stay hospital review (screening criteria to assist PSROs in quality assurance), 1976, The Association.
4. U.S. Dept. of Health, Education, and Welfare, Office of Professional Standards Review: PSRO program manual, Washington, D.C., March 1974, U.S. Government Printing Office.

12

Information systems and
peer review

MARSHA A. BREMER
VERGIL N. SLEE

Hospitals today are increasingly concerned about quality assurance. The reasons for this growing concern are many and include the ethical and professional concerns for providing optimal care, the growing problem of liability, and the legal responsibility contained in statutory and case law. The Darling case established that there is a "contract" between the hospital and society requiring *reasonable* diligence regarding the quality of care for *all* the patients *all* the time. This concept is restated in the standards of the Joint Commission on Accreditation of Hospitals: The hospital shall demonstrate that the quality of care provided to all patients is consistently optimal by continuously evaluating it.[1]

There is a well-recognized need for a systematic and visible hospital quality assurance function.

THE QUALITY ASSURANCE FUNCTION

The hospital's quality assurance function has five components:
1. Planning for quality
2. Structure control
3. Quality control
4. Quality improvement
5. Accountability

Planning for quality. Quality does not just happen; it requires planning, which includes a budgetary commitment.

Structure control. Structure control refers to the mechanisms employed to ensure a sound fiscal organization, responsible and effective governing bodies and management, efficient and responsive medical staff organization, delineation of privileges, and credential review.

Accountability. Accountability involves providing to all concerned the evidence needed to establish confidence that the quality assurance function is being performed.

The remaining two components, *quality control* and *quality improvement,* relate directly to controlling the quality of care provided to patients. Both are essential and require identical steps:
1. Setting standards: statements of what ought and ought not to be done
2. Surveillance: observation of what actually is done
3. Analysis: does what is done conform to the standards?
4. Action: taken when performance does not conform to standards
5. Follow-up: to ensure that the action worked

While the steps involved in the two components are the same, their timing, targets, application, and purposes are very different: quality control refers to the concurrent activity performed to provide each patient with care that conforms to standards; it provides a quality "floor," maintaining the quality of care. Quality improvement is the retrospective review of the care provided to groups of patients to detect chronic problems and to improve the care of future patients; it provides a quality "staircase," improving the quality of care.

This chapter deals specifically with quality improvement as a component of the hospital's quality assurance function and with the role that information systems can play in it.

QUALITY IMPROVEMENT

The first principle of quality improvement is that it applies to all aspects of the hospital and to all patients all the time. The traditional approaches to quality control have fallen far short of that goal.

While the first formal quality assurance effort in hospitals was begun in 1919 by the American College of Surgeons (ACS) through the establishment of its Hospital Standardization Program, the first modern quality control effort (that is, a review of actual care provided) appeared in the 1940s when ACS called for tissue committees.

This was followed by committees to review specific aspects of the care given in hospitals: for example, deaths, transfusions, infections, and antibiotics. In the average hospital such committees managed to review the care of between 10% and 15% of all patients.

In the 1950s the concept of the medical audit began to gain acceptance as a unified method of replacing these one-target committees and looking retrospectively at various groups of patients to determine patterns of care. At this point the powerful tool of statistics was added to the armamentarium. The significance of death rates, complication rates, and normal tis-

sue rates were seen, and hospitals began to introduce systematic efforts to improve care by changing patterns of behavior.

In most hospitals this review focuses on diagnoses and procedures, and a common list includes acute myocardial infarction, pneumonia, congestive heart failure, hernia, appendectomy, cesarean section, cholecystectomy, and tonsillectomy and adenoidectomy. In the average hospital this list accounts for approximately 12% of all patients, again leaving the care of 80% to 90% unexamined.

The question then is how to move from between 10% and 15% to 100%. An obvious approach might be to lengthen the list of reviewed diagnoses and operations, but this would soon prove futile, for increasing the list from 8 topics to 50 would only increase the percent of patients reviewed to 50% (given that the 50 topics include normal deliveries and newborns).

To expand the percentage to 90% would require between 700 and 1000 studies. It is obvious to anyone with experience in doing medical audit studies that the time and resources required would by far exceed those devoted to patient care. Furthermore most of the groups would contain only one or two patients, hardly enough to establish a pattern.

Yet the moral, ethical, and legal commitment to all patients remains the same. How then can this commitment be met?

MONITORING

The solution to the problem lies in comprehensive, retrospective, statistical monitoring.

Monitoring is the continuous examination of routinely collected data on selected critical parameters to see if the observed pattern of care matches preestablished standards. A monitor has five requirements:

1. Continuousness: the monitor must be on-going; that is, it must examine the data at reasonable and regular intervals.

2. Grouping: patients must be grouped in appropriate ways, and all patients must be examined in at least one group. Monitor (or study) groups are not restricted to diagnosis and operation. In fact, at least six ways of grouping patients are possible:
   a. All patients (excluding newborn) require certain elements of basic care (temperature and weight recorded, minimum laboratory standards met); thus all patients can constitute a valid group at this level of detail.
   b. Narrowing the focus to specific clinical departments within the hospital reveals additional elements such as preoperative workups for surgical patients.

For the entire hospital and within clinical departments, groups may be defined to reflect

   c. The practice of basic preventive medicine, for example, routine examinations for detectable malignancies.
   d. Response to findings, for example, follow-up and treatment of elevated blood pressure.
   e. Control of therapeutic measures, for example, appropriate use of antibiotics.
   f. Finally, groups defined by diagnosis and by operation where enough cases occur to show patterns of care.
3. Parameters: once groups have been identified, monitor parameters must be selected. A parameter is simply the "thing" measured—survival, complication, and so on. Monitor parameters are those key critical elements (things) that, when balanced to include indicators of the outcome and the process of care, can reveal care "in control" or "out of control." A specific diagnosis or operation can be monitored in relation to
   a. Justification for hospitalization
   b. Justification for therapy
   c. Validation of diagnosis
   d. Outcome (for example, mortality,

complications, condition at discharge)
   e. Critical investigation
   f. Critical management
4. Performance: data on hospital performance must be provided for all parameters in all groups. These data will typically be expressed as percentages, for example, the percentage of patients who had minimum laboratory workup. Taken together, these percentages create a hospital-wide profile that is in a sense a multichannel one, for patients may be included in many groups.
5. Standards: to evaluate performance, comparison must be made to standards—statements of desired optimal performance. Comparison to previous performance may also prove useful as an indicator of trends. In addition, norms—statistical representations of usual, observed behavior—may provide valuable assistance in interpreting one's own performance.

INFORMATION SYSTEM

The sine qua non for monitoring in a quality control system is a well-designed medical record information system. The number of items on which data must be collected to monitor effectively is of course very large. (CPHA's Quality Assurance Monitor, QAM-3—described below—contains over 750 parameters.) In even the smallest hospital, retrieving the data by hand becomes a burdensome and time-consuming task, since a number of items must be retrieved from every medical record. By its very nature such a manual process must eventually fail.

This then makes evident the need for the technology of the computer.

In addition to being automated, the information system, to fulfill its monitoring function, must meet several more requirements:

1. The data collected must pertain to the quality of care given, reflecting both the outcome and the process of

care. The minimal information required for indexing of records will not suffice, for data on case management are essential.

2. The data must be collected routinely and uniformly; all patients must be covered in the data collection; and the data elements needed for monitoring must be entered into the information system for all patients all the time.

3. Reports must be generated often enough to enable continuous (periodic) evaluation of hospital performance.

PROFESSIONAL ACTIVITY STUDY (PAS)

The Professional Activity Study (PAS), the principal program of the Commission on Professional and Hospital Activities (CPHA), meets the above requirements. PAS began in 1953 as a cooperative study among 13 southwestern Michigan hospitals. Its purpose was and remains the study of hospital and professional activities for the improvement of patient care. Now 2200 hospitals throughout the United States, Puerto Rico, Canada, and several foreign countries participate. PAS hospitals treat over 40% of all patients in the U.S. and nearly a third of all patients in Canada.

Data are routinely and uniformly abstracted from the medical records of all patients discharged from PAS-participating hospitals. The information is processed by computer at CPHA and returned to the hospitals in the form of graphs, statistics, indexes, and listings of individual patients—data displays. The data also are collected to form a library that currently consists of over 130 million hospitalizations and are used to provide comparison information.

The data elements collected and reported are designed to reflect the outcome and the process of each patient's care and to aid in the evaluation of the quality of care.

Fig. 12-1 is a reproduction of the 1977 PAS case abstract. The types of information collected include basic identifying information, diagnoses and procedures, investigation and management data, and areas to be used at the option of the participating hospital.

The data items in PAS provide virtually all the data needed to monitor the quality of care of all patients and were used to develop the only comprehensive retrospective monitoring device now in use in hospitals. This device, called the Quality Assurance Monitor (QAM), is an optional extension of PAS.

In accordance with the requirements for a monitor, QAM

1. Reports continuously (quarterly).
2. Groups patients in increasing levels of specificity, from hospital-wide groups (all patients excluding newborn, all newborn) to department-wide groups (for example, all surgical service patients) to groups by specific diagnosis and operation.
3. Reports hospital performance on carefully chosen monitor parameters specific to each group.
4. Includes groups designed to evaluate how well the hospital practices basic preventive medicine, responds to findings, and controls therapeutic measures.
5. Provides standards set by national specialty organizations, and space for standards set by the hospital's own medical staff. Three other bases for comparison are included: the hospital's own past performance, regional norms derived from the performance of other hospitals, and thresholds for investigation.

QAM is continually improved. Development of the current phase, QAM-3, was aided by special advisory committees appointed by the American Academy of Pediatrics, the American College of Obstetricians and Gynecologists, the American College of Physicians, and the American College of Surgeons. The committees

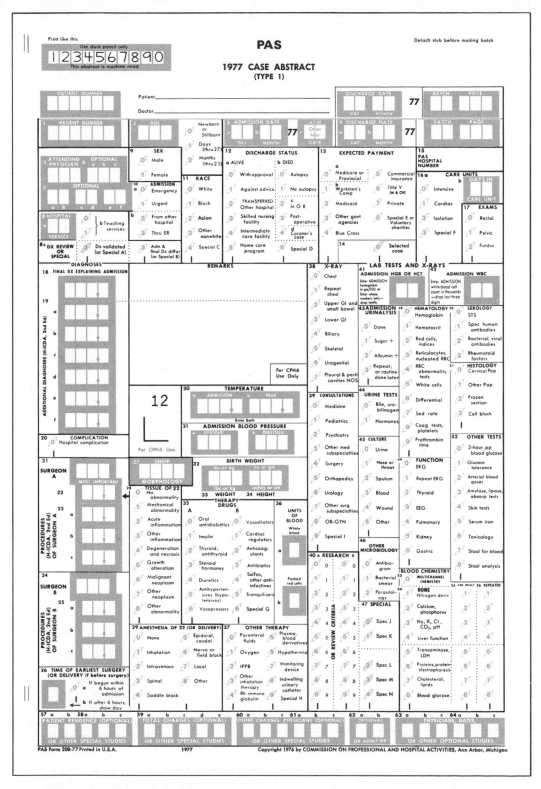

Fig. 12-1. Example of a 1977 PAS system case abstract. A variant of this document contains space for documenting concurrent review activities and for the entire PSRO Hospital Discharge Data Set (which includes the UHDDS).

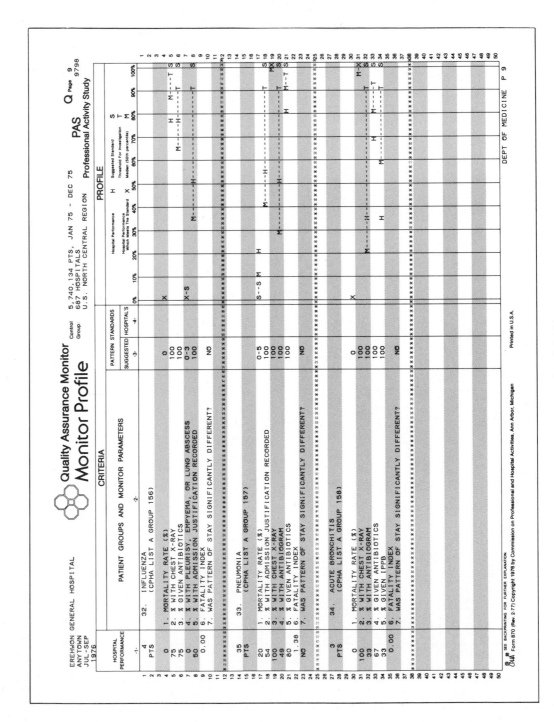

Fig. 12-2. Example of QAM report.

helped refine patient groups and monitor parameters and provided standards for the parameters. These suggested standards are presented in QAM-3 as a prime basis for comparison.

Fig. 12-2 shows a sample of a QAM report from an actual PAS hospital. Shown are third-quarter 1976 data for medicine service patients. The hospital's own performance can be readily compared to its own and suggested standards and, through the profile at the right, to thresholds for investigation and to the median performance of hospitals in the same region.

MEDICAL CARE EVALUATION STUDIES (MCE)

Comprehensive retrospective statistical monitoring is a powerful tool in the hospital's quality assurance system because it enables review of all patients all the time. But it also adds a side benefit—that of providing a technique for setting priorities for in-depth MCEs. How to choose objectively what medical audit studies to undertake is a problem all medical staffs face.

Regardless of the method, in-depth MCEs are time and resource consuming, and the number that can realistically be undertaken in any hospital is limited. Because of this there is an obvious need for a selection technique.* The technique must assure a high probability that those topics which most need it are chosen for review and that resources are not likely to be expended in areas where care is already being delivered in conformance with standards.

The monitor does this by producing a signal when care delivered does not match predetermined standards. In effect the monitor sorts care that is in control from that which appears to be out of control.

---

*JCAH and PSRO have requirements for the number of MCEs a hospital must complete. Both call for between 4 and 12 studies per year. It is possible for a hospital to meet these requirements without reviewing more than 3% or 4% of its patients. This makes it even more imperative that an objective selection technique be employed.

Once identified, these apparent problem areas can be evaluated in greater detail. While in some cases some limited form of inquiry may suffice, an in-depth medical audit (medical care evaluation) study will be called for in others.

The last few years have seen a proliferation of methodologies for performing medical audit studies or MCEs. We will deal not with a specific methodology but with the six essential characteristics of any method as defined by the Joint Commission on Accreditation of Hospitals. These six requirements are

1. Valid criteria that permit objective review of the quality of care provided to all patients are established.
2. Measurement of actual practice against the criteria produces reliable data.
3. Results of measurement are analyzed by peers.
4. Action is taken to correct the problems identified.
5. Action is followed up.
6. The results of patient care evaluation, that is, general findings and specific recommendations, are reported.[2]

Requirements 2 through 5 either rely totally on the information system or can be greatly helped by it.

Requirement 2, measurement of actual performance, is the retrieval of data on hospital performance for each criterion included in the study. To support this activity the hospital's information system must meet requirements in addition to those that support monitoring. First, it must collect and efficiently report the majority of indicators of the quality of patient care, allowing rapid retrieval of those indicators. The words *majority of indicators* constitute an important qualifier. While this means that for some of the criteria for some studies the system will not contain needed information, a closer look tells us that we would not want it to do so. The reason is that to collect all the information that might ever be needed would result merely in duplicating patient records. Then the system would be burdened by all the well-recognized drawbacks of those records. The optimal system is one that achieves the best cost-benefit ratio; that is, that carries the greatest number of relevant data items at an acceptable cost. Rarely needed data can be more inexpensively retrieved manually.

This points up a second additional requisite of the information system: it must produce an audit trail; that is, a trail from statistics that reveal patterns of care to identification of the patients who make up those statistics, and finally to the original medical records of those patients.

An information system that contains most of the information needed for measurement of practice for MCEs and that links this information to the original records is an invaluable tool in the measurement step.

Requirements 3 and 4, analysis of results of measurement and recommendation of corrective action, can logically be discussed together because the recommendations must derive directly from the analysis.

Analysis of the findings of the data retrieval (measurement) really involves two interrelated functions. First, one must determine whether problems exist in the care of the patients under study. Then those problems must be traced to their source so that the next task, recommendation of corrective action, will be on target.

Again, the information system can play a major role in these tasks through the reports it provides.

By uniformly arranging data previously scattered throughout (or buried in) stacks of patient records, these reports can reveal patterns among the study patients— patterns that in turn will point to the source of the problems. To put it another way, the information system must arrange the trees so that the forest becomes visible.

Uniform data display helps determine whether problems are atributable to the hospital as a whole, to a single subspecialty,

or to a few individuals, thus enabling objectives for corrective action to be directed exactly to the level where they are needed. Hospitals can ill afford to expend resources on an education program directed to the entire medical staff when only one area is involved.

Requirement 5, follow-up on corrective action, is done to ensure the action has been effective and continues to be so. Perhaps the most important step in medical care evaluation, follow-up is frequently overlooked. This need not be true. With an efficient information system and the support of nonphysician personnel, it is the easiest task of all.

Vital characteristics of the information system that permit this follow-up activity are

1. Routine collection and reporting of information on all patients: this permits immediate access to data about patients currently under study as well as those previously studied.
2. Flexibility: as well as containing routinely collected data, the system must have the capability of adapting to local, hospital-based needs.

SUMMARY

Today there is a recognized need for a systematic and visible quality assurance function in the hospital. The quality improvement component of this function can be successful if

1. It continuously monitors the quality of care provided to all patients.
2. It includes in-depth evaluation of problem areas.
3. Programs for corrective action are targeted at the causes of problems.
4. The results of corrective action can be shown to be effective and continuing.

A sound information system is essential to a successful quality assurance system.

PAS, which provides QAM, is used extensively by hospitals because it meets the requirements discussed. PAS provides virtually all the data needed for retrospective statistical monitoring and a large percentage of that needed for in-depth studies. A uniform abstract is completed for each patient discharged from a hospital so that data collection is efficient and information is routinely available. Generous optional data capacity is provided for specially targeted data collection. PAS is now used for about 42% of the short-term hospital discharges in the United States and 28% in Canada. Norms of practice, nationwide and regional, are readily compiled.

REFERENCES

1. Accreditation manual for hospitals, March 1975, Joint Commission on Accreditation of Hospitals.
2. Perspectives on accreditation, Jan.-Feb. 1975, no. 1, supplement, Joint Commission on Accreditation of Hospitals.

ADDITIONAL READINGS

Bremer, M. A.: JCAH audit using PAS—a handbook for health record analysts, Ann Arbor, Mich., 1975, Commission on Professional and Hospital Activities.

Guidelines for hospital patient care evaluation, June 1975, California Medical Association and California Hospital Association.

Juran, J. M., editor: Quality control handbook, ed. 3, New York, 1974, McGraw-Hill Book Co.

Perspectives on accreditation, July-Aug. 1975, no. 4, Joint Commission on Accreditation.

The quality assurance monitor report book, Ann Arbor, Mich., 1974, Commission on Professional and Hospital Activities.

Slee, V. N.: Quality control in quality assurance, Paper presented at the Estes Park Institute Hospital Medical Staff Conference, Asilomar, Calif., November 17, 1975.

Slee, V. N.: PSRO and the hospital's quality control, Ann. Intern. Med. **81:**97-106, 1974.

Slee, V. N.: How to know if you have quality control, Hosp. Prog., January 1972.

Slee, V. N.: How can you audit *all* the care? Mod. Hosp., vol. 97, no. 1, November 1961.

U.S. Dept. of Health, Education, and Welfare, Office of Professional Standards Review: PSRO program manual, Washington, D.C., March 1974, U.S. Government Printing Office.

Waldman, M. L.: A progress report on the medical audit study, Hosp. Prog., August 1975.

Waldman, M. L.: The medical audit study—a tool for quality control, Hosp. Prog., February 1973.

Williams, K. J.: Beyond responsibility: toward accountability, Hosp. Prog., January 1972.

13

Assistance for hospital informational needs: the health data broker

JAMES P. COONEY, Jr.

A health data broker has been defined as "an organization possessing the technical resources including manpower to facilitate the collection and processing of health statistical data to meet common information needs among multiple users at various geopolitical levels (local, state, and national)."[1]

It is anticipated that the trend toward health data brokers operating in designated service areas (normally a state) will accelerate under the pressure of growing demands from

1. Multiple users for common sets of health information in terms of both the quantity and quality of such information
2. Increasingly scarce fiscal and manpower resources to develop and continuously support duplicative health data collection and processing organizations

Certain existing health data brokers have demonstrated a capacity to assist many hospital data-based functions including peer review. Therefore it is predicted that as data brokers expand both geographically and in terms of service capacity, they will become an increasingly common resource for hospitals. In anticipation of the brokerage trend the purpose of this chapter is threefold:

1. To discuss the patterns and reasons for anticipated changes in demands for medical information in reference to hospital-based care
2. To explore the data-broker concept as a logical response to the expected changes
3. To outline areas where the data-broker organization can assist the hospital

In reading the subsequent material it should be kept in mind that the hospital assistance role is only one of many roles most data brokers fulfill, and that hospital-related medical information is only one of the informational sets the broker handles. We are discussing here only one small piece of the overall broker activity.

MEDICAL INFORMATIONAL CHANGES: PATTERNS AND REASONS

Increasing criticism is voiced to hospitals and their medical staffs on issues of expense, poor quality, inefficiency, and disorganization. At the same time, increasing and duplicative demands are being made on hospitals and their staffs by both governmental agencies and nongovernmental third parties for information for purposes of quality control, cost control, planning, and reimbursement. Faced with the increasing demands and criticisms, hospitals and medical staffs frequently find themselves in a defensive position because the very information by which criticisms could be answered is only sporadically available or altogether unobtainable.

While there are many things in health delivery that need improvement, there are also a great many things that are being done well. However, without solid data to speak for it, all too often what is done well is not communicated to those decision makers for whom it is important to demonstrate effectiveness. In areas where effectiveness could be improved, the ability to see what is needed to solve the problems is compromised because of incomplete information or a total lack of it.

Hospitals often unknowingly contribute to their problems by a failure to understand or appreciate the collective performance of hospitals and medical staffs. This situation is brought about by

1. Limited perspective: self-evaluation of performance by those responsible for it tends to lack objectivity. An individual or an institution, by its focus on self, often is not in the best position to define what it really does well and what it does not do well enough.

2. Lack of information: hospitals often lack the security of a quantitative information base for decision making. This does not necessarily mean that bad decisions are consistently made but rather that consistency of decisions can be improved over the long run by working from a constant and orderly fact base.

3. Uneasiness with large quantities of data: by the nature of professional work and the educational process required to support and improve it, hospital professional staffs have generally not had the experience of working with and deriving the maximum value from large masses of numbers. As a consequence there is a tendency to resist them, to be uncomfortable with them, and to work without them.

4. Externally imposed need to justify performance: today external comparisons are becoming a norm of analysis, but this required analytic approach is new and still resisted or unacceptable to a segment within an institution.

5. Insular nature of the hospital: in the past hospitals have been individual, self-contained institutions, and their focus properly tended to be restricted within their own walls; therefore the service and performance of other hospitals within a common health service area was not germane to their frame of reference.

Admittedly the preceding observations are generalizations and are not necessarily to be expected in all hospitals and among all medical staffs, nor in the same degree where they do occur. However, to a greater or lesser degree these are among the major factors that have contributed to the problems of institutional accountability and the availability and usability of institutional information.

Irrespective of the factors involved, the end product is all too often a lack of quantitative information on performance. This absence of facts forces staff into the area of assumptions to identify problems and support their resolution. Such a direction for decision making can result in actions that are not in the best interests of medical staffs, hospitals, and the communities they serve. The problems of decisions based on assumptions are unnecessary today given the resources available for the development and maintenance of a solid base of facts.

The most solid basis for improved decisions and program development begins with a uniform base of facts. From this fact base, properly interpreted, comes knowledge; and from the knowledge, properly handled, comes the power to influence the effective development of both the care and the educational programs of the hospital.

As things typically exist today, the hospital is full of bits and pieces of scattered facts and data. These bits and pieces require organization to be of maximal use internally, to be interrelated with each other, and to permit comparisons among hospitals.

The utility of the isolated or disorganized facts is largely limited to the benefit of individual patients and staff members. However, once organized, a statistical interrelationship can be established, and the benefits of data can extend to patients as a group, present and future, physicians, hospitals, and the health services delivery system as a whole.

The development of an organized fact base should not and typically does not require the collection by the hospital of more or new information. It merely capitalizes on the information that already exists, links pieces of information together within the institution, and interrelates them for maximal comparability.[2] This leads to the following benefits:

1. The understanding and improvement of the internal management of patients in a clinical sense and an enhancement of hospital management in a business sense
2. Development of a common statistical comparative base with other institutions to permit the recognition of areas that are most promising for improvements in the delivery of patient care
3. Improved communication and education of relevant staffing and patient groups both within and external to the hospital(s) to further assist the constructive evolution of the care system

Clearly one of the most valuable single informational resources within any hospital is the patient medical record. From its inception the medical record represented a complete and chronologic history of an individual's course of care in an institutional setting. Seen in this light the medical record is an important and basic document for ensuring the present and future medical welfare of the individual patient. The focus and role of the medical record more recently has rapidly broadened beyond concepts of relevance limited to an individual patient to those relevant to numbers of patients present and future, abstract and real. Medical records, once their informational content has been accumulated and systematized, have become the necessary and basic tools for a host of important secondary functions ranging from training of medical and paramedical personnel to preparation of bills and claims forms. In addition to the growing recognition of the value of case information in staff development for medical professionals, the increasing value of an expanding fact base is becoming recognized as relevant for research.

With these evolutionary trends in the use and utility of medical information from clinical records, concomitantly occurred developments of systems for and standards of recording and retrieval. These mechanical-type developments have been accelerated under the impact of medical, institutional, and legal requirements.

As the environment of health care funding and support surrounding hospital operations began to change and the vague outlines of a national health system began to appear over the horizon, the relevance and utility of information components of the medical record were seen to take on growing importance for purposes of utilization and peer review and long-range institutional and community health planning, in addition to the already recognized financial claims administration related to third-party payors of the institution.

The medical record today is still basically what it started out to be: a complete and chronologic history of an individual's course of care in an institutional setting. Through the application of modern information technology, the same information typically contained in the document intended for the care of an individual can be made into multifunctional data for a broad range of use within and external to the institution. While the handwritten record and its information are passive, with systematized and standardized data-handling techniques coupled with controlled indexing and abstracting, the once inert record content can be an active tool in the evaluation of the quality of patient care, the assessment of community and institutional health services availability and utilization, and health care delivery effectiveness.

Growing interrelationships and needs for comparisons among hospitals, educational concerns emerging from recognized problems in the quality of care, and rising costs in the institutional delivery of health care combined with rising expenses of health data retrieval have jointly led to the development of hospital discharge abstract systems. While varying combinations of factors may have contributed to the development of a variety of these data systems in various geographic areas, the systems generally share similar basic characteristics. The abstracting service is usually an organization whose principal, if not sole purpose, is to collect data abstracted from medical records for a group of hospitals, process these data on a scheduled basis, and return reports to the institutions in a series of analytic and standardized formats. Hospital participation in these systems is voluntary, and the institution is normally charged at a set rate per discharge. These services generally work with the hospitals in terms of developing a standardized means of abstracting of the data and assisting with the education of relevant personnel in the use and application of the reports containing the processed data. Discharge abstract systems currently in existence are beginning to serve as the catalyst for the development of health data brokers (if not serving as the broker themselves), which carries the service concept a step beyond previous activity. Specifically the scope of service has expanded beyond hospital use of hospital data to multiple organizational (that is, fiscal intermediaries, PSROs, and so on) use of hospital data.

Hospital and medical staff functions in the past did not necessitate the development and use of an extensive quantitative information base from which to measure group performance either within or among institutions. However, developments largely external to the hospital already alluded to have changed this pattern. Performance of the individual hospital or provider must be measured and evaluated against comparisons among relevant others. Paralleling this changing need for data analysis and reporting has been a rapid proliferation of recognized needs to assist medical staffs and hospitals with their internal informational handling. This assistance is at the base mechanical: the collection and processing of information. However, added to this base is an increasing technical assistance service in the use of information within the hospital and by organizations external to the hospital. The data broker is thus emerging as the logical organizational response to both the mechanical and technical assistance, with a spectrum of information-related functions.

THE HEALTH DATA BROKER CONCEPT AND OPERATION

It is increasingly apparent that the informational needs of hospitals, medical staffs, and a variety of third parties center around a common minimum set of data.[3] These organizational groupings having common data requirements exist at all geopolitical levels and include but are not limited to professional standards review organizations (PSRO), the planning-oriented health systems agencies (HSA), state legislative and regulatory bodies, licensure and accrediting organizations, third-party payors, and rate review bodies. While these groups do not all share the same common total informational needs, they do share a need for a minimum set of common information.[4]

The principal diagnosis is cited as but one example of an element of information that is required by virtually all organizations, and there are many such items. In the past each group requiring that particular element of information established its own methods for collecting it on their own separate forms, establishing individual and varying definitions of the same element, and processing the data in each of their many computers. The process meant that the hospital was required to provide the same item or slight variations on the same item to each of several external groups at varying times and on painfully unstandardized forms. In addition to the cost diseconomies inherent in these multiple demands, there were inherent problems of data quality and comparability once the data were dispersed.

Discharge abstract systems emerged to assist the hospitals and their medical staffs to meet internal informational needs and to offer the hospitals comparative information on the performance of similar other institutions. The functions of the discharge data abstract systems have now been extended for reasons of economy, flexibility, and data quality into brokerage functions. Data brokers not only return to the hospital and its medical staff the reports of required information as is presently done, but they also, with consent of the hospital and its staff, provide elements of the same information to those other groups external to the hospital that require the information. They thus serve as the conduit of data flow in many directions.

As noted previously the brokerage service is not limited in concept nor in actual operations to only hospital medical information, but information sets beyond those normally contained and provided through a hospital are also serviced such as vital statistics, health manpower, health service analyses other than hospitals, the monitoring of health care expenditures, and so on.

Existing health data broker organizations normally have a service area that is conterminous with state geographical boundaries. However, it is anticipated that economies of scale and informational requirements that extend across geopolitical boundaries will necessitate the development of area brokers in certain parts of the country having service areas either larger or smaller than the state unit. The ultimate service area of brokers will be dictated by a compromise between the need to provide a low-cost service and the need for flexibility to respond comprehensively to local informational needs.

In any given service area the collection and processing role of the broker can be expected to (and will) vary. This variation results from the capacity of already existing collection and processing resources within the area. The broker does not duplicate existing resources (for example, a discharge abstract system). Rather the broker expands on such existing resources to meet multiple needs, such as the channeling of existing data to multiple users. The broker only develops its own collection and processing capacity in the absence of existing resources.

Regardless of a variation in collection and processing roles among brokers, all ultimately will have the responsibility within their service area for assuring uniformity in data collection and output accuracy, completeness, validity, and reliability. These responsibilities can be expected to be governed by nationally developed standards and guidelines that assure the quality of data, economy of collection, and preservation of confidentiality.

The collection and flow of information abstracted from the patient record is presented in Fig. 13-1, using selected medical information.

In those areas where brokerage functions exist, several attributes have been demonstrated:

1. A reduction in the cost of collecting and processing information occurs. This reduction affects the provider of the data by reducing multiple demands for the same information to but one request for a standard set of data input. Further, extraneous data requests are eliminated or significantly reduced. The reduction affects the receiver/user of the data in that his costs of data collection and processing are now shared among several groups.

2. Through the development of com-

monly acceptable guidelines and standards and a monitoring system, the quality and quantity of the required information are significantly improved.

3. Since all data users are sharing a uniform base of information, then each can deal with the issues inherent in the information. They need not contend with problems raised by variation in the numbers that nonuniformity generates among multiple users and the confusion and error this provokes at the hospital level where the data are generated.

4. There is greater opportunity to protect confidentiality in the centralization of potentially sensitive information in that its release can be controlled through uniform and more elaborate control mechanisms.

5. Most existing data brokers generate a technical assistance capacity to serve hospitals. This capcity is also of significant value to the users of information in that the availability of analytic assistance provides more productive and focused use of the processed information.

These generally helpful attributes accrue to all users of fully developed brokerage services. Specific assistance to the hospital and its medical staff is discussed below.

Broker assistance to the hospital

In terms of service on behalf of the hospital, as illustrated in Fig. 13-1, the broker acts primarily as a data intermediary between the individual hospital and those agencies or organizations having common information needs, but it may also deal with information-handling problems that arise wholly within the institution. The operation of both broker roles will be described by focusing on those clinical and sociodemographic data most commonly required among organizations. At present a minimum set of patient data*[2] has been defined and has generally been accepted by a majority of national programs (in-

cluding those of HEW) that require such information.[5]

Before these data requirements can be met the hospital may find it needs assistance in abstracting the minimum required data set from the patient record. The nature of such assistance varies to match the specific needs and resources of the individual institutions. The spectrum of the brokerage services can include any or all of the following:

1. Assisting in the development of a data collection system within the hospital to assure economy, accuracy, and completeness of primary source data

2. Furthering the economic organization of the medical record (as a primary source document) to promote efficient and accurate data abstracting and clinical utility of the information it contains

3. Providing continuous technical assistance to the data abstracting process including education and training of involved personnel, diagnostic and and procedural coding service, and special problem resolution

Once the data are abstracted, the broker edits and organizes the information to assure accuracy and completeness. In this process the broker works directly with the hospital in the correction of errors and assists in developing accuracy control measures necessary for maintaining the quality of the hospital system.

While a minimum data set has been defined and accepted, additional data elements over and above the minimum are nearly always required by the hospital to facilitate its internal operations and by other users at the local level. Because of this built-in variation in the total information set and the confidential nature of any information that pertains to individuals or to identifiable episodes, guidelines have been developed for governing data release by the broker to agencies and organizations other than the contracting hospital or providers. Governed by the policies and guidelines, the broker in effect

*The Uniform Hospital Discharge Data Set (UHDDS).

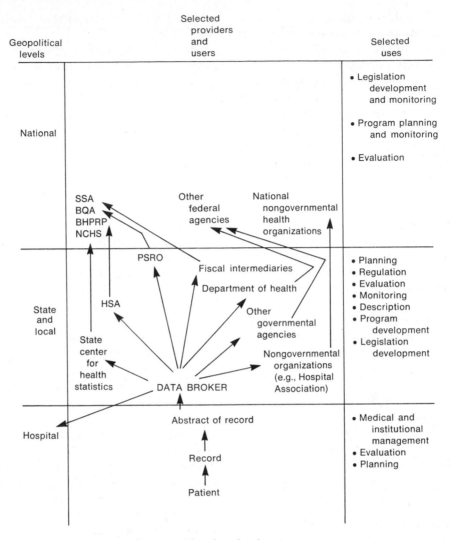

Fig. 13-1. The data broker system.

becomes a data trustee on behalf of the hospital.

Those agencies and organizations requiring processed data on a routine basis direct their requests to the broker. The routine information requests of major user organizations are established in advance through national and local negotiations. The requests that are approved by the hospital are then processed by the broker and provided to the users in the format specified.

In reference to ad hoc requests for information the broker in effect assumes those functions and complies with those requests for hospital statistics that the individual institutions and their organizational representatives approve.

The intermediary role of the broker as outlined above offers significant cost savings to both the providers and users of information not only through economies of scale but also through effective system designs that eliminate duplicative data handling and capitalizes on the efficiencies of highly mechanized collection-processing systems. In effect the providers and users pool their combined collection and processing operations into a single system operated by the broker. By this action the unit cost is lowered to providers and users alike. In addition the brokerage function itself promotes the uniformity of the fact base among multiple users.

Through the trustee role and the provision of technical assistance, the broker can do much to increase the appropriateness of data analyses. This occurs through the staff of the broker organization, which in aggregate represents far more competent technical knowledge than any individual hospital could afford to hire and support. This staff can identify and encourage appropriate data use and decrease inappropriate data use. The broker functions as a neutral base for multiple providers and users; therefore as it is viewed as having no vested interest, it can freely assist all parties to meet their analytic needs without compromising self-interests or investments.

Institutional uses of patient data appear to be expanding as rapidly as external uses, especially in the areas of performance monitoring, evaluation, and planning. The nature of these uses coupled with the growing volume of clinical data accumulating in the record of the individual patient call for steps to render more efficient the use of the patient record as the principal tool of review. Using the entire patient chart as the primary method for performance monitoring simply is no more practical than reviewing all items on individual patient bills as a means of assessing institutional financial stability. Data must be abstracted from records, processed, and grouped into information displays relevant to hospital goals and objectives and medical staff needs. An abstracting and aggregating data service is at least the minimum required by the hospital.

Abstracting services performed by and within many hospitals cannot help but feel the pressures of growing external requirements for data. Technical skills and resources needed to meet expanded requirements for information handling are increasingly scarce and expensive. These factors have led a majority of hospitals to seek data services outside the institution, and it is anticipated that the remaining hospitals will rapidly seek such services also.

Institutional performance is now continuously compared against other institutions by external agencies and organizations. Hospitals must learn and use such comparative methods to make their own comparisons to gauge progress from their own perspective. Internal abstracting and processing services cannot provide comparative data on other institutions, but the external processer can.

The major purpose of any data collection and processing system is ultimately to provide useful information for a variety of purposes. There is no point to collecting and processing any data unless resultant information displays are useful and are used. A good deal more is involved in doing this than meets the eye, and a good broker would perform a real service for hospitals by developing data displays tailored to individual needs and readily understandable, so the professional staff will put them to effective use. There is literally no limit on how information can be displayed, and for this reason reports to hospitals can be developed in specific reference to that institution's needs. Brokers today have staff complements with the necessary technical expertise to work closely with the hospital staff in identifying their real, as opposed to perceived, informational requirements and in developing reporting mechanisms relevant to those specific requirements.

Beyond this service, brokers should be expected to provide technical assistance to hospital staffs in interpreting the information they receive as a kind of continuing education and whenever special problems need to be addressed. Data analysis is a specialized skill just as is caring for patients. The more complex the problem, the greater the need for expertise and teamwork, and these technical strengths of data brokers are being increasingly and productively used by the hospital. It must be stressed, however, that the broker staff does not interpret data and makes no decisions on behalf of the hospital. Rather the broker assists the hospital staff in fully appreciating the meaning, patterns, and consequences inherent in their own data.

In summary it is noted that the existing data brokers have developed and are developing in response to and as an organizational solution to the problems inherent in the following trends:

1. The number of organizations and agencies external to the hospital requiring the same patient data from all institutions is large and increasing at all geopolitical levels.
2. The amount of information required on given patient episodes is also large and increasing.
3. Hospitals currently need a quantitative base from which to accomplish institutional goals and manage a host of internal functions, and this is also increasing.
4. External data needs are being standardized in terms of content of a uniform data base for multiple users.
5. Data abstracting, collection, processing, and use costs are high and continue to increase but can be shared for lower unit costs to individual institutions. Skilled technical assistance personnel are in increasing demand while becoming increasingly scarce.
6. Comparison of performance among hospitals is becoming a standard method of evaluation.
7. Sharing existing services and sharing the development costs of new ones is more economical for a group than is the independent development and maintenance of individual services.

The health data broker is a service shared by both provider and user. It is therefore neutral to both while also in a favorable position to understand the needs for both and how these needs can be most equitably met. The pooled resources and experiences of many hospitals can work toward improvement of data quality, usability, and most importantly, toward a legitimate payoff to the hospital for all the time, effort, and money it invests in meeting data requirements imposed both from without and within. While existing data brokers have demonstrated their capacity, the further development of this capacity requires extensive and continual cooperative work among the broker, data providers, and data users.

REFERENCES

1. The United States National Committee on Vital and Health Statistics: Interim report on the uniform hospital discharge data set, February 1976, The Committee.
2. Uniform hospital abstract—minimum basic data set, Vital and health statistics series 4, no. 14, Rockville, Md., 1973, U.S. Dept. of Health, Education, and Welfare.
3. Hospital discharge data, report on the conference on hospital discharge abstract systems. In Murnaghan, J. H., et al.: Medical care, vol. 8, no. 4 (supplement), Philadelphia, 1970, J. B. Lippincott Co.
4. Cooney, J. P., Jr., and Crosby, E. L.: The use of a common data set for hospital management, guidelines for health services research and development no. 6, Rockville, Md., 1971, U.S. Dept. of Health, Education, and Welfare, National Center for Health Services Research and Development.
5. Hodgson, D. A., et al.: The uniform hospital discharge data demonstration, publ. no. HRA-74-3102, Rockville, Md., 1973, U.S. Dept. of Health, Education, and Welfare.

Functioning systems

14

The Medical Care Foundation of Sacramento

JAMES J. SCHUBERT

The Medical Care Foundation of Sacramento was established in 1958 by the Sacramento County Medical Society to develop a management system for individual practitioners. Specifically it set its sights on improving the efficiency of health care delivery, developing and improving minimum standards for private health insurance plans, improving the quality of the health care delivery within the community, and minimizing the system's deficiencies.

The Foundation is governed by a board of trustees, the members of which are either appointed or elected from nominees provided by the medical societies and hospital and pharmacy associations. There are seats on the board for consumers, hospital administrators, and pharmacy representatives in addition to physicians. The foundation currently has a membership of over 1000 physicians and covers a geographic area of five counties in northern California surrounding Sacramento, the state capital. Approximately 1 million people reside in this area, including numerous Medicaid beneficiaries, 80,000 Medicare eligibles, 50,000 people under the CHAMPUS program, and 210,000 privately employed individuals. The health service population totals approximately 100,000. The Kaiser-Permanente health system operates within this same five-county area

and currently has enrolled some 180,000 people in its program.

The foundation, with 200 employees, operates as the economic arm for the member physicians of the three medical societies in its five-county service area. The foundation has a service provision contract with the local PSRO, which evolved from the Certified Hospital Admission Program (CHAP), a creation of the foundation.

The success of any concept, no matter how creative, innovative, or valuable it may be, is greatly dependent on people who care enough to make it work. The foundation is fortunate to have experienced the dedication of many such individuals. Two in particular, the late Kathleen O'Connor Henwood, R.N., and H. John Rush, M.D., must be credited with responsibility for the success of CHAP. The foundation board of trustees gratefully acknowledges their unfailing interest, effort, and participation in the development and functions of CHAP and their belief in its purposes, principles, and intrinsic capabilities, with a spirit of compassion for patient needs.

THE FOUNDATION'S PEER REVIEW SYSTEM

CHAP is the hospital utilization program operated by the Medical Care Foundation of Sacramento. The foundation also operates a large peer review program, stimulated by the physician service claims coming to the foundation for payment. These combined programs impact not only hospital practices but office practices as well.

CHAP operates independently with a staff distinct from that of the claims peer review program. CHAP is a preadmission and concurrent review program. The claims peer review is a retrospective review program. Each program is supported by its own professional and technical staff composed of registered nurses, professional review analysts, statisticians, data systems personnel, and clerks.

Contributing clinical skills to both review programs are individual physicians appointed by the board of trustees who serve as advisors in their field of practice. Each in turn is a member of a specialty committee made up of other practitioners in that medical specialty, and each committee elects its own chairman. A given specialty committee is not only responsible for the retrospective analysis of physician claims coming through the foundation for payment, but is also responsible for setting medical policies to be utilized by CHAP.

CHAP has a separate executive committee made up of physicians who are responsible for conducting day-to-day activities and decision making.

Generally speaking, this group is comprised of internists and general practitioners. When necessary they may call on the individual specialty committees for advice and cooperation in reviewing any particular case in which such clinical expertise is needed. The individual members of the CHAP committee work independently as clinicians on a day-by-day basis in various community hospitals. At least monthly, and frequently weekly, the committee meets to discuss particular problem cases or to review any policy decision that should be implemented. Overall the committee is responsbile for the review

of admissions to both hospitals and skilled nursing facilities.

Supervising the activities of the claims peer review specialty committee and the CHAP committee is the Medical Review and Appeals Committee appointed by the board of trustees and made up of senior practitioners in various specialties. It approves all new medical policy guidelines and hears and reviews appeals from the various committees involved with CHAP and with the peer review program. The vice president of the board of trustees of the foundation chairs the committee, and several other trustees staff it. The board of trustees must approve monthly all actions of the Medical Review and Appeals Committee.

THE CERTIFIED HOSPITAL ADMISSION PROGRAM (CHAP)

CHAP, conceived by Sacramento area doctors, is now widely known and duplicated by foundations throughout the country. The purpose of CHAP is to monitor hospital bed utilization and, as with claims peer review mechanisms, to assure quality care. The foundation believes so strongly in its plan for preadmission hospital screening that it has copyrighted the CHAP program to ensure that other organizations do not use the same name for programs that do not measure up to the foundation's standards.

CHAP began in 1969 as an outgrowth of an attempt by the Medical Care Foundation of Sacramento to reduce total insurance policy costs by improving efficiency in the use of the acute hospital. In 1965 the Kaiser-Permanente hospital and medical system became established in Sacramento County at the request of the California State Employees' Association, under special provisions of state law. Because a great number of patients who had been previously treated by private practitioners on a fee-for-service basis enrolled into the prepaid Kaiser system, a great deal of anxiety and apprehension emanated from the individual practitioners.

Subsequently the foundation was asked to develop a competitive program. Mr. Leon Hyman of California Western States Life Insurance Company was approached concerning the feasibility of developing a program competitive to the Kaiser program in Sacramento. He suggested the use of some method of monitoring statistically determined lengths of stay utilizing the PAS (Ann Arbor, Michigan) data that recently had been developed. At that time the physician members of the foundation board of trustees who were involved in research and development activities felt that any imposition of a time limit on covered hospital benefits through such a mechanism might prove to be repugnant to the practicing physicians and hence unacceptable not only to the physicians but probably to their patients as well. After some deliberation of the problem, it was felt that perhaps another form of monitoring system could be developed in which the participating practitioners would set the length of stay guidelines on the basis of the medical needs of their own individual patients and practices. An arbitrary length of stay would not be assigned to each patient; rather, a standardized monitoring system to demonstrate the necessity of hospital admissions would be put into effect.

It was from this broad range of discussion that the concept of CHAP evolved. The aim was to eliminate acute hospitalizations where outpatient treatment could be substituted and to eliminate unnecessary days from a hospitalization period. The methodology decided on was to establish a system of preadmission notification so that a screening process would be carried out prior to nonemergency hospitalization to determine whether an admission is required for the given illness or whether it could be managed on an outpatient basis. Briefly stated, this approach works as follows: on preadmission notification, a nurse review coordinator who is an employee of the foundation under the supervision of physician advisors and attending physicians would monitor the length of stay of the patient.

With the cooperation of Mr. Hyman and the Printers' Union of Sacramento County, CHAP was initiated in 1969. The 800 members of the group, which carried a foundation-sponsored health plan, were used in a test program to refine the proposed methodology. Initial experiences were excellent in that the system was able to identify some unnecessary diagnostic admissions. The health plan itself was modified to provide 100% coverage for outpatient physician and laboratory evaluation. Monitoring by the nurse coordinator was low key and, because of the low volume of study patients, had little impact on any one particular physician's practice. Initial response from the physicians was satisfactory, and no hostility developed. Despite the general inflationary trend within the community, this program did indeed save a substantial amount of money. Savings from hospital expenses in turn were used to pay for the outpatient benefits of the program. Overall premiums in the program were kept low, and during an open enrollment period very few patients switched into the prepaid Kaiser program.

Some time later the state of California Medicaid program experienced a substantial deficit. Accordingly, regulations were issued requiring prior authorization for all acute, nonemergency admissions to hospitals. Dr. Earl Brian, director of the Department of Health Care Services at that time, was approached by several physicians within the community to indicate how he would view applicaton of CHAP to the Title XIX beneficiaries in lieu of the state's prior-authorization program. Dr. Brian and his staff examined CHAP and felt it was a reasonable program that could be implemented for Title XIX. Accordingly, in April 1970 a contract was negotiated between the Department of Health Care Services and the Medical Care Foundation of Sacramento to apply CHAP to all Title XIX hospital admissions in the counties of Sacramento and El Dorado.

At that time there were 100,000 Title XIX beneficiaries within that area. Obviously such an immense number of patients requiring certification under CHAP at one time brought on a series of growing pains and operational experiences that were invaluable to the Medical Care Foundation of Sacramento during subsequent years. The number of nurse coordinators had to be increased virtually over night from 1 to 20, and the number of staff people supporting the 20 nurses and various physician reviewers also increased proportionately.

It should also be noted here that when CHAP was first conceived, the administrators of area hospitals having the largest numbers of beds were approached to obtain their reaction to a hospital utilization program of this magnitude. Their cooperation and enthusiasm really provided the impetus that made this program move. Many of the hospitals had been financially hurt because of Title XIX and Title XVIII services in their hospitals, and thus the administrators were anxious to eliminate any retroactive denials. An understanding was reached with Dr. Brian that retroactive denials under Title XIX would be eliminated as part of the conditions for operating CHAP in the community. With that assurance the hospitals put in a major effort in implementing CHAP. They were extremely cooperative in providing necessary space within the hospitals for CHAP clerical people and in meeting other requirements necessary for an orderly development of the program. To this date CHAP has almost unanimous support of the hospital administrators of the area. This program was expanded subsequently to include the Medicare population (Title XVIII), which could only be done with hospital administrator support.

The overall configuration of this system then was based on an areawide hospital utilization program made up of physician reviewers and registered nurse coordinators working within the structure of a medical foundation but with the cooperation of area hospital administrators. There is no formal relationship required with the hospital utilization committees of the individual hospitals. Essential support functions are coordinated through a centrally organized administrative system funded entirely through foundation contracts. The cost of CHAP varies from group to group depending on the demographic composition of the patient population served.

CHAP system requirements

The foundation defines three specific requirements for a preadmission hospital screening system:

1. The first requirement is the preadmission notification and evaluation of elective hospital admissions along with a concurrent review of emergency admissions by local practicing physicians. This means that physician-consultants must be available in each field of practice and used as reviewers when indicated before elective and after emergency hospital admissions.

2. The second requirement calls for centralized, responsible, professional management by a recognized county, district, or state medical society, or a subsidiary foundation acting as an independent administrator. In short, doctors must run the review program completely independent of hospital administration and utilization committees. Reviewers must be appointed by and responsible to the society or foundation. The professional society (or component) must provide an appeals mechanism that provides due process or a second opinion for patient, hospital, physician, and fiscal agent.

3. Nurse review coordinators, as employees of the administrative agency, are required to follow the course of patients in the hospital to help determine the necessity of admission and certified length of stay. The review coordinator, the key element in the entire CHAP review process, must be a registered nurse experienced in hospital patient care as well as

one with the personality and insight needed to work smoothly with physicians and patients who might have conflicting attitudes toward utilization control. A number of registered nurses are utilized in the central office to screen admission notification and coordinate activity between physician advisors and on-site reviewers in their attempts to obtain further detailed information on certain hospital cases when indicated. Other nurse reviewers are assigned to the various hospitals where they make daily ward rounds to review patients under CHAP contract coverage. They are allowed to review and extract information from the hospital charts for use in review process and to consult with the attending physician and with their own physician advisors when necessary. The nurse coordinator does not make decisions to deny payment to any physician nor to deny certification of any hospital admission. Only a physician advisor can make such a decision.

Admission notification for eight to ten procedures is isolated to trigger the request for additional information, consultation, and patient examination by a physician advisor. These include (1) multiple tonsillectomies in one family, (2) hysterectomies in patients under age 30 (the consultation must justify this procedure), (3) hospitalization for procedures that could be done on an outpatient basis, (4) requests for more than one preoperative hospital day, (5) all plastic surgeries that could be classified as being cosmetic (photographs must be presented to the advisor for review), (6) ileojejunal bypass, (7) dental extractions requiring hospitalization, (8) requests for umbilical herniorrhaphies on patients under 6 years of age, and any other procedure that may be questioned by the CHAP coordinator at the initial screening of the requests for hospital admission. A certain number of physicians have been identified in the community as having aberrant practices along these lines, and in many cases the board of trustees of the foundation has placed these physicians on total prior-authorization review. In these cases the physician is not guaranteed payment for any of his services, nor is the hospital guaranteed payment for the patient stay until such time as the foundation has reviewed the case in detail, which in some cases requires a confirming consultation.

Once an admission of any type is reviewed in the central office and the approved length of stay is assigned, the hospital is then guaranteed payment for that hospital admission up to that given length of stay. The admitting physician is also guaranteed payment for his services, assuming that they meet all of the medical policy guidelines. These guidelines were developed over the last 3 years by all of the various specialty groups in the Sacramento area. They are designed to be used by the claims examiners in the claims peer review activity, by the professional review analyst, and by the physician advisor as he performs retrospective review.

The CHAP committee, as mentioned previously, is made up of practicing physicians usually in the field of general practice and internal medicine who are assigned on a rotating basis to function within the central office or are assigned to review the admissions of a particular hospital. Very commonly these reviewing physicians are members of the hospital utilization committee, but this is not a requirement of the CHAP system. It is desirable that they be senior physician advisors who have had past experience within the peer review and hospital utilization systems and are of unquestionable ability. Again, as mentioned earlier, the various specialty committees are available to them as resource committees in case of clinical problems arising within a specific specialty.

Supporting the CHAP review program is a computer system. The input document for the computerized data system is the CHAP Initial Certification Request form generated either at the hospital admission office in case of emergency admissions or by the attending physician's office staff

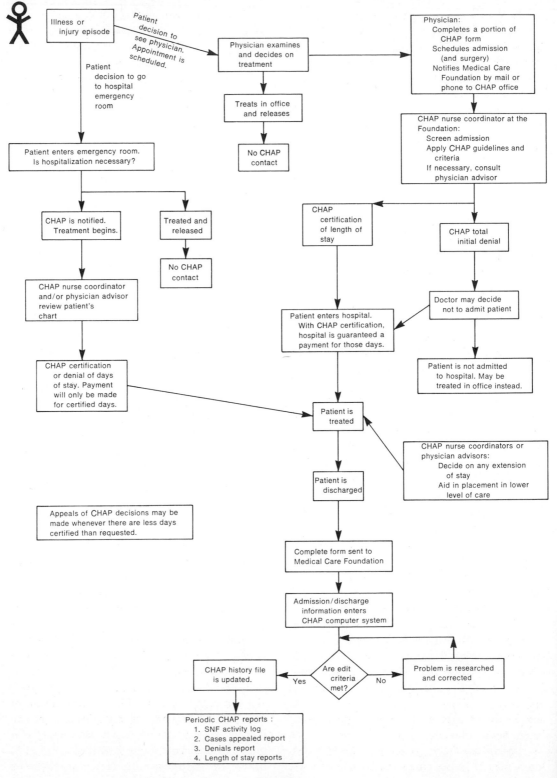

Fig. 14-1

in the case of elective admissions. The data on this CHAP form meets the PSRO requirements now in effect in the five-county area surrounding Sacramento. From this form sufficient data are obtained to provide management reports to the foundation and CHAP such as physician and hospital profiles, diagnostic and surgical categorical information, lengths of stay, utilization trends, and patient profiles. Such reports are not only necessary to the CHAP program but also essential to the insurance programs administered by the foundation. For example, the data generated on length-of-stay reports make it possible to compare by diagnoses the lengths of stay of local hospitals. This report is also used by CHAP management to locally set criteria for lengths of stay and to update the CHAP coordinators' coding manual. The reports that show utilization trends are used to show the effectiveness of CHAP when securing new business or renewed business with the sponsored insurance plans. Various inpatient management reports from CHAP are integrated with management reports coming from the claims peer review departments that monitor ambulatory practice (Fig. 14-1).

Over 100 physicians now participate in the peer review functions of the foundation, including CHAP, and they participate in the day-to-day management of these programs.

Setting CHAP in motion

Since it is the elective admission that triggers the preadmission CHAP mechanism, let's take a look at the usual routine involved in the certification process.

1. Typically the patient is seen and evaluated in his personal physician's office. When the clinical evaluation leads to a decision to admit the patient to a particular hospital for treatment, the physician's office fills out a CHAP Initial Certification Request form, which then becomes a source document for the review of that particular patient's hospital stay. Fig. 14-2 shows how this form would be filled out

for a patient with pneumonia. The data required on that portion of the form completed by the physician's office include physician's identification, patient identification, and illness identification information.

2. Concurrently the physician's office makes arrangements for the admission with the hospital admission office and completes the form as to the anticipated date of admission and, in surgical cases, the scheduled date of surgery and informaton pertaining to the procedure. If the hospital admission is to take place at least 5 days from that time, the form is mailed to the foundation. Should admission be required earlier than that, verbal notification is made by telephone to the CHAP office on scheduling the admission. The form is then completed as usual and mailed for regular processing.

3. On arrival at the foundation's CHAP office the form is screened by nurse review coordinators experienced in CHAP procedures. They use local criteria and guidelines established by the CHAP committee in addition to those of physician advisors, special review committees, and the Medical Review and Appeals Committee that have evolved from previous experience. Assuming that the admission data on the CHAP form meets the required screens and criteria, an expected length of stay is assigned to that admission. A copy of the processed form is sent by the CHAP review personnel to the hospital admissions and business office. The hospital is then guaranteed payment for that admission up to the expected length of stay. The review coordinator assigned to that hospital will then utilize the original CHAP document as a case review document within the hospital and record the patient's clinical progress as shown in Fig. 14-3. Should the patient be discharged before the expected length of stay expires, the form is simply validated by the nurse reviewer at the time of discharge by certifying the number of days the patient was

Text continued on p. 318.

**MEDICAL CARE FOUNDATION
OF SACRAMENTO**

650 UNIVERSITY AVE.

SACRAMENTO, CALIFORNIA 95825

PHONE (916) 929-3221
INITIAL CERTIFICATION

**CERTIFIED HOSPITAL ADMISSION
PROGRAM**

CHAP STAMP

BATCHING

No. C

MCF

OFFICE USE ONLY   OFFICE USE ONLY

SECTION A (SHADED) FOR DOCTOR AND HOSPITAL USE

PATIENT NAME (LAST)	(FIRST)	(M.I.)	ADMITTING PHYSICIAN (LAST)	(FIRST)	LICENSE NO.
Doe Jane			Doe John		

ADDRESS 650 University Ave   ADDRESS 650 University Ave

CITY	COUNTY	STATE	ZIP	CITY	COUNTY	STATE	ZIP
Sacto	Sacto	Cal.	95825	Sacto	Sacto	Cal.	95825

BIRTHDATE MO DA YR	SEX	MEDICAL RECORD NO.	RACE 1 ☐ BLACK 2 ☐ WHITE 3 ☒ OTHER
11 11 11		111 111	

PATIENT PROGRAM IDENTIFICATION (CHECK ALL THAT APPLY)

ADMITTING DIAGNOSIS
Pneumonia

1 ☒ MEDICARE   1 2 3 4 5 6 7 8 A
2 ☐ FCHP
3 ☐ MEDI-CAL
4 ☐ TITLE V
5 ☐ SPONSORED

PROPOSED PROCEDURE OR TREATMENT

NAME OF EMPLOYER   NAME OF INSURED
GROUP NO. ➞
SSA NO. ➞

6 ☐ OTHER SPECIFY

DAYS REQUESTED	ADMISSION DATE MO DAY YR	SURGERY DATE MO DAY YR	PROCEDURE DATE MO DAY YR
	04 30 76		

I. D. NO.

FACILITY NAME	FACILITY NO.	PHYSICIAN SIGNATURE	DATE
MCF	000000		

SECTION B - ADMISSION INFORMATION

ADMISSION DATE MO DAY YR	PRIMARY ADMITTING PROGRAM TYPE (1-6) ▶	MCF COVERAGE VERIFIED MO DAY YR DATE:	INITIAL DAYS CERTIFIED	ADMISSION CHAP RN. NO.	REVIEW PHYSICIAN I.D. NUMBER	I.C.D.A. ADMIS. DIAG. CODE	I.C.D.A. SURG.	OTHER PROC.
4 30 76			5	123		1	1	1
LEVEL OF CARE ▶ 1 ☒ ACUTE 2 ☐ S.N.F. 3 ☐ I.C.F. 4 ☐ L.T. / CUSTODIAL						2	2	2
ADMISSION STATUS 1. ☒ MEDICAL 3. ☐ OBSTETRICS 5. ☐ PEDIATRICS 7. ☐ NEWBORN 9. ☒ EMERGENCY 2. ☐ SURGICAL 4. ☐ GYNECOLOGY 6. ☐ PSYCHIATRY 8. ☐ ELECTIVE 10. ☐ URGENT						3	3	3

SECTION C - DISCHARGE INFORMATION

DISCHARGE DIAG. CODES	SURGERY PERFORM.	SURGERY DATES MO. DAY. YR.	OTHER	PROCEDURE DATES MO. DAY. YR.	COMPLICATIONS	RECODE INITIAL DAYS	O.B. DELIVERY DATE	MO	DAY	YEAR
1	1	05 05 76		1		3				
2	2	05 04 76		2		ATTENDING PHYSICIAN	(LAST)	(FIRST)	(MI)	
3	3	05 06 76		3		LICENSE NO.				
4	4	05 09 76		4		PRIMARY OPERATING PHYSICIAN	(LAST)	(FIRST)	(MI)	
5	5			5		LICENSE NO.				

TOTAL INITIAL DENIAL	REASON CODE ▶	DECISION APPEALED (√) ☐	DECISION REVERSED (√) ☐	REVERSAL CODE	DAYS CERTIFIED ON REVERSAL		DATES OF DAYS DENIED		

TOTAL EXTENSIONS DENIED	TOTAL NO. DENIED 1	REASON CODE (1) (2)	DECISION APPEALED (1) (2)	DECISION REVERSED (1) (2)	REVERSAL CODE (1) (2)	DAYS CERT. ON REVERSAL (1) (2)	DATES OF DAYS DENIED FROM	THRU

EXTENSIONS	TOTAL NUMBER OF EXTENSIONS REQUESTED 3	TOTAL NUMBER OF EXTENSIONS APPROVED 2	TOTAL NUMBER OF EXTENSION DATES REQUESTED 13	TOTAL NUMBER OF EXTENSION DAYS GRANTED 10	FINAL HOSPITAL DAYS CERTIFIED ▶	ACUTE DAYS 18	S.N.F. DAYS	OTHER DAYS

SUMMARY	HOSPITAL DAYS REQUESTED 21	HOSPITAL DAYS CERTIFIED 18	DAYS OF STAY OTHER THAN WARD (1) (2) (3) (4) (5) SPECIFY:	CHAP DAYS DENIED	NON CHAP DAYS	DISCHARGE DATE MO DAY YEAR 05 19 76

DISCHARGE CODES
1. ☐ OTHER HOSPITAL
2. ☒ S.N.F.

PROVIDER NO. 000000
PROVIDER NO.

3. ☐ TO HOME   6. ☐ TO STATE HOSPITAL   9. ☐ EXPIRED
4. ☐ I.C.F.   7. ☐ L.O.A.   10. ☐ STILL IN
5. ☐ B & C   8. ☐ TO HOME AGAINST MED. ADVICE   11. ☐ OTHER

REMARKS:

RETROACTIVE ☐ YES	REV. PHYSICIAN I.D. NO. (DENIAL)	DISCHARGE R.N. NUMBER 123
SPECIAL REPORTS ▶		DATE TO REVIEW DATE TO HOSPITAL

Z-002 3/76 COPYRIGHT APPLIED FOR   PLEASE SEND ALL 6 COPIES TO M.C.F.   S

Fig. 14-2

MEDICAL CARE FOUNDATION
OF SACRAMENTO

CHAP STAMP

№ C

BATCHING

650 HOWE AVE.
SACRAMENTO, CALIFORNIA 95825

PHONE (916) 929-3221
INITIAL CERTIFICATION

CERTIFIED HOSPITAL ADMISSION
PROGRAM

OFFICE USE ONLY   OFFICE USE ONLY

SECTION A (SHADED) FOR DOCTOR AND HOSPITAL USE

PATIENT NAME (LAST)   (FIRST)   (M.I.)   ADMITTING PHYSICIAN (LAST)   (FIRST)   LICENSE NO.

Doe   Jane

ADDRESS   ADDRESS

CITY   COUNTY   STATE   ZIP   CITY   COUNTY   STATE   ZIP

4/30/76   75 yr. old female   adm. from c̄ chest pain; SOB.
↑ Temp 101⁶   P₁₀₀   R 26

Amp: pneumonia

Plans: C + R
        I/m antibiotics
        observe

5/1   Temp 100   I/m Pen. G. Q
      BRP c̄ help

5/3   Con't c̄ SOB
      Temp 101 P₁₀₆

(5/4   Recoded 3 days)
      Plan Thoracentesis → done 5/4 - 5/5
                           fld to lab for culture ⟩
                                         Sens.

5/7 Pleural cavity irrigated c̄ Pen. Sol.
     c̄ Thoracentesis-
     temp 100²

CX R -
pneumonia
? pleural fld.

CBC -
    WBC 11.5
    Hgb 12.2

RPT   CBC
    WBC 16.5 ↑
    leukocytes ↑

CX R -
    ↑ pleural fld.

Reviewed c̄ advisor
Ext. 4 days

Continued.

Fig. 14-3

5/8   No improvement in condition   C X R
       T 101   P 112   No change
       Some SOB → ? Pulmonary abcess
    ? Plans - Insertion of chest tube &
       surgical drainage

5/9   In surgery — I + D → pleural cavity   WBC 15.6
                 Chest tubes

5/11   Temp 100
       To ↑ activity   Con't c̄
(PO#2) Chest tube intact   i/v antibiotics   C X R
       liq diet

                                              (Extension
                                              + 5days)

5/13   amb. c̄ help   i/v is dc'd
(PO#4) Temp 99   P 88   started po antibiotics
       Chest tubes removed

5/15   Up ad lib   (5/14) C X R
PO#6   No chest pain   clearing - small
       diet - TWR   am't fld in pleural
       Temp wnl   cavity

5/16   Arrangement started for SNF   ⎰ 7days with SNF coverage
       ? transf.   5/17   (Rev c̄ adv) → ⎱ Plan observation → pulmonary
                                                      disease.

5/17   Family does not want pt. to go
       to an SNF. Would like for pt. to   (Reviewed c̄ adv.
       stay in acute hosp. until the daughter,
       that would be caring for her, returns   No further
       from vacation.   coverage in
                                                    acute hosp.
       PT's MD agrees → No further time needed in acute hosp.

Fig. 14-3, cont'd.

MEDICAL CARE FOUNDATION OF SACRAMENTO

650 HOWE AVE.
SACRAMENTO, CALIFORNIA 95825

PHONE (916) 929-3221
INITIAL CERTIFICATION

CERTIFIED HOSPITAL ADMISSION PROGRAM

CHAP STAMP

Nº C

BATCHING

OFFICE USE ONLY   OFFICE USE ONLY

SECTION A (SHADED) FOR DOCTOR AND HOSPITAL USE

PATIENT NAME (LAST) (FIRST) (M.I.)   ADMITTING PHYSICIAN (LAST) (FIRST)   LICENSE NO.

Doe   Jane

ADDRESS   ADDRESS

CITY COUNTY STATE ZIP   CITY COUNTY STATE ZIP

5/17 cont

Hospital's business office (mr —) notified of denial
2 copies of denial letter To hospital

attending MD notified of denial → Copy of
denial letter to MD (attending).

5/18 Ambulatory
Temp WN

5/19 Disch To SNF

Fig. 14-3, cont'd.

actually hospitalized. A copy of this validated form is used for billing the fiscal intermediary or the foundation and therefore is returned to the business office.

4. Should the diagnosis change during the course of the hospitalization or some clinical event occur to the patient that a prolonged hospitalization becomes necessary, arrangements to extend the length of stay are made by the review coordinator on request initiated by the attending physician and with the approval of a physician advisor. Fig. 14-4 shows how this form would be filled out if it appeared

Fig. 14-4

that a clinical complication was developing. Extensions to the lengths of stay are handled after a brief review of the case conducted between a nurse coordinator and the physician advisor and usually without any need to contact directly the attending physician. Figs. 14-5 and 14-6 illustrate the sequence for further extensions and show reviews that might take place in a case of pneumonia complicated by empyema. In those cases where the need for extension of length of stay is unclear and when the patient's condition appears not to warrant an extension of length of stay,

MEDICAL CARE FOUNDATION OF SACRAMENTO
CERTIFIED HOSPITAL ADMISSION PROGRAM - EXTENSION REQUEST
CHAP

MCF

PATIENT NAME (LAST) (FIRST) (M.I.): Doe Jane
FACILITY NAME | FACILITY NO.
SEX | ADM. DATE | PATIENT I.D. NUMBER
ADMITTING PROGRAM: 1. MEDI-CAL ☐ 2. MEDI-CARE ☐ 3. F.C.H.P. ☐ 4. COMMERCIAL ☐ 5. OTHER ☐
LENGTH OF EXTENSION REQUESTED ► p̄ 5/11
REASON FOR EXTENSION REQUEST

Dx: Empyema-
I-D pleural cavity - Insertion chest tube 5/9

RECERTIFICATION SIGNATURE (MEDICARE ONLY) — DATE / /
ATTENDING PHYSICIAN'S NAME
RECERTIFICATION SIGNATURE (MEDICARE ONLY) — DATE / /
ATTENDING PHYSICIAN'S SIGNATURE — DATE

APPROVED ☒	FIRST EXTENSION ☐ / SUBSEQUENT EXTENSION #2 ☒	NUMBER OF DAYS APPROVED ► 6	THROUGH ►	DATE 5 /16 /76
DENIED ☐	FIRST DENIAL ☐ / SUBSEQUENT DENIAL ☐	NUMBER OF DAYS DENIED ►	REASON ►	
DENIAL APPEALED ☐ YES ☐ NO	REASON ►	DATE / /	DECISION UPHELD ☐ YES	DECISION REVERSED ☐ YES
IF DECISION REVERSED GIVE REASON CODED ►		ADDITIONAL DIAGNOSIS CODES		ADDITIONAL DIAGNOSIS CODES

EXPLAIN

APPROVED BY: MD advisor
CHAP R.N. SIGNATURE: RN coordinator — DATE / /

Z-003 Rev. 3/76 $

Fig. 14-5

direct contact between the nurse coordinator and the attending physician is made for the purpose of obtaining more information. Infrequently contact between the attending physician and the review physician may become necessary to expedite the process. Following clarification of medical information concerning the patient, a decision is then made by the physician advisor to extend the length of stay based on established medical necessity or to deny extension of length of stay based on a lack of substantiation. Fig. 14-7 displays the denial letter that is received by the patient,

MEDICAL CARE FOUNDATION OF SACRAMENTO

CERTIFIED HOSPITAL ADMISSION PROGRAM - EXTENSION REQUEST

CHAP

PATIENT NAME (LAST)	(FIRST)	(M.I.)	FACILITY NAME	FACILITY NO.
Doe	Jane			

SEX	ADM. DATE	PATIENT I.D. NUMBER
	/ /	

LENGTH OF EXTENSION REQUESTED ► $\bar{p}$ 5/16

ADMITTING PROGRAM

1. MEDI-CAL	☐	4. COMMERCIAL	☐
2. MEDI-CARE	☒	5. OTHER	☐
3. F.C.H.P.	☐		

REASON FOR EXTENSION REQUEST

Pneumonia - Empyema

chest tube insertion

RECERTIFICATION SIGNATURE (MEDICARE ONLY)	DATE	ATTENDING PHYSICIAN'S NAME	
	/ /		
RECERTIFICATION SIGNATURE (MEDICARE ONLY)	DATE	ATTENDING PHYSICIAN'S SIGNATURE	DATE
	/ /		

APPROVED	☐	FIRST EXTENSION	☐	NUMBER OF DAYS APPROVED ►		THROUGH ►	DATE 5/16/76
		SUBSEQUENT EXTENSION	☐				
DENIED	☒	FIRST DENIAL	☒	NUMBER OF DAYS DENIED ►	3	REASON ►	
		SUBSEQUENT DENIAL	☐				
DENIAL APPEALED	☐ YES ☐ NO	REASON ►	DATE / /	DECISION UPHELD	☐ YES	DECISION REVERSED	☐ YES
IF DECISION REVERSED GIVE REASON CODED ►			ADDITIONAL DIAGNOSIS CODES			ADDITIONAL DIAGNOSIS CODES	

EXPLAIN

See nurses notes for explanation date 5/17/76

APPROVED BY

MD advisor

CHAP R.N. SIGNATURE	DATE
RN coordinator	/ /

Z-003 Rev. 3/76

1

Fig. 14-6

the attending physician, and the hospital.

5. Awareness of social problems related to the financing of care play an important part in the nurse coordinator's role. For example, if a patient's hospitalization has been certified for a period that may make him or her ineligible for postacute care, the hospital, the patient, and the attending physician are all advised what the financial implications are to the patient. Because of their vast experience in the management of this program, the nurse coordinators anticipate potential placement problems and begin to look into

---

GSPSRO

GREATER SACRAMENTO PROFESSIONAL STANDARDS REVIEW ORGANIZATION

P.O. BOX 13978   SACRAMENTO, CA 95813   (916) 929-3221

DATE OF ADMISSION _04-30-76_

DATE OF NOTIFICATION _05-17-76_

HOSPITAL _MCF_

☐ ACUTE   ☐ SNF

To _Jane Doe_ :
    (Patient)

PATIENT'S MEDICARE NUMBER _12345678A_

The Greater Sacramento Professional Standards Review Organization (GSPSRO) has reviewed your:

☐   Pending admission.

☐   Admission to the hospital on _____ .

☐   Continued stay at the hospital after _5/16/76_ .

GSPSRO has determined that the above is not certifiable for payment under the Medicare program.

The basis for this determination is as follows:

No further need for acute hospitalization

You (the beneficiary, patient's representative, physician, or facility) have a right to appeal and request a reconsideration of this determination. A request should be made in writing to the GSPSRO at the captioned address no later than two months from the date of this notice.

Sincerely,

James Bramham M.D

JAMES C. BRAMHAM, JR., M.D.
Interim Medical Director

cc: Attending Physician
     Provider
     CHAP Office

Dr notified 5/17/76

Hosp notified 5/17/76

SERVING THE FIVE COUNTIES IN CALIFORNIA PSRO AREA IV: SACRAMENTO • EL DORADO • NEVADA • PLACER • YOLO

Fig. 14-7

them early in the course of admission. The hospital administrators in each of the major hospitals have consequently assigned special staff nurses to work with the nurse review coordinators to arrange for the placement of these patients in the proper environment following completion of an acute hospital stay.

6. It must be noted here that during the course of the initial development of the Medicare CHAP program, it became apparent that the placement problems of elderly individuals were of a serious nature because of the magnitude of their frequency. The attitude of CHAP to the elderly was that they deserved the same compassion and understanding as all other patients. Every effort is therefore made to minimize placement problems for these individuals to keep certification within contractural obligations.

7. In a case where an attending physician disputes the decision of a review physician, either one may ask for an additional review of the case by yet another physician or a review by the CHAP committee itself. Occasionally the CHAP committee in its deliberations might ask for an opinion from the hospital utilization committee. This is particularly necessary in instances where several physicians, who because of philosophical differences, deliberately defy CHAP by refusing to discharge patients despite the fact that the medical necessity for their continued hospitalization has long since expired.

8. Following a review by the CHAP committee, final appeals may be made to the Medical Review and Appeals Committee of the foundation. Typically several CHAP appeals are heard monthly. The final review authority rests with the fiscal intermediary, the government agency, or the insurance program involved in the particular patient's case.

Overt opposition to CHAP did develop in certain hospitals, particularly after the Medicare program came under CHAP jurisdiction. Most of the physicians in opposition to the foundation program are not members of the foundation and, when the review of Title XIX patients became effective in 1970, indicated they were not amenable to taking care of welfare patients. When this review program was extended also to Medicare, the opposition became overt.

Emergency admissions do not require preadmission certification, but the nurse coordinator does monitor the patient's hospital course after the admission has occurred. It is the responsibility of the attending physician, the hospital, or the patient or relative to notify the CHAP office at the time of or within 48 hours of an emergency admission to have that patient's hospital stay monitored and certified. Following notification of the admission, the same general procedures take place. The initial review of the chart by the nurse coordinator is made at the hospital, and an initial length of stay is applied to the case. Following this, the review procedures are identical to those of the elective admissions.

Assessing the CHAP system

The strength of the CHAP system is based on its central organization. Physician reviewers and nurse coordinators work outside the hospital environment, permitting maximum objectivity. The preadmission notification system is particularly important in dealing with those physicians who have had long-standing problems with unestablished medical necessity for their hospital admissions and unnecessary admissions for diagnostic purposes in particular. Monitoring the length of stay is perhaps even more essential and is a strong aspect of the CHAP system. It is undoubtedly that aspect that is the most cost saving.

The system, however, has inherent limitations and weaknessess just as any system does. The necessity to generate a separate piece of paper from the doctor's office or hospital for a patient covered by CHAP is a significant problem in duplication of data requirements and in logistics of routing the forms. It has also built up the need for additional personnel within the foundation. Although the program can run adequately without extensive computer support in data management and the like, the vagaries of various government program demands mandate the reporting of major amounts of information that probably will never be used. This has caused resentment among both nurse coordinators and physicians within CHAP as well as from the hospital administrators and on-site physician reviewers in the hospitals and doctors' offices. Another weakness is the failure to develop an adequate exception report system where preadmission notification applies only to those physicians who have clearly demonstrated a pattern of practice other than that which is commonly acceptable in the community.

Coding presents another problem. Obviously diagnostic and procedural coding is a necessity for adequate and efficient data processing and as such has presented a problem because of the individual coding inconsistencies. Originally the registered nurse coordinator was responsible for coding, and this added a great burden to professional activities. Coding has since been brought into the central office and is now done by specialized coding clerks.

Operational and technical problems

Operational and technical problems are difficult to resolve. The integration of results from MCEs, that is, medical audit with results from the utilization program of the CHAP system, is essential. Rather than create a central medical audit system, however, it is the feeling of CHAP that medical audit should be done by hospital committees. A technical problem lies in developing an exception report system for length of stay certification that is selective for only those physicians who have demonstrated uncorrected problems with length of stay. Such physicians need to have their cases reviewed before lengths of stay are extended. The exception report system for preadmission notification is likewise not yet completed.

Meeting new needs

A PSRO recently has been developed in Sacramento County. At the present time it involves utilizing the CHAP system under subcontract. Over a period of time there will be an evolution from the current CHAP to one that is guided by new incentives for physicians and that can become more integrated with hospital politics and clinical activities.

The effectiveness of CHAP in saving money is expected to diminish while the cost of managing it increases because of overriding governmental regulations and data-reporting requirements. As stated earlier, the data collected on the CHAP form does meet the requirements of the PHDDS; however, the form had to be modified to collect this information. The existing data system had to be modified because of the federal reporting requirements (additional copies of reports have to be generated and forwarded to state and federal authorities, and the data must be analyzed by inhouse statisticians prior to release to the governmental agencies and the like), which has a tendency to increase the cost of utilization review. One overriding governmental regulation that is of particular concern is the Waiver of Liability provision, a provision under section 213 of the 1972 Medicare amendment. In brief, this states that a patient is entitled to at least 3 more days of hospitalization after CHAP has issued a denial letter. This only serves to increase the lengths of stay, thus increasing the cost of care. Another area of concern is the reimbursement of a facility for what is termed "administrative days." CHAP certifies those days considered to be medically necessary, and any additional time the patient remains in the facility can be declared as administrative days. The facility is reimbursed for those days. Another major thrust of CHAP in the next several years will likely be that of supporting the health maintenance organization that is being developed by the Medical Care Foundation of Sacramento. Over a period of 3 to 4 years an enrollment of somewhere between 50,000 to 100,000 people is expected to be achieved by the foundation's HMO (health maintenance organization). This prepaid concept will demand extensive peer review utilization control, including CHAP, to make it successful.

The current CHAP system, which is essentially unchanged from the day of its inception in 1970, is expected to undergo some changes in the future because (1) some of the CHAP functions will be taken over by the PSRO and (2) because of the need for a prepaid health program. The imposition of a large bureaucracy in Washington for managing the PSRO program undoubtedly will have an effect on CHAP and will decrease its efficiencies because of the immense required reporting system and the use of professional personnel in nonprofessional activities as a result. There has been and undoubtedly will continue to be some loss of local autonomy. Undoubtedly these peer review systems will be gradually replaced in methodology as the organization of medical care delivery in the community changes. The government is increasing its regulatory emphasis on medicine with the result that we are now approaching the advent of national health insurance financing.

CHAP was originally designed to develop a utilization program that could effectively reduce insurance plan premiums so they could become competitive with closed panel programs. The added costs of inflation and malpractice insurance premiums have minimized the apparent fiscal effects of these CHAP savings within the community, but nevertheless such savings continue to exist.

The CHAP system is a common-sense approach to monitoring the use of the hospital. It can be viewed as one dramatic step by local practicing physicians to demonstrate their public accountability. With the advent of the health maintenance organization other bold changes can be expected in medical care delivery by fee-for-service private-practicing physicians that will continuously cause some disruption in the minds of opponents to change. It is the feeling of the Medical Care Foundation of Sacramento and CHAP that orderly change guided by the medical profession itself and based on the needs of the patient will successfully prevent a total nationalization of the medical industry.

15

Quality assessment and utilization review in a functioning peer review system

ALAN R. NELSON

Prior to the establishment of the Utah Professional Review Organization (UPRO) in 1971, most operational peer review projects dealt either with utilization review or with quality assessment. No broadly organized operation combined the two aspects of peer review into an integral process. Thus claims review was performed in San Joaquin, hospital admission certification was developed at Sacramento, and several schools of public health conducted a variety of quality assessment projects without regard to utilization review.

As the design for the UPRO's various projects took place, it became clear that a new approach was needed if local groups of physicians were to manage peer review systems, as was being contemplated in proposed PSRO legislation. Several new concepts emerged:

1. An ideal quality assessment and utilization review program is managed at the level of the physician community. Organization at this level permits the application of criteria across the various institutions within the community and permits comparisons to be drawn among hospitals and regions.

2. Such a system may employ a screening structure for utilization review that is also used to collect data for quality assessment programs and ultimately provides screening for quality assurance.

3. Ideally this community-based peer review system (as opposed to hospital-based) looks at all levels of care, permitting integration of ambulatory care review with institutional review and review of long-term care. By broadening the scope of review efforts, epidemiologic data may be collected as part of the long-term assessment program.

4. By linking quality assessment to utilization review in an inextricable fashion, a funding source is provided for quality assessment that had heretofore been lacking. Stated otherwise, payment sources that stand to benefit from improved utilization practices subsidize quality assessment, since they buy a single review package. Ultimately this subsidization extends to continuing physician education, since the review organization also conducts an educational program based on its review findings.

In incorporating these concepts into program design, UPRO has developed and implemented two general peer review projects: the On-Site Concurrent Hospital Utilization Review (OSCHUR) program, which conducts utilization review and quality assessment activity in all major hospitals in the state, and the Physician Ambulatory Care Evaluation (PACE) program, which assesses quality and utilization patterns for ambulatory services under Medicaid. While each of these projects was developed simultaneously, they have somewhat differing theoretic bases and marked operational differences; hence they will be discussed separately.

THE OSCHUR PROGRAM

The OSCHUR program, the first UPRO project, was begun in 1971. By June 1974, 34,000 hospital admissions had been reviewed concurrently; with the OSCHUR system serving as the field audit mechanism for the UPRO, 30,000 hospital stays are now being reviewed annually.

The OSCHUR program was designed to provide effective review and, at the same time, avoid or eliminate the undesirable features of alternative review plans (Table 15-1).

The OSCHUR process involves review of admissions covered by subscribing payment sources (private as well as under PSRO) for the necessity of admission, appropriate length of stay, level of care,

ancillary services, and, for selected cases, an assessment of quality.

Screening process

All screening by the nurse coordinators is supported by criteria that have been developed by physician panels, organized at the state level, and representing each of 17 specialties. The nurse coordinator, referring to criteria, either certifies the admission need or submits the case to peer review by the utilization review committee member who serves as the UPRO consultant. After consulting UPRO norms the nurse coordinator applies an indicator of expected length of stay, which can be extended if necessary without a formal request by the attending physician. If an extension beyond the norm is not clearly indicated, the case is submitted to the UPRO consultant for peer review.

Approximately 90% of hospital admissions and stays require only screening review and data collection by the nurse coordinator rather than full peer review by a physician consultant. The nurse coordinator's screening and skill in synthesizing the relevant information in profile form minimizes the time commitment by the medical consultant, and his time is spent

Table 15-1. Comparison of OSCHUR review program with alternative review plans

Alternative review plans	OSCHUR review program
1. Review is punitive via retroactive denial.	1. All hospital care is reviewed and certified concurrently with no retroactive denial.
2. Review requires an increased physician time commitment.	2. Nurse coordinators are utilized to screen cases for peer review and synthesize chart data to make review more efficient.
3. Review requires increased physician paperwork.	3. All data are collected by nurse coordinators; physicians are not required to fill out recertification request forms.
4. Physician reviewers are not compensated for hours spent reviewing.	4. Physician reviewers are compensated as consultants on an hourly basis for actual review time.
5. Preadmission certification of hospital need poses a bureaucratic obstacle to legitimate patient entry into the hospital.	5. Admission certification is conducted within one working day after hospital admission.
6. Quality of medical care suffers as a result of attention to cost containment.	6. Quality of patient care is always first priority, and utilization review is linked to a system of quality assessment.

largely in making review decisions. UPRO data show that an average of 0.16 physician hours are spent per patient screened for review. This is equivalent to about 1.3 minutes of physician review time per hospitalized UPRO patient. In the rare instance where the dialogue between the physician reviewer and the attending physician fails to resolve the question of utilization appropriateness, UPRO certification is withdrawn and payment for continuing care is at risk.

Improved screening capability results from the nurse coordinator's clinical skills and synthesizing ability. The nurse coordinator also effects more accurate data collection than other systems have usually possessed. In addition to collecting the uniform data set shown in the adjacent box, the nurse coordinator encodes the discharge diagnosis on the last hospital day and adds precision and uniformity to the application of diagnostic nomenclature by selecting the appropriate code for the discharge diagnosis and clinical condition (based on guidelines developed by UPRO). Thus, while the physician may apply an ambiguous discharge diagnosis of chronic lung disease, the nurse coordinator is permitted to assign the code for chronic obstructive emphysema or, alternatively, bronchial asthma, based on the clinical information on the chart and instructions developed within the guidelines.

Quality assessment

Quality assessment under the OSCHUR program has involved the retrospective analysis of aggregate disidentified data collected against process criteria for selected diagnoses. Diagnoses are chosen for audit based on an inference of quality deficit, adequate case volume, and geographic and specialty breadth. Data are collected that express compliance with criteria elements regarded as critical to ideal care. Where areas of substantial noncompliance exist, an attempt is made to link the information with continuing education programs. For instance, when data

---

OSCHUR PROGRAM
Data elements collected by
nurse coordinator

1. Hospital
2. Nurse coordinator
3. Data first review
4. Patient's hospital number
5. Birthdate
6. Sex
7. Marital status
8. Race
9. Zip code
10. Source of payment
11. Patient's insurance number
12. Indications for admission
13. Emergency/elective
14. Documentation: history and physical
15. Documentation: progress notes
16. Admitting problem or diagnosis
17. Therapy
18. Complications
19. Final diagnoses (3 maximum)
20. Primary physician and specialty
21. Consultant 1 and specialty
22. Consultant 2 and specialty
23. Admission date
24. Anticipated discharge date
25. Surgery date
26. Extension granted to date
27. Actual discharge date
28. Patient disposition
29. Level of care
30. Medical advisor review
31. Certification granted/denied

---

showed approximately 40% noncompliance for criteria specifying the need for a prothrombin time and partial thromboplastin time in patients with gastrointestinal bleeding, communication to chairmen of each hospital's quality audit committee urged discussion of the data with the hospital staff. Report forms were requested to provide UPRO with information on the effectiveness of the meetings. Finally, reaudit confirmed the success (or lack of success, in certain hospitals) of the education effort. An article describing physician performance for these (and other) criteria was also published in the *Bulletin* of the Utah State Medical Association.

Since this type of quality assessment consists only of providing answers to questions posed by peer committees, there is no implication of "cookbook medicine" or challenge to the physician's authority to deliver care to individual patients.

In addition to the process audit conducted for selected diagnoses, UPRO is implementing a type of outcome audit in which management objectives are defined for clinical conditions or diagnoses, and the success of the physicians in attaining the management objectives is measured. This appproach to outcomes assessment was selected because physician panels often find it difficult to discriminate between outcome quality assessment and traditional clinical research that seeks to link an action with an expected outcome. Following is an example of management objective criteria (for bacterial and viral pneumonia):

1. Identified causative organism (does not require specific identification, may be tentative but provides a basis for logical therapy)
2. Afebrile or improving febrile course
3. Absence of complications (empyema, lung abscess, or increasing pleural effusion)
4. Follow-up outpatient visit arranged
5. Stable or improving x-ray picture (must be at least two studies on separate occasions)

The advantages of retrospective aggregate data analysis are clear: enhanced confidentiality, lessened liability, and preservation of individualized care based on each physician's understanding of each patient's unique needs. The disadvantages in such quality assessment are the dependency on effective education programs and the lag time inherent in behavior modification. Quality assurance programs, on the other hand, intervene in the direct care of an individual physician with his patient, with peer review seeking to modify the physician's action on a concurrent basis. UPRO has been cautious as it approached the question of intervention in direct care but

has begun a pilot project that will attempt to test the physician acceptance of such intervention by the peer review program and will measure the impact on patient care. A medical care evaluation study will provide concurrent peer review for all whole blood administration that does not meet the UPRO criterion of anemia plus hypovolemia. Intervention criteria, as well as management objective criteria, are publicized widely in the physician community before the peer review program implements the study.

Special projects

Additional MCEs have been conducted as special projects by UPRO. One such study tabulates all complications occurring during the hospital confinement, divides the complications into ten categories (Table 15-2), and permits comparison between hospitals in the system for each of the complication categories. When an area of complication occurrence appears particularly prominent in this report, more intensive investigation can be undertaken. Thus, when adverse reactions to medications appear particularly common in an institution, a detailed analysis of the type of adverse reaction is made. The results are then linked to continuing physician education programs.

While it has seemed appropriate to design criteria on a statewide basis, utilizing panels representing each of the 17 major specialties in the state, it has become apparent that each hospital must identify an individual with the responsibility to receive the data derived from the peer review projects and disseminate the information and educational efforts throughout the hospital staff. Frequently this individual is the chief medical advisor representing UPRO within the hospital. Often he also serves as chairman of the quality audit committee. UPRO has made an effort to integrate the peer review activity with the hospital's own quality audit structure to avoid duplication. The committee with the responsibility for complying with JCAH standards also has the responsibility

Table 15-2. OSCHUR program complication study, January 1975 to June 1975

Complication	Reviewed patients (%)
Adverse reaction to surgery	2.27
Adverse reaction to medication	2.37
Urinary tract infection	0.92
Accident unrelated to therapy	0.72
Wound infection	0.33
Postoperative temperature	0.43
Refused medical care	0.50
Thromboembolism	0.28
Obstetric complication	0.26
Pneumonia	0.25
Other complication	0.07
Total	8.40

for modifying UPRO criteria, if it wishes, and for analyzing and acting on the data supplied by UPRO audit.

Review of ancillary services

UPRO has conducted a series of studies monitoring the utilization of laboratory and x-ray services. One such study attempted to identify the norm for utilization of arterial blood gases, electrocardiograms, and blood chemistries for patients with selected diagnoses during the hospital confinement. On analysis of the data, however, meaningful frequency-distribution curves did not emerge, and while it is possible to define modal behavior, review of the exceptions beyond the mode has usually shown extenuating circumstances. In summary then UPRO's studies of ancillary service utilization have not been effective in identifying targets for physician education; physician behavior in the study population has been surprisingly appropriate.

Data needs

The data needs for the OSCHUR program are relatively unsophisticated and the programming task simple. Nonetheless the data system capability for internal management (physician hours, nurse coordinator patient load, and so on) provides significant assistance to staff (see boxed material). In addition, the ability to identify percentiles for lengths of stay for selected diagnoses, hospitals, and individual

---

UPRO MONTHLY ACTIVITY REPORT
April 1975

Time expended		
Medical advisor	90.5	hours
Nurse coordinator	2980	hours
Hospital activity		
Total discharges	3440	
Average length of stay	7.5	days
Discharges/workday	156.4	
Average workday census	1165.3	
Medical advisor activity		
Number of patients reviewed	515	
Percentage of patients reviewed	15.0	
Hours per patient reviewed	.18	
Hours per discharge	.026	
Nurse coordinator productivity		
Full-time equivalents employed	17.0	
Average workday census/FTE	68.8	
Nurse coordinator hours/discharge	.87	
Discharges/workday/FTE	9.2	

physicians is helpful in analyzing changes in behavior derived from peer review. Finally, the ability of the system to provide each practitioner in the state with his own performance in complying with criteria for each of the diagnoses studied will likely have educational benefit.

Evaluation

Evaluation of the effectiveness of OSCHUR in curtailing unnecessary utilization relies on analysis of multiple factors across time periods before and after implementation.

Admission rates, length of stay, and hospital days per thousand per year must all be studied; a decrease in average length of stay does not necessarily reflect improved utilization, since elimination of unnecessary short-stay admissions will result in a longer average length of stay. In addition to gross measurement of these factors, a study of selected diagnoses may provide a clearer idea of program impact. Rates of admission and length of stay for disease entities subject to greater peer review impact (that is, back pain, pneumonia, or hypertension) will likely show more change than will those conditions for which the hospital confinement is more stereotyped (normal obstetrical delivery or acute appendicitis). For example, the average length of stay for patients with psychosis decreased from 18 days to 13 days after OSCHUR was implemented in Utah's major hospitals.

It has also become clear that the impact of the review program varies according to the subject population. The impact of the OSCHUR program was negligible for patients covered by Educators Mutual Insurance Association; the utilization rate of approximately 450 bed days per thousand per year may be an irreducible minimum. The data for Title XVIII and Title XIX recipients will probably not be available until implementation of the PSRO evaluation protocol, since neither accurate identification of the denominator population nor accurate baseline data have been available to UPRO.

The Hawthorne effect

Subtle but definite enhancements of medical care quality accompany the mere presence of a peer review system. The simple act of defining process criteria for psychosis resulted in higher compliance with the critical care criteria and presumably better patient care. Aggregate compliance for 20 criteria elements considered to be critical to ideal care (see boxed material) was 64% before criteria setting and 88% afterward. Fifty hospital stays were audited in each time period.

Medical record keeping has improved substantially, especially in the rural setting, since the attending physician must define a management plan for the expected length of stay to be assigned.

Linkage to continuing medical education

Much has been written about the difficulty in translating peer review findings into changes of physician performance. The experience of UPRO suggests that the breadth of acceptance of peer review data as valid is directly correlated with the level of participation of the reviewees in criteria generation or formal adoption. UPRO has also found that multiple structural efforts at physician education must be employed: individual mailings, hospital staff meetings, specialty organization efforts, statewide medical information organs such as journals and bulletins, and cooperative efforts with medical schools. Finally, direct communications between the reviewer in the hospital and the attending physician may be the most effective device if objective criteria accepted widely by the community form the basis for the interaction.

THE PACE PROGRAM

The Physician Ambulatory Care Evaluation (PACE) project grew out of a joint interest of UPRO and the National Center for Health Services Research in exploring methods for evaluating the medical care of patients in physician offices. The purpose of PACE is to test the degree to which

---

OSCHUR PROGRAM
Major psychoses

History: elements critical to ideal care
 1. Age
 2. Sex
 3. Severity of symptoms
 4. Duration of symptoms
 5. Progression of symptoms
 6. Environment (home, work, school, institution)
 7. Precipitating event
 8. Prior similar illness
 9. Prior treatment
10. Use of drugs (prescribed or illicit)
11. Social class (economic status, race, religion, education)
12. Patient's insight
Physical exam: elements critical to ideal care
13. Organic status should be described by a physician (for example, psychiatrist, referring M.D.), especially with psychotic depressions or severely disorganized personalities.

Procedures: elements critical to ideal care	When:
14. Psychiatric evaluation (includes mental status)	Onset of hospitalization
15. Laboratory screening (multiphasic)	Onset of hospitalization
16. Laboratory, blood, CBC	Onset of hospitalization
17. Laboratory, urine routine	Onset of hospitalization
18. Laboratory, VDRL	Onset of hospitalization
Therapy: elements critical to ideal care	When:
19. Alleviate symptoms (for example, use of drugs, ECT, and psychotherapy)	Ongoing
20. Specific posthospital care to be provided	Prior to discharge

---

peer review can evaluate physician office practice through analysis of the information present on Medicaid billing forms. Expressed otherwise, the thesis PACE attempts to test is that the information present on the billing form (which includes diagnoses, investigative procedures, and therapy) can be used to build profiles of physician performance based on individual patient histories. These profiles and histories may be passed against screening guidelines (criteria) to determine those cases where care seems to fall outside expected quality levels (see boxed material on p. 332, top).

Ambulatory care criteria

The same specialty panels that wrote the criteria for the OSCHUR program also wrote or approved criteria for PACE.

The criteria were written on the "critical to ideal care" format and consisted of combinations of diagnoses, therapy, or investigation that were either critical to ideal care or inconsistent with ideal care. Not only was it possible to identify claims as exceptional if the criteria were not met, but it was also possible to construct time-span criteria that linked two or more events over a specified time interval. For instance, the PACE data system may be asked to report for review those patients consulting a physician for diarrhea more than three times within a 3-month period without a stool culture or examination for ova and parasites having been performed.

As an exceptional claim is reported, the physician reviewer may use the cathode ray terminal to display the physician's

---

PACE PROGRAM
Sample criteria

Premalignant dermatoses (1508)
 Report surgical excision of premalignant dermatoses. (125)
 Report cases involving more than three uses of cryotherapy/chemotherapy/electro-
  dessication per 90-day period for premalignant dermatoses. (170)
Diarrhea and related disorders (2001)
 Report if three visits occur within 90 days without proctosigmoidoscopy or colon-
  oscopy being performed. (068)
 Report if three visits occur within 90 days without a stool examination. (069)
 Report cases involving more than four visits in 90 days for the treatment of lower
  gastrointestinal disorders. (070)
Diabetes mellitus (2005)
 Report cases involving more than four visits within 180 days. (030)
 Report cases in which no urine analysis is performed within 1 year. (031)
 Report cases in which no blood sugar analysis is performed within 1 year. (032)
 Report cases involving more than two blood sugar analyses within 180 days. (033)
NOTE: Numbers following titles are guideline set numbers. Numbers following de-
 scriptions are guideline reference numbers or audit numbers.

PACE PROGRAM
Sample physician communication

Dear Doctor _____:
 As you probably know, UPRO conducts professional review of ambulatory care services rendered to Utah Medicaid recipients, under contract with the state. The program is built on a computerized screening process which reports variations from guidelines expressing peer expectations regarding appropriate medical care in *the general case*. Physician reviewers examine these instances of variation in the context of associated medical care, with the idea that unusual patterns of practice may be indicative of areas where exchange among the professional community would be constructive.

 We are writing you regarding an aspect of your practice which seems unusual: we have noted five instances between January and June 1975 where your patients received injections of corticosteroids apparently as therapy for acute upper respiratory disorders. The present PACE guideline is that injections of steroids are not generally medically indicated for the treatment or in the presence of acute upper respiratory infections and related symptoms. We do not expect that guidelines will apply in every case. However, we thought you would want to know that your rate of variation in this regard is exceptional.

 If you feel that your rationale would be helpful to peers considering this or other guidelines, we invite you to write.

           Respectfully,

          _____, M.D.
          for the PACE Review Committee

profile (to see if the exception occurs frequently within the practitioner's recorded experience) or may also see the patient profile, revealing such habits as doctor shopping or drug abuse.

A core of reviewers (all practitioners) assist the PACE project by reviewing exceptional claims and profiles and activating a series of educational measures designed to correct deficiencies. The essential feature of the corrective efforts relies on notification of deviant physicians rather than retrospective denial of claims. While a front-end interdiction of claims payment lies within the capacity of PACE, it is seldom invoked. Rather, PACE relies on notification of aberrant behavior through a graded series of communications (see boxed material).

Optimum Systems, Incorporated, was selected in 1972 to provide the data system support for the PACE project. Currently 335,000 claims have been entered into the system, and exceptions are being reported at the rate of approximately 1600 per month. Besides reviewing the exceptions (both for quality and utilization), the reviewers periodically review sample patient and physician profiles. In so doing, patterns emerge that lead to the formation of additional criteria for programming. An example is the identification of a patient who received prescriptions for Percodan simultaneously from several physicians. After identifying this pattern for a single patient, an exception criterion was programmed that will display for review all patients receiving more than 50 narcotic units per month.

Over the 3 years of development of the PACE project, review physician productivity has also been documented. Contact with other ambulatory care review projects similar to PACE, particularly the program at the Santa Clara Foundation for Medical Care, indicated that a physician could review 20 to 30 cases per hour. The Utah PACE experience tended to confirm that this rate was reasonable once the reviewer had been exposed to the report formats

and disposition choices for 1 or 2 hours.

Data validity has also been a concern of UPRO. A random sample of claims was selected, the diagnosis and procedure information were re-encoded, and accuracy of the input and reporting thus verified. Some 2000 claims were reviewed as an audit check, and the rate of agreement was 95%. Considering the intensity of the audit and the fact that some items of disagreement represented rather fine distinctions, UPRO considers these results acceptable. Reviewer confidence in the accuracy of the PACE data appears well founded.

Current developmental activities

Current PACE developmental activity is directed toward providing a module for quality assessment and utilization review linked to the Medicaid management information system operated by the state agency. This development, since it is replicable, could serve to facilitate peer review of ambulatory services by other PSROs, subject to their individual modification of criteria.

The results of efforts to alter physician behavior are only now becoming available through continuing audit of the PACE data. Currently 197 exception criteria are programmed into the system. A typical example of these criteria is shown in the boxed material on p. 332. The review of exceptions and profiles continues in an ongoing fashion. Communications between the peer review organization and the physicians being reviewed help make criteria responsive to real situations and the profession's best judgment. The first 17 physicians to whom corrective letters (see boxed material on p. 332) were directed had (together) 214 exceptions in the 3 months prior to July 1, 1975 (Table 15-3). Between July and November 1975 only 3 of these 17 physicians have exceptions reported (four total). Thus preliminary data suggest that peer review with PACE system support can alter physician behavior.

Table 15-3. PACE program educational letters*

Criteria	Number of exceptions
Injectable estrogen	63
Injectable antibiotics/penicillin	31
Excessive visits for flu	8
Failure to follow up otitis media	64
Injectable steroids given to diabetics	12
Excessive urinalyses performed	20
Injections for URI	10
Excessive visits for URI	6
Total	214

*Eighteen corrective letters covering eight criteria were sent to 17 physicians who together had 214 exceptions in the 3 months prior to July 1, 1975.

LOOKING TO THE FUTURE

The current operational success of the OSCHUR and PACE projects leads to some speculation about the future. The peer review system in Utah ideally should continue to be managed at the level of the physician community rather than independently by each hospital. A continuum of patient care should be subject to review, extending from ambulatory services into the hospital setting and again to outpatient review. The PACE project, when linked to OSCHUR, will permit assessment of duplication of studies as well as deficiencies in follow-up or prehospital care. In the near future all hospital care, both privately and publicly funded, should come under UPRO scrutiny. Ideally the payment source should serve only to establish the eligibility of the patient for the services offered and as a fund disbursement agent. All review, whether related to utilization or quality and whether inpatient or outpatient services or drugs, should be conducted by a review organization managed by physicians. In so doing, a conflict of interest inherent to the insurer acting as the reviewer is avoided. The only question will be the diligence of the medical profession in providing critical self-analysis. UPRO continues to be optimistic.

16

Research in quality assessment and utilization review in hospital and ambulatory settings

BEVERLY C. PAYNE

Except for the results of insights, hunches, untested trials, and professional intuition, the cause of peer review has had little solid foundation in methodology, theoretic construction, controlled field trials, or reliable results to develop new hypotheses and establish new valid correlations and conclusions until recently.

The research basis for measures of medical care quality and effective use of health care institutions began in 1956 with the personally developed criteria of Paul Lembcke.[1] This evaluation has since evolved into the consensus development of criteria for utilization of the hospital and medical care quality. It is now proposed as the process and outcome measures appropriate for monitoring medical care delivery by the JCAH and PSROs.

Elaborations of the criteria approach to medical care evaluation (including quality and effectiveness measures) with firm research protocols, careful analyses, and statistically validated results are found in the research of Fitzpatrick, Reidel, and Payne in *Hospital and Medical Economics,*[2] Payne and Lyons in *Method of Evaluating and Improving Personal Medical Care Quality,*[3] and Brook and Appel in "Quality of Care Assessment: Choosing a Method for Peer Review."[4]

The careful correlation of outcome measures of medical care to process measure has been the contribution of John Williamson,[5] and his success in developing outcome measurement models has influenced the development of outcome criteria in the research to be described.

The use of implicit rather than explicit criteria for evaluation of medical care has been the mode of operation of hospital tissue and audit committees. In a research context, Trussell and Morehead utilized implicit criteria in a series of quality of care studies characterized by the Teamsters study of 1964. In the past several years Dr. Morehead[6] has made liberal use of explicit criteria in various studies of hospital and ambulatory medical care.

The methodology proposed and described for the research conducted in diverse settings (Michigan, Nassau County, Hawaii, and again Southeast Michigan) is retrospective, based on explicit consensus criteria, derived from data routinely and regularly recorded in the medical records of hospitals and ambulatory care settings, and collected by trained abstractors on PAS abstracts. The data are analyzed by computers programmed to produce various analyses to evaluate critically the multiple variables suspected or proven to have potential to explain the differences in quality or utilization patterns among various hospitals, physicians, specialties, methods of payment, and organization of medical care delivery.

EXPLICIT HOSPITAL CARE CRITERIA

The initial research use of explicit consensus criteria was reported in *Hospital and Medical Economics,* a study of utilization patterns of a representative sample of Michigan short-term general hospitals. The criteria for hospital admission, length of stay, complications prolonging the expected length of stay, and appropriate use of hospital facilities are expressed as effective or appropriate use of the hospital.

The criteria of central importance in the research or operational assurance of quality were developed by panels of carefully selected Michigan physicians. They were outstanding clinicians from community hospitals and teacher-clinicians from the two medical schools in Michigan. They composed seven panels, averaging three members addressing their consensus opinion to the diagnosis-specific requirements for admission to the hospital and the expected length of stay.

The following admission criteria in surgical diagnoses (from *Hospital and Medical Economics,* 1962) were usually the accepted indications for the elective surgical procedure.

CHOLECYSTITIS AND CHOLELITHIASIS[2]

I. Indications for Admission
   A. Acute abdomen requires hospitalization for evaluation
      1. Nausea, vomiting, dehydration, pain of gallbladder, colic
      2. History of recurrent pains or gall bladder attacks
      3. Fever, associated with above symptoms
      4. Jaundice
      5. Present tenderness and pain in right upper quadrant
      6. Leucocytosis
   B. Diagnosis of gallstones or non-functioning gallbladder already established; patient is admitted for cholecystectomy.

In some medical diagnoses the indication for admission was absolute, as in known or suspected acute myocardial infarction (100%), or in others were related to the severity of the pathologic process as in the following (from *Hospital and Medical Economics,* 1962).

DIARRHEA (UNDER TWO YEARS)[2]

I. Indications for Admission
Diarrhea, severe, with any one or more of the following:
   A. Weight loss
   B. Lack of oral intake as evidenced or accompanied by
      1. Nausea
      2. Vomiting
      3. Abdominal distension
   C. Oliguria
   D. Fever

The length of stay criteria were given usually as a range of days in uncomplicated cases and recognized many contingencies, as in the following (from *Hospital and Medical Economics,* 1962).

FRACTURE OF THE NECK OF THE FEMUR[2]

IV. Probable Length of Hospital Stay
   A. Two weeks if
      1. Patient can swing injured leg over side of bed and
      2. Can transfer to wheelchair with help of one other person and
      3. Has sufficient care at home to absolutely prevent necessity of weight bearing on injured leg
   B. Average length of stay: 4 weeks (with surgery)
   C. Stay of 4 to 6 weeks plus period for physical therapy may be expected if conditions under A do not prevail, and depending on indications for discharge
   D. When no operation is done:
      1. Expected length of stay is 3 to 4½ months if treated with bed rest and traction
      2. Expected length of stay is 3 to 6 months if treated with spica hip cast and bed rest

The complications that extended the expected length of stay are both specific to the condition under consideration but also common to all hospitalized patients, as in the following (from *Hospital and Medical Economics,* 1962).

ACUTE MYOCARDIAL INFARCTION[2]

V. Complications Extending Length of Stay
  A. Shock
  B. Original pain of unusually long duration
  C. Cardiac failure at any time
  D. Serious arrhythmias
    1. Ventricular tachycardia
    2. Fibrillation, ventricular or atrial
    3. Heart block
    4. Frequent premature ventricular systoles (early in hospital stay)
  E. Previous myocardial infarction
  F. Angina before infarction
  G. Other heart disease
  H. Previous cardiac decompensation
  I. Unusually large myocardial infarction
  J. Persistent S-T segment deviation
  K. Extension of the infarction
  L. Embolic phenomenon
  M. Recurrence of original pain
  N. Difficulty in regulation of anticoagulant therapy
  O. Absence of laboratory facilities for prothrombin determinations after discharge
  P. Other important disease

The length of stay criteria were difficult in some instances to apply to cases of shorter or longer than expected stay. A definitive end point would assist in evaluation of the length of stay, and consequently the panel further considered the specific indications for discharge. An example of this indication for discharge is the following (from *Hospital and Medical Economics,* 1962).

URINARY TRACT CALCULUS[2]

V. Indications for Discharge
  A. No sepsis
  B. Kidney functioning
  C. Absence of pain and discomfort
  D. Temperature normal 24 hours
  E. No draining wound or other postoperative complication

The evaluation of appropriateness of admission and length of stay requires data and analysis from these four criteria sections, that is, from admission criteria and

length of stay, complications and discharge criteria. Fortunately the computer programming, though complex, is thoroughly competent to analyze the retrospectively collected data with accuracy. Further study allows exploration of differences in performance between hospitals, between physicians by a number of characteristics, and among sources of payment.

STUDY 1: UTILIZATION STUDY (1958)

Using such criteria from panels of physician experts, data from 5750 cases representing 18 diagnoses and 49 hospitals in Michigan in 1958 were analyzed for appropriateness of admission and length of stay.

Appropriateness of admission was found to occur in 97.1% of all cases.

Appropriateness of length of stay occurred in 83.4% of cases; 6.8% were considered understay, and 9.6% were considered overstay. Only slight differences were found between six regional areas of Michigan.

The patients were found to pay more out of pocket, proportionately and absolutely, in instances of understay and appropriate admission, and pay less out of pocket in instances of overstay and inappropriate admissions. Overall there were no differences of importance in appropriate admissions (1.1% only) between sources of payment (Blue Cross, commercial insurance, and patient only).

There were no substantial differences (0.9%) in appropriate admissions between various specialty categories of physicians. Likewise there was little difference (4.2%) in appropriateness in length of stay evaluation between various specialty physician categories for all diagnoses.

STUDY 2: QUALITY CARE FEASIBILITY (MICHIGAN)

Following completion of this first Michigan study, several developmental substudy projects were undertaken. One was to expand the evaluation of effectiveness of use of the hospital to adequacy or quality of medical care, and the second to develop experience in application of the criteria methodology to other geographic areas (Nassau County, New York,[7] in 1963, and western Pennsylvania[8] in 1961).

The Nassau County study[7] was initiated by the County Medical Society and included five hospitals in Nassau County. Panels of physicians adapted the Michigan study criteria for use in evaluating care. Few modifications were made, and the results obtained from reviewing retrospective hospital data were similar in every respect to those described for the Michigan study.

The experience in western Pennsylvania was substantively different. The Hospital Utilization Program of western Pennsylvania was only beginning to function in 1963. They were receptive to the methodology, described in a workshop atmosphere, utilized in the Michigan study. The criteria developed in Pennsylvania followed the same format and content but were expanded to include many more than the original 19 diagnostic categories. These criteria were then used in an operational rather than a research setting. Many hospitals in Pennsylvania subscribed or cooperated in the Hospital Utilization Program to demonstrate the effectiveness of professional accountability in this non-government, voluntary effort.

Criteria developed for measurement of the quality or adequacy of medical care was predicated on the finding that about 30% of the services expected to be performed in the Michigan study were not done. Specific diagnostic observations were added to the existing criteria. Recorded observations were expected of the physician in obtaining specific historical items, physical examination findings, laboratory and radiologic examinations, and special studies appropriate for diagnosis.

Analysis of feasibility studies in acute myocardial infarction, urinary tract infection, cholecystitis, and bronchitis demonstrated significant deficiencies in the recording of history items, physical examination findings, and laboratory and

radiologic studies. Important for the future applicability and acceptability of such studies was the positive response and behavioral change in the participating physician performance that followed a dissemination of the findings of the research studies conducted in the hospital setting of St. Joseph Mercy Hospital in Ann Arbor, Michigan (1961 to present).

STUDY 3: MEDICAL DATA COLLECTION (MICHIGAN, 1970)

A feasibility study[9] was conducted in four Michigan hospitals with the full cooperation of the medical staffs to assess the utility of those methods of collecting and evaluating medical data from medical records of a fifth hospital. The cooperating physicians, in a setting simulating an audit committee, were asked to use an entire record, an abstract of a record, and then each method with explicit criteria to evaluate the effectiveness and quality of medical care in three diagnoses. The results suggested that by any of the methods (record with implicit criteria, record with explicit criteria; abstract with implicit criteria, abstract with explicit criteria; record, abstract and explicit criteria) the physicians' evaluations were undifferentiated. That is, the ability to agree on whether medical care was adequate or inadequate was not achieved by any of the methodologies. The degree of inter-rater agreement was 50% or the same results one would have from flipping a coin!

This experience convinced us that collection of data by trained observers instead of physicians, computerization of the criteria, and data analysis were preferred for objective evaluation. Physicians would then develop the criteria and interpret the results of the data processing.

HOSPITAL UTILIZATION REVIEW CRITERIA (1965)

In 1965, representatives of Michigan physicians, 75 specialists and family practitioners and academic and community clinicians convened in panels for an ambitious plan to develop criteria for over 100 diagnoses. These criteria were published as the *Hospital Utilization Review Manual* in 1968.[10] All aspects of hospital, medical, surgical, and obstetrical care are included in the manual, but no psychiatric diagnoses were attempted due to the editors' uncertainty about the development of measurable criteria in this field.

These criteria contained the fruits of the previous feasibility studies and brought us nearer to reliable measures of physician hospital performance, quality of care, and effectiveness of hospital use.

STUDY 4: HAWAII STUDY (1970 TO 1972)

In 1970 the Hawaii Medical Association entered into a research alliance with the University of Michigan for the purpose of evaluating the quality of medical care in Hawaii. The study was accomplished in three integrated parts: (1) Episode of Illness Study, (2) Office Care Study, and (3) Continuing Education Study and is fully reported in *The Quality of Medical Care: Evaluation and Improvement.*[11] The Episode of Illness Study measured the quality of medical care in 22 general hospitals using 21 diagnostic categories and the medical records of 3316 patients discharged from Hawaii hospitals in 1968. The opportunity to review the hospital record was assured by cooperation of the Hawaii Hospital Association, the administrative staffs of the 22 hospitals, and their medical staffs. The further opportunity to review 2886 (87%) of these medical records from the physicians' private offices was an expression of commitment to the study by Hawaii physicians; only 5% of the physicians declined to allow our examination of their office records.

It was then possible to document the entire episode of illness from physician office to hospital and back to physician office for a follow-up period as long as 2 years in some instances.

A unique opportunity was available in Hawaii to compare the medical behavioral characteristics of three systems of medical care delivery, that is, prepaid multispecialty group practice, fee-for-service multispecialty group practice, and solo medical practice. The analyses of the performance of these different types of medical care delivery will be presented (see p. 343), as they contain policy related conclusions.

The second part was an Office Care Study of a different group of diagnostic categories seen in ambulatory settings. This study involved 93 volunteer primary care physicians (family practitioners, pediatricians, gynecologists, and internists). Ten diagnostic categories were chosen for study in three distinct practice settings— solo practice, fee-for-service multispecialty groups practice, and prepaid multispecialty group practice. In these sites, primarily in Honolulu, 1675 cases were examined according to the established criteria.

Analyses of the data in each study compared the performance of physicians by their several characteristics, for example, time in practice, type of practice, specialty, board certification, the hospitals by size, and source of payment for care.

Development of criteria

The criteria for both the Episode of Illness and Office Care studies were developed by panels of Hawaii physicians selected by the Hawaii Medical Association as highly respected, experienced clinicians capable of acting to create acceptable peer consensus criteria for evaluation of quality of medical care and effectiveness of hospital use.

Eight panels of physicians averaging five physicians per panel developed the Episode of Illness criteria, and four panels of physicians averaging four physicians per panel developed the Office Care Study criteria. These criteria were not subject to ratification by the total physicians represented.

Abstracting

Trained abstractors, following verbal and written instructions, collected medical data from the sampled medical records. Their accuracy and reliability was tested periodically during the data collection and was highly satisfactory.

After the initial development of skill and abstracting ability, the five abstractors were able to collect data at a rate of 20 minutes per record over all diagnoses. Obviously some disease categories were more complicated (cerebrovascular accident) than others (tonsillectomy) and required more time for data abstracting. The ability of the abstractors was challenged by some of the physicians, and the doubters were supplied with the records for their own observation. They subsequently affirmed that the reported findings were verified by their own review.

The entire 3316 hospital records and the 2881 ambulatory records in the Episode of Illness Study were abstracted over a 4-month period by the five abstractors traveling throughout the seven inhabited Hawaiian Islands.

The medical information indicated as necessary for the criteria was recorded on Professional Activity Study abstracts, and the initial computer-programmed analysis was accomplished by special arrangement with the Commission on Professional and Hospital Activities. Subsequent special analyses have been programmed for University of Michigan computers.

In the Episode of Illness Study the sampling of records from the total of patients discharged was designed to be representative of the total universe of patients in each diagnostic category. Since the numbers of patients differed widely among the diagnoses, the interval of case selection also varied, from 1:1 in cerebral vascular insufficiency to 1:48 in full-term deliveries. The chance of a case being selected from the records of each hospital was therefore a reflection of the frequency with which patients in that diagnostic category were discharged from all 22 hospitals in Hawaii.

Sampling of records in the Office Care Study began with the participating physicians keeping a 6-week log of all cases seen with any of ten diagnoses. From the 12,000 patient visits so identified, a sample drawn on a random basis resulted in the 1675 cases finally abstracted.

Weighting or scoring of physician performance

In previous studies, both our own and others, the evaluation of medical care has been expressed in an all-or-none manner. Either an admission is appropriate or inappropriate, the length of stay appropriate or inappropriate, and the services supplied (the physician performance) is adequate or inadequate. This black and white designation of physician performance is unrealistic, fails to quantify performance or quality of care, and provides no descriptive analysis of the strengths or deficiencies in medical care delivery as a basis for positive response to the research findings.

Weighting of the criteria items provided at least a partial response to the above recognized defects in research design. The panels of Hawaii physicians were asked to develop importance weights for each process item that related to quality assessment, that is, history, physical examination, laboratory, radiology, or special examinations. These weights were graduated from the lowest (1) to the highest (3). The physicians, in objectively weighting each item, found this confining and frequently gave weights of less than 1 (0.5 or 0.3) to less important items.

From this system of weights a scoring scheme was derived to express a weighted percentage of service criteria items recorded on hospital and ambulatory care records. A simple formula explains the physician performance index (PPI):

$$\text{PPI} = \frac{\text{Observed weighted criteria items}}{\text{Optimal weighted criteria items}} \times 100$$

With this quantitative measure a convenient means of expressing performance is devised to compare performance between hospitals, across all hospitals, and between physicians of various characterizations such as specialty, time in practice, organization of medical care delivery system, and methods of payment.

Of even greater usefulness for our research purposes, it provides a listing of weighted criteria items for the physician, or the audit committee, or the responsible administrative hospital personnel to review and determine exactly what process items were omitted in the delivery of care to one patient or to the universe of patients studied. A more complete discussion of this potential occurs on p. 344.

There are at this time no absolute reference points for the measurement of the PPI. A similar observation can be made for all cognitive written examinations. What do they measure? We do, however, use these examination results to screen medical school applicants, to promote them from one year to the next, and to qualify them for medical practice, and after a period of postgraduate training, another cognitive examination certifies the candidate as a specialist.

Comparisons of the PPI to a golfer's par is improbable until we determine what par is in physician performance, and comparisons of the PPI with baseball batting averages will make most physicians national sports heroes.

The PPI does in the most appropriate analogy closely resemble the scoring of cognitive written examinations. The advantage, and we feel this is an extraordinarily important one, is that the PPI is a measure of performance, of the recorded evidence of the skill and care taken by the physician in the delivery of medical services to his patients. It is therefore a measure of both his knowledge of what should be done, diagnostically and therapeutically, and his effectiveness and efficiency in intervening responsibly in the health problems of his patients to apply that knowledge.

Results in the Hawaii study

Table 16-1 is a summary of the most important findings of the Hawaii study. It demonstrates that the composite perfor-

mance index for all physicians in all hospitals and all diagnostic categories was 71.2%. This means that according to the medical records the average patient in this study received 71.2% of the weighted optimal care criteria items specified by the physician panels. This ranged from 88.6% in full-term pregnancy to 48.2% in chronic urinary tract infection. A 10% difference is statistically significant.

There is a difference in PPI between large hospitals and small hospitals (less than 4000 discharges per year) of almost 10%. There is also a difference in PPI between different sites of medical care delivery. The prepaid multispecialty group practice scored 79.4%, fee-for-service multispecialty group practice scored 74.2%, and solo practitioners scored 69.5%.

The most important difference in performance was found between modal specialists and the colleagues. The total score for all diagnoses by modal specialists was 77.9%; for others (specialists in other fields or general practitioners) it was 64%.

The PPI for modal specialists was nearly eight percentage points higher in large hospitals than in small hospitals. Nonmodal specialists performed at a lower scoring level, but there appeared to be no significant difference in nonmodal specialist practice between large and small hospitals. The greatest difference in the PPI was between modal specialists in large hospitals and nonmodal specialists in small hospitals, a difference of over 15 percentage points. Also there was a difference of 13.8 percentage points between scores of modal specialists and nonmodal specialists in large hospitals.

It thus appears that the specialist, doing the task he understands best, in a large hospital performs in a manner most in conformity with standards established by his peers. But even in small hospitals he also performs better than his nonmodal specialist colleagues—a difference of 7.4 percentage points.

Finally, the comparisons between the three practice settings reveal that the de-

Table 16-1. Summary data, episode of illness study*†

Study variable	Physician Perfor- mance Index‡	Percent ap- propriately admitted‡	Percent of appropriate admissions with appro- priate length of stay‡	Patients with ap- propriate admission and length of stay, a percentage of total patients admitted
All variables	71.2 (3316)	89.9 (3316)	82.3 (2573)	74.5 (3316)
Hospital size§				
Large	73.7 (2560)	91.4 (2560)	84.7 (2019)	71.8 (2560)
Small	63.8 (756)	85.5 (756)	76.5 (554)	66.5 (756)
Specialty				
Modal specialists	77.9 (1851)	94.0 (1851)	88.0 (1497)	83.0 (1851)
Others	64.0 (1455)	85.4 (1455)	75.6 (1072)	65.3 (1455)
Hospital size and specialty				
Modal specialists in large hospitals	78.4 (1720)	94.7 (1720)	89.1 (1397)	84.7 (1720)
Modal specialists in small hospitals	70.7 (131)	86.6 (131)	77.6 (99)	69.5 (131)
Others in large hospitals	64.6 (833)	86.0 (833)	74.8 (620)	65.4 (833)
Others in small hospitals	63.3 (622)	85.1 (622)	76.3 (452)	65.7 (622)
Practice setting				
Prepaid multispecialty group	79.4 (679)	96.9 (679)	90.3 (565)	87.8 (679)
Fee-for-service multispecialty group	74.2 (581)	93.5 (581)	85.2 (467)	79.3 (581)
Solo practice	69.5 (2045)	88.2 (2045)	80.6 (1537)	71.7 (2045)
Large hospital, modal specialists by practice setting				
Prepaid multispecialty group	80.4 (610)	97.6 (610)	90.8 (512)	88.9 (610)
Fee-for-service multispecialty group	77.7 (385)	91.6 (385)	87.8 (315)	82.1 (385)
Solo practice	78.4 (725)	94.4 (725)	89.4 (569)	85.0 (725)

*From Payne, B. C.: The quality of medical care: evaluation and improvement, Chicago, 1975, Hospital Research and Educational Trust.
†A 10% difference in any of these statistics is significant at the 0.01 level.
‡Numbers in parentheses indicate total number of cases used in determining values of variable.
§Large hospitals are defined as those that discharged over 4000 cases in 1968; small hospitals are those that discharged fewer than 4000 cases in 1968.

scribed differences disappear (that the PPI showed no important difference) when the modal specialist in the large hospital performance is analyzed. If modal specialists behave in an identical manner in the large hospitals, what then is the explanation for the good performance of physicians in the prepaid setting when large and small hospitals and modal and nonmodal specialists are included in the indexes?

The difference must lie in the ability of physicians in prepaid multispecialty practice to direct a patient with a specific problem to the proper modal specialist. This hypothesis is supported by the finding that the percentage of patients cared for by the modal specialists in all hospitals differed strikingly—93% in prepaid multispecialty group, 71% in fee-for-service multispecialty groups, and 34% in solo practice.

Examination of physician performance related to board certification shows that only in 3 of the 23 diagnostic categories did board-certified specialists demonstrate statistically better performance than nonboard certified specialists.

Number of years in practice correlated with PPI in 5 of the 23 diagnostic categories. In 4 of these 5 categories, physicians with fewer than 20 years practice scored higher than those with 20 or more years.

Table 16-2. PPIs for office care study by practice setting*

Study variable	Prepaid multi-specialty group practice† (%)	Fee-for-service multispecialty group practice† (%)	Solo practice† (%)	All practice settings† (%)
Condition/diagnosis:				
Essential benign hypertension				
Follow-up	49.3 (82)	54.9 (20)	49.6 (89)	50.2 (191)
Acute tonsillitis				
Adult	37.0 (81)	40.8 (12)	33.8 (33)	35.8 (126)
Child	26.5 (19)	24.8 (30)	32.0 (37)	28.8 (86)
Menstrual disorders	30.8 (24)	30.6 (32)	29.2 (78)	29.6 (134)
Arteriosclerotic heart disease				
Follow-up	39.9 (71)	44.9 (27)	29.7 (98)	34.1 (196)
Urinary tract infection				
Acute	52.7 (40)	51.7 (15)	54.6 (55)	53.8 (110)
Chronic	19.8 (26)	32.4 (8)	25.6 (21)	26.0 (55)
Diabetes mellitus				
Follow-up	44.3 (60)	49.3 (29)	39.8 (94)	42.5 (183)
Periodic examination:				
Internal medicine				
Initial	39.2 (27)	48.2 (20)	28.2 (19)	38.4 (66)
Return	40.0 (55)	45.6 (26)	35.9 (24)	40.3 (105)
Preemployment or university entrance	45.6 (12)	44.9 (24)	30.5 (42)	35.3 (78)
Gynecology	44.2 (52)	39.4 (29)	40.7 (65)	41.1 (146)
Pediatrics	49.4 (69)	35.1 (67)	38.4 (63)	39.3 (199)
Total weighted PPI	44.8 (618)	40.9 (339)	39.2 (718)	40.9 (1675)

*From Payne, B. C.: The quality of medical care: evaluation and improvement, Chicago, 1975, Hospital Research and Educational Trust.
†Numbers in parentheses indicate number of cases observed.

Office care study

Details of the Office Care Study are contained in *Quality of Medical Care: Evaluation and Improvement;* a brief summary will describe the criteria approach to medical care evaluation in the ambulatory setting.

In Hawaii 93 physicians volunteered cooperation in a retrospective review of office medical records. Ten diagnostic categories were selected for study in three practice sites described in the Episode of Illness Study. Primary care specialists were involved, including gynecologists, pediatricians, general practitioners, and internists.

Table 16-2 lists the diagnostic categories studied, the sites evaluated, and the PPIs of the physicians' professional activities in 1970. The performance between sites is remarkably similar for these volunteer physicians. The greatest difference occurs between fee-for-service multispecialty group practice and solo practice in the diagnostic category arteriosclerotic heart disease (15.2%) and between prepaid multispecialty group practice and solo practice in return periodic (internal medicine) examinations (14.1%).

The overall office care PPIs of 40.9% compare unfavorably with the Episode of Illness PPIs of 71.2% derived from hospital and ambulatory records.

When physician performance was examined by specialty, significant differences were found in 10 of 12 diagnostic categories. In nine of these the modal internist, gynecologist, or pediatrician scored higher than the general practitioner. In one category (tonsillitis in children) the internist scored higher than the pediatrician.

Specialists without board certification had statistically significant higher performance indexes than did board-certified specialists in 4 of 13 diagnoses. In one diagnosis board-certified specialists' PPIs were higher than non-board-certified specialists.

The experience had demonstrated that with cooperation, appropriate criteria, and suitable conventions for collecting data, the feasibility of studying ambulatory medical care characteristics and quality of care is possible.

CONSENSUS CRITERIA DEVELOPMENT

Repeated references have been made to the criteria for admission, length of stay, and quality of care, with sidelong glances at the process of developing these criteria.

Because it is apparent that this method requires the most valid, practical, and yet concise description of medical criteria, a more searching description of consensus criteria is presented.

The reader should understand that this is a distillation of many efforts at developing consensus criteria. Many blind alleys have been entered, many learning experiences have tempered the next effort, and many mistakes must still be corrected or items for analysis improved.

The first decision to be made concerns the diagnostic categories to be studied. Our research projects have sought diagnostic categories (1) of high incidence in either hospitals or ambulatory setting, (2) representing multiple medical specialty activities, and (3) reasonable responsiveness to therapeutic manipulation, (4) not self-limited, and (5) not unduly dependent on patient cooperation.

Data on incidence of disease or discharge diagnoses may be found in the Commission on Professional and Hospital Activities annual report of the most frequent discharge diagnoses from their hospital data base. Also, data is available from federal sources—the Health Insurance Bureau and Social Security Administration. Ambulatory physician office visits are reported by the National Disease and Therapeutic Index from Ambler, Pennsylvania.

With diagnosis or condition, surgical procedure or therapeutic agent chosen for study, a panel of physicians recognized by their peers as capable clinicians and familiar with the diagnostic category chosen are convened. They should be properly prepared with a description of the task to be performed and examples of previous criteria to illustrate past efforts on which to build. With this preparation, panels can develop excellent criteria for rather straightforward conditions, such as appendicitis, in about 1 to 2 hours. Complicated or multiple branching criteria, such as urinary tract infection, acute and chronic, adult and children, male and female, may take 3 to 4 hours of concentrated effort to reach consensus.

In medical criteria for hospitalized patients it helps to follow the logic of, How did they get there? When do they leave? What services should they receive? It is impressive to observe clinicians draw on the combination of research-based evidence, personal experience, pragmatic needs of the patient, and social needs of the health delivery system to arrive at useful and acceptable criteria for medical care. A consistent thread had been maintained in these panel criteria meetings. Often debated but always uniform is the decision to create optimal criteria, as opposed to minimal criteria. This is consistent with the professional goals of better diagnostic and therapeutic techniques and instrumentation throughout time. It also provides physicians with a goal of excellence to be achieved rather than mediocrity and better tools to understand differences in performance between physicians and among sites of medical care delivery.

The development of criteria begins with indications for hospital admission and proceeds to ranges of length of stay, indications for discharge and of services recommended (all for specific diagnostic categories), the enumeration of complications extending length of stay, and the description of optimal outcomes. Finally the panel will deal with identifying the factors that prejudice the optimal outcomes described and will develop the weights on the process items (history, physical examination, laboratory examinations, and therapeutic items) that make possible the scoring of performance.

In surgical diagnoses, especially for elective surgical procedures, the indications for operation are the indications for admission. Such indications are multiple in criteria for admission, for example, in hysterectomy. Medical diagnoses as well as surgical diagnoses are frequently emergencies, and as such the suspected or proven diagnosis is indication for admission, for example, acute myocardial infarction, fracture of the hip, diabetic coma, or bacterial meningitis. Frequently the diagnosis alone is not sufficient for appropriate admission, and the panel must recognize and categorize the reasons that made admission appropriate. For instance, admission for established diabetes mellitius is unusual, but in the presence of ketoacidosis, cellulitis, or vascular complications the admission is appropriate. Acute bronchitis is not considered appropriately admitted unless the patient has chronic obstructive pulmonary disease, or is alone and elderly, or is in precarious cardiac compensation. Diagnostic admissions are appropriate given certain circumstances that make outpatient procedures difficult, hazardous, or when time does not permit deliberate diagnostic behavior.

Length of stay determination should in my opinion be related to the medical needs of the recuperating patient and not to statistical norms developed by cumulative data relating length of stay to a specific diagnosis. The hazard of the statistical approach is the elevation of the median or mean or percentile of the usual to the level of expected, even ideal, behavior. An example is the declining length of stay in acute myocardial infarction from 4 to 3 to 2 weeks, as medically desirable and always in advance of the statistical norms.

Length of stay determination by statistical norms is convenient, but it denies the value and logic of determination of length of stay by the discharge status of the individual patient and the length of stay determined by medical necessity—not custom. We now know it was wrong to keep all acute myocardial infarctions hospitalized for 4 weeks. On the basis of new medical information we may decide, in the patient's best interest, to permit discharge when the probability of ventricular arrhythmias has disappeared.

Physician panels usually identify an appropriate range of days of stay and then modify this with discharge status criteria. This allows the panel to specify that the patient is ready for discharge when he has achieved a recuperative stage in the illness or condition that permits discharge to home or to a suitable extended care facility. This discharge status may be achieved before or after the expected length of stay in range of days.

Medical services recommended for optimal care include physician-delivered and physician-initiated services. The recording of critical items of the history, critical observations in the physical examination, and critical laboratory and radiologic examinations is an example of the optimal medical care criteria we will discuss.

It is in these areas that the most significant evaluation of quality of care delivered is accomplished, and it is the area of greatest interest to the criteria panels of physicians.

The physicians are asked to list those items they consider essential to the accurate process of diagnosis, therapy, or prognosis of the condition under consideration. These are the critical items in the criteria. Lively debate usually characterizes this activity, and consensus is reached by accord, but sometimes by realistic compromise between optimal and ideal expectations. All participants have agreed that this is a useful learning experience as well as a means of developing useful peer evaluation tools.

Earlier criteria were concerned primarily with the diagnostic process. These alone were found incomplete when related to the outcome of care. Subsequent criteria have shown the utility of developing therapeutic criteria as well.

We have not been concerned with a validation of the physician's final diagnosis. This is a second-guessing effort on the basis of a medical record completed by another physician or physicians, frequently with incomplete data, and dependent on subjective individual interpretation. Later a careful validation schema may be developed experimentally.

We are concerned with the diagnostic and therapeutic activities appropriate to the diagnosis the physician has recorded as the results of his investigation. Since the cost of collecting data in time and money requires that trained nonphysician abstractors may be employed instead of physicians, the requirements of the criteria must be in terms readily understood and readily available from the medical record free of interpretation by the abstractor.

The criteria must be arranged in a pattern or tabular form to serve as an abstract sheet for use of the abstractors. We have used worksheets specifically designed for the diagnosis to be studied (Fig. 16-1). This allows the abstractor to enter such numbers as are needed and otherwise to record the presence or absence of each criteria item in yes or no form. We have also used the Professional Activities Study Abstract (Commission on Professional and Hospital Activity, Ann Arbor, Michigan) by exploiting the 36 cells provided for research data sprinkled throughout the abstract. For this we have assigned certain criteria items to companion abstract cells and instruct the abstractor to enter numbers that have specific assigned meaning (for example, 1 = yes, 2 = no, 3 = not recorded), or numbers to record certain

laboratory values, such as blood sugar values, or serial blood pressure recordings, or other values for which no usual PAS cell is suitable.

Uniformity of abstractor recording is assured by use of a manual that describes each item, where it is found, what abbreviations or expressions are recognized, the conventions for observing data collected prior to hospital admission, or in ambulatory records the period of time before or after the sampled visit that observations can be accepted. For example, it is acceptable to record a chest x-ray as performed within 1 year in hypertension, but it must be for the sampled visit in pneumonia.

An example of ambulatory care criteria that embodies the quality measures described in the above are taken from a current, continuing research project funded by the National Center for Health Services Research, *Evaluation and Improvement of Ambulatory Medical Care* (see boxed material on pp. 350-351).[12]

In these criteria we see the items considered critical in diagnosis and therapy of essential hypertension, initial visit, and the weights given by the panel to each item. The weights are developed by first considering the relative importance of diagnosis and therapy and arbitrarily assigning a total weight of 100 to each diagnosis. These weights allow the panel to emphasize the relative value of each item in diagnosis or treatment. Once a weight is assigned to the diagnostic category it is apportioned to history, physical examination, and radiologic and laboratory examination. Then the individual items within each category are assigned a value to reflect the total weight of each component area of the criteria. The assignment of weights in essential hypertension, initial, is 40% to diagnosis and 60% to therapy. In follow-up hypertension, however, the weights are different, 30% to diagnosis and 70% to therapy. The panels thus recognized the burden of skill and knowledge to be differentially applied to

BASIC DATA

    Patient number   _____   Age   _____

    Date of admission   _____   Sex   _____

    Date of discharge   _____   Payment (check one):

      For deaths only (check one):   Private   _____

        Autopsy   _____   Blue Cross   _____

        No autopsy   _____   Commercial insurance   _____

    Days of stay   _____   Other (specify)

    Physician number   _____   _____

DIAGNOSES

    Primary (check one):

            _____   Pyelonephritis (600.0)

            _____   Cystitis (605.0)

            _____   Urinary tract infection (609.0)

            _____   Prostatitis (611.0)

    Secondary: _____

             _____

ADMISSION DATA

	Yes	No
Was there acute or severe illness?	_____	_____
Was there obstruction requiring treatment?	_____	_____
Was this the initial episode?	_____	_____
Was the infection recurrent or resistant?	_____	_____
Was admission for cystoscopy and retrograde pyelography?	_____	_____
Was admission for preplanned therapy with Kantrex, Polymyxin, or Neomycin?	_____	_____
Was admission for another reason?	_____	_____
If yes, specify _____		
Was renal failure present?	_____	_____

HOSPITAL SERVICES

    Specific reference to the following was made:

      1. Frequency of urination?   _____   _____

      2. Presence of obstructive symptoms?   _____   _____

Continued.

Fig. 16-1. Urinary tract infection worksheet. (From Payne, B. C., editor: Hospital utilization review manual, Ann Arbor, Mich., February 1968, University of Michigan Medical School, Dept. of Postgraduate Medicine.)

 3. Characterization of pain (if present)? _____ _____

 4. Presence of hematuria? _____ _____

 5. Pattern of incontinence (if present)? _____ _____

 6. Chronology of symptoms and signs? _____ _____

 7. Previous urologic disease? _____ _____

 8. Rectal examination? _____ _____

 9. Bladder examination? _____ _____

10. Pelvic examination? _____ _____

11. Neurologic examination? _____ _____

12. Determination of residual urine? _____ _____

13. Urinalysis with stain of sediment? _____ _____

14. Urine culture done prior to treatment? _____ _____

15. Sensitivity test with culture done prior to treatment? _____ _____

16. CBC? _____ _____

17. Intravenous pyelogram during or immediately prior to

    admission? _____ _____

18. Cystoscopy? _____ _____

    Within 72 hours? _____ _____

19. Retrograde pyelogram? _____ _____

    Within 72 hours? _____ _____

20. Chest roentgenogram? _____ _____

21. Tuberculin skin test? _____ _____

22. Acid-fast stain of urine for tubercle bacilli? _____ _____

23. Antibacterial therapy instituted within 12 hours of ad-

    mission? _____ _____

24. Blood sugar?

COMPLICATIONS (specify) _____

_____

Fig. 16-1. cont'd.

DISCHARGE CRITERIA

	Yes	No
1. Resolution of spesis?	_____	_____
2. Obstruction requiring further treatment?	_____	_____
3. Complication requiring further treatment?	_____	_____
4. Temperature normal for 24 to 48 hours?	_____	_____

EVALUATION

Type of admission (check one):

Diagnostic _____

Therapeutic _____

Admission was:

Appropriate _____

Inappropriate _____

For appropriate admission only:

Length of stay: appropriate _____

inappropriate _____

If understay, how many days? _____

If overstay, how many days? _____

Hospital services were:

Adequate _____

Inadequate _____

(Specify) _____

_____

OTHER COMMENTS

_____

_____

_____

_____

_____

Fig. 16-1. cont'd.

AMBULATORY CRITERIA
Hypertension—initial evaluation
HICDA 401, 403

Definition: Three or more blood pressure measurements (unless prior hypertension is established) in excess of 140/90, sitting position. It is recommended that blood pressure be measured in both arms, standing and sitting, with a cuff size proportional to the size of the arm, properly positioned, and diastolic sound recorded at the fifth phase or disappearance of sound, unless audible down to 0, in which case fourth phase should be used.

(Weight) A. History: observations recommended recording
(3)   1. Previous blood pressure measurement and/or diagnosis or treatment of hypertension
(2)   2. Family history of hypertension
(3)   3. Previous renal disease or renal trauma
(1)   4. In women, oral contraceptives
       In women, previous toxemia of pregnancy
     5. Cardiovascular or cerebrovascular events
       a. Cardiovascular events (for example, myocardial infarction, angina, congestive heart failure)
       b. Cerebrovascular events (for example, stroke, transient ischemic attacks)

   B. Physical examination: observations recommended recording
(7)   1. Blood pressure taken in each arm in sitting and standing position initially, in one arm during follow-up visits
(0.4)   2. Height
(0.4)   3. Weight
(3)   4. Funduscopic examination
(0.4)   5. Radial-femoral pulse lag
(0.4)   6. Major arterial pulses
(0.4)   7. Arterial and abdominal bruits
(2)   8. Heart size, gallop sounds, rate, rhythm, characteristic of apex impulse
(0.4)   9. Physical indications of endocrine causes for hypertension (for example, cushingoid facies, facial flush, sweating, tremor)

   C. Laboratory
(2)   1. Urinalysis
(3)   2. Serum potassium
(3)   3. Serum creatinine or blood urea nitrogen
(1.6)   4. Urinary catecholamines—metanephrine or vanillundelic acid in young, severe hypertensives

   D. Radiology   Consistent with diagnosis:
(1)   1. Chest x-ray   1. IV pyelogram
       (PA and lateral)   2. Renogram

   E. Special examination   Consistent with diagnosis:
(3)   1. Electrocardiogram   1. Renal arteriogram
                              a. Renin determination
                              b. Aldosterone determination
                              c. 17 hydroxysteroid determination
                              d. 17 ketosteroid determination

---

AMBULATORY CRITERIA—cont'd

F. Outcome goal
  1. Normalize the blood pressure by sequential management approach, with caution in the presence of suspected cerebrovascular disease and with tolerable adverse drug effects
  2. Substantial reduction of the blood pressure when normalization not possible or in presence of intolerable adverse effects
G. Treatment: sequential management
  1. Sodium restriction
(60) 2. Diuretic
  3. Vasodilators*—no required order
    a. Reserpine
    b. Hydralazine
100   c. Propranolol
    d. Guanethidine
    e. Alpha-methyldopa
H. Factors that prejudice good outcome
  1. Initial blood pressure in excess of 200/120
  2. Hypertension in a black male
  3. Cushings syndrome
  4. Malignant hypertension
  5. Intolerance for prescribed antihypertensive drugs
  6. Renal failure
  7. Lack of patient compliance

*Full weight is given for any drug combination that controls blood pressure, provided sequential pattern is followed.

---

the problem of management of the hypertensive patient at different times in the course of treatment.

The outcome or end result of treatment is unweighted. Presumably this is a reflection of the adequacy of the process measures. Outcomes are usually intermediate in terms of time. Immediate outcomes of treatment are inconclusive in chronic disease and in some acute processes as well. Ultimate outcomes of care may require years of observation, such as cancer therapy or organic heart disease. Even intermediate outcomes cannot be said to be the result of good medical care alone. The ability of the patient to sustain and recover from injury, whether of traumatic, surgical, bacterial, viral, or immune causation, is a highly individual expression. Recognizing this, the panel provides us with risk factors or factors that prejudice

a good outcome. This list is not exhaustive but reasonable, diagnosis-related possibilities that should be considered in evaluating the outcome of medical intervention.

There are few diagnoses that can be evaluated for quality or effectiveness of care from the ultimate outcome alone. Among these are tetanus, cardiopulmonary arrest, anaphylactic shock, and cardiac tamponade. If one accepts this, then evaluation of a combination of process and outcome of care is a reasonable approach to the assurance of medical care of optimal quality.

CONTINUING EDUCATION STUDY

You will recall that we mentioned Continuing Education Study as the last part of the Hawaii study (p. 339). It is my thesis that the entire purpose of peer review is an improvement in medical care delivered

Table 16-3. Acute urinary tract infection, percentages of criteria items observed

	Weight	Criteria item	All hospitals (%)	Referent hospitals (%)	Hospital (%)
History	0.5	Urination frequency	14.0	17	12
	0.5	Obstructive symptoms	26.4	60	25
	0.5	Pain	70.7	92	62
	0.5	Hematuria	29.3	70	38
	0.5	Pattern of incontinence	11.6	38	38
	0.5	Chronology	86.4	100	100
	0.5	Previous urologic disease	56.2	88	88
Physical examination	1	Digital rectal and/or pelvic examination	36.8	62	25
	1	Bladder examination	26.7	38	25
	1	Kidney area examination	59.1	77	62
Laboratory	3	Urinalysis with stain sediment or culture	74.0	100	100
	1.5	Urine culture	70.2	100	100
	1.5	Sensitivity	49.2	80	75
	1	CBC	86.8	100	100
	1	Renal function test	42.1	100	100
	1	IV pyelogram unless prostatitis	36.2	62	29
	3	Antibacterial therapy within 1 hour	67.8	100	62
		Number of cases	98		8
		Weighted criteria items observed	56.0	70.7	66.5

to the patient. The Hawaii Medical Association concurred with this goal and assured us of the cooperation of Hawaii physicians in responding to the findings of the research activities. The feedback of medical and questionnaire data to four participating hospitals' medical, nursing, and administrative staffs was accomplished in a series of seminars described in *The Quality of Medical Care: Evaluation and Improvement.*

In this study five diagnoses chosen from the Episode of Illness Study formed the basis for comparison between performance in the initial data collection period (1968) and subsequent data collection periods in 1970 and 1971.

Criteria item tallies (Table 16-3) were prepared for each diagnosis and each participating hospital. These tallies were a statistical reporting of the observed criteria-related items of medical care. As such they represented the adherence to standards expressed by the diagnosis-specific criteria. The physicians could then evaluate their own joint performance and the PPI scores attached and compare this performance with the total of 22 hospital performances and to the referent hospital. The referent hospital is a statistical construct of the best performance in each item from all the participating hospitals.

In small groups and representative hospital medical staff groups, physicians identified areas of strength and weakness in performance. On this basis they developed action plans that could be instituted with administrative assistance to improve performance throughout the hospital, usually on a departmental basis.

Table 16-4, displaying the percentages of criteria items observed from the Hawaii study, compares the recording of the specific items of the criteria for cholecystitis in four large hospitals over the three data-collection periods, with performance

Table 16-4. Chronic cholecystitis and cholelithiasis, percentages of criteria items observed

	Criteria item	Total local hospitals (%)			Hospital A		
		1968	1970	1971	1968	1970	1971
History	Food intolerance	64	72	76	61	66	92
	Previous attacks	86	91	93	87	93	100
	Jaundice	46	67	70	42	62	72
Physical examination	None critical						
Laboratory	CBC	81	88	92	95	100	100
	Urinalysis	97	98	94	97	100	100
X-ray	Chest x-ray within 1 year	2	17	9	0	21	4
	Cholecystography	75	82	77	87	90	92
Special	ECG *if* over 50 years old	47	36	41	44	33	70
	Normal gallbladder	3	0.5	0	3	0	0
	Number of cases	552	184	194	76	29	85
	(Age >50)	(106)	(87)	(88)	(38)	(12)	(10)
	PPI	57	74	73	68	76	87

within one of the participating hospitals, hospital *A,* over the same data-collection period. Of particular interest is the observation that jaundice, either present or absent, is made in only 46% of patients in 1968 and 70% of patients in 1971. Chest x-rays are performed in only 2% of patients within 1 year of the cholecystectomy in 1968 and slightly more, 9%, in 1971. Pathology documentation of a normal excised gallbladder was found in 3% of 106 patients in 1968 and none of 88 patients in 1971. The PPI in all hospitals for care of cholecystitis improved from 57% in 1968 to 73% in 1971, and for hospital *A* from 68% in 1968 to 87% in 1971, a change that reflects the vigorous response of the chief of surgery to the research data.

In four participating hospitals we were able to document a 4% to 7% improvement in overall PPIs over the period of observation. We considered this inconclusive and at least in part attributed the minor change to the brief period, only 5 months, of educational activity within the medical staff between the first feedback seminars in February 1971 and the follow-up data collection.

Many of the changes initiated in the seminars were not possible to document in the medical data collected. Organizational changes within one hospital reassigning admitted patients to floors staffed by nurses specifically trained for expert attention to the needs of particular diseases is one such change. Development of a transport system to relieve nurses of the duty of transporting patients or laboratory specimens is another. In still another hospital the criteria-based assessment of medical care was extended by the staff into review of appendectomy, herniorrhaphy, and hemorrhoidectomy. They were also successful in implementing an assessment of blood transfusions and to reverse completely the previous pattern of administration of packed red blood cells from 10% to over 95% of all transfusions.

The greatest changes (7%) in PPI occurred in two hospitals in which there was a close functional and administrative relationship between medical staff and the hospital administration. General practitioners also show the greatest (7%) degree of improvement in PPI between 1968 and 1971. No other measured variable was found to exhibit this influence on the PPI.

OFFICE CARE ASSESSMENT STUDY (ONGOING)

The research activity described deals primarily with the hospitalized patient. These patients are served by the highly organized, secondary- and tertiary-oriented, costly element of modern hospital medical practice. For these reasons the focus of research and now practical implementation of the peer review process begins with the hospital system of care.

It is estimated that only 20% of medical care is delivered in the hospital, and with growing emphasis on surgical centers for ambulatory care, HMOs, and multispecialty group practices (both prepaid and fee-for-service), this percentage may become even less. Such a shift in emphasis makes an old observation more imperative. If physicians have found it difficult to monitor quality of care in an organized setting, what is the situation in the world of ambulatory care, and how should we go about improving it?

I consider the office care section of the Hawaii study a feasibility measurement of the climate, the available tools, and the methodology for evaluating ambulatory medical care. A 4-year project, now 1 year underway, extends and expands these concepts into a study of ambulatory medical care in six different sites. The sites include two private solo practice sites of about 60 physicians, multispecialty group practice (prepaid and fee-for-service), and two medical school ambulatory medical care delivery sites. Data has been collected for evaluation of the quality of medical care in 23 diagnostic categories and compared to the optimal criteria developed for these diagnostic categories by physicians representing the six sites.

Preliminary analyses of the data indicates that the overall weighted PPIs for all diagnoses in all sites and all specialties is 68%. That is, the average patient in this study received 68% of the optimal medical care described in the criteria. Outcome determinations, relationship of process to outcomes, risk factors, specialization, pay-ment mechanisms, and other physician and patient characteristics will be analyzed to understand the complex relationship we recognize as the medical diagnostic and therapeutic process.

CONCLUSIONS

We now view the criteria-based method of quality of medical care assessment and utilization review as validated by the series of research and demonstrations projects described. It has been validated in the most functional terms:

1. That it is practical to establish consensus process and outcome criteria at an optimal and peer accepted level
2. That the logistics of data collection by trained nonphysician abstractors have been proven manageable, successful, reliable, and accurate
3. That the assessment of quality of medical care can and, from a practical point of view, should be accomplished on a suitable sample of the total universe of cases available for review
4. That analysis of the data is accomplished by computers programmed to display the data in any and every way possible to enhance ready understanding of the variables
5. That the analyses presented in a proper format to the receptive audience of participating physicians and allied professionals can lead to positive, constructive change in the delivery of medical care that is more effective as well as more efficient
6. That continued monitoring of this process is desirable to achieve the maximal effect and to sustain the changes initiated

The pattern then becomes criteria, sampling, abstracting, analysis, feedback, behavioral change, criteria, sampling, and so on.

REFERENCES

1. Lembcke, P.: Medical auditing by scientific methods, J.A.M.A. **162:**646-655, 1956.

2. Fitzpatrick, T., Reidel, D., and Payne, B. C.: Effectiveness of hospital use. In Hospital and Medical Economics, Chicago, 1962, Hospital Research and Educational Trust.

3. Payne, B. C., and Lyons, T.: Method of evaluating and improving personal medical care quality, Report to National Center for Health Services Research, 1972.

4. Brook, R., and Appel, F.: Quality of care assessment—choosing a method for peer review, N. Engl. J. Med. **288:**1323-1329, 1973.

5. Williamson, J.: Evaluating quality of patient care—a strategy relating outcome and process assessment, J.A.M.A. **218:**564-569, 1971.

6. Morehead, M.: The medical audit as an operational tool, Am. J. Public Health **57:**1643, 1967.

7. Payne, B. C.: Pilot study of hospital use in Nassau County, New York, 1963, Hospital Insurance Association of America.

8. Hospital Utilization Project of Pennsylvania, 3530 Forbes Avenue, Pittsburgh, Pa. 15213.

9. Taylor, F. C., Payne, B. C., Mann, F. C., and Birch, L.: Medical record review in a hospital committee setting (a feasibility study), University of Michigan, Ann Arbor, Mich., April 1970, Center for Research on Utilization of Scientific Knowledge, Institute for Social Research.

10. Payne, B. C., editor: Hospital utilization review manual, Ann Arbor, Mich., February 1968, The University of Michigan Medical School, Dept. of Postgraduate Medicine.

11. Payne, B. C., and study staff: The quality of medical care: evaluation and improvement, Chicago, 1975, Hospital Research and Educational Trust.

12. Evaluation and improvement of ambulatory medical care, contract no., HSM-110-70-69, National Center for Health Services Research, 1972, U.S. Dept. of Health, Education, and Welfare.

17

The quality assurance system

CLEMENT R. BROWN, Jr.
ROSEMARY McCONKEY

Quality assurance differs as a system importantly and essentially from (medical) peer review systems, which only assess the quality of care. To us, medical peer review means review by physicians of the care provided by physicians. Medical peer review involves the assessment of care through a process usually called medical audit. Quality assurance includes both quality assessment through medical audit *and a change program based on medical audit or medical peer review.* Thus a quality assurance system not only assesses the quality of care but more importantly and essentially assures the quality of care.

Essential to the definition of a quality assurance system for health care are the following assumptions:

1. The system begins and ends with the patient because he is ultimately responsible for his health.
2. The patient or potential patient is the final arbiter of quality.
3. The patient ultimately has responsibility for assurance of the quality of his health care.

Given the above assumptions that the patient has the major and ultimate responsibility for his health, the practicing physician or other health professional shares responsibility with the patient for care. Currently much euphemistic discussion and verbal commitment is given to patient or consumer participation in health affairs, to patient rights, and to other representations of involvement. However, focusing patient responsibility in the perspective and purview of quality assurance affords the opportunity to rethink and to initiate new thinking on the shared roles and responsibilities of patients and practitioners for health care. Any system that goes full circle to assure quality health care must, by definition and commitment, place the ultimate responsibility for health and health care with the patient or potential patient.

SYSTEM ELEMENTS

Assurance of quality of health care. The ultimate goal of the quality assurance system is to assure that the patient and community receive quality health care. This goal requires the system to maintain the delivery of quality health care and to achieve those changes necessary to improve the delivery of health care and the intended outcome—good health. Anything less than this goal does not represent a quality assurance system. Quality assessment or medical peer review is a part of the quality assurance system.

Patient and community responsibility. The quality assurance system begins and ends with the patient, who in aggregate constitutes the community. The patient and community share ultimate responsibility for maintaining health and for the quality of care they receive to help maintain health. The patient and community must join with health professionals to define the level of health they wish to achieve, but the patient and community must be the final arbiters or evaluators of health care.

Components. The quality assurance system is a total system that includes component subsystems necessary to assure the quality of health care. For example, education or change is a critical component of the total quality assurance system. The education or change program must be based on sound principles for achieving behavioral change and for achieving the desired health care outcomes.

Accountability. The quality assurance system provides for two-dimensional accountability. The patient is ultimately accountable to himself, and health professionals are accountable to the patient and to the community. The patient or community delegate authority to the health professionals to perform certain functions that help the patient to maintain or achieve optimal health.

Patient data base. The quality assurance system requires that an age-, sex-, and race-standardized data base be acquired on each patient. Such a data base assures identification of health care problems, potential problems, and risks for each patient.

Problem-oriented medical record. The quality assurance system utilizes the problem-oriented record as the most effective and efficient system for the patient's health record.

Change. This system mandates that all those whose behavior may need to change to achieve quality health care participate in the development and ratification of criteria for such health care. This includes participation of patients.

There must be a precommitment by health professionals and patients to participate in change or educational programs to improve both the processes and outcomes of health care when this is found necessary.

The quality assurance system can achieve significant change where necessary to improve patient care. Significant change and how it occurs will be described later in this chapter.

Health manpower rules. Data concerning actual health care outcomes and processes must be collected, abstracted, and displayed by medical record practitioners or health record analysts for those health professionals who will evaluate the degree to which preagreed criteria have been met. An automated or computerized medical record abstracting system may be used.

Evaluation. The ultimate evaluation of a quality assurance program will be documentation that change where necessary to improve health and health care has occurred. In this way the program that begins with the patient ends with the patient. Is his health improved? Is he receiving quality health care? Is he meeting his health goals? Is he receiving the assistance necessary to meet his goals with a quality program?

System implementation. A total system should provide mechanisms to operationalize the system. Implementation of a quality assurance system requires both knowledge and specific skills. Workshops can be designed to provide health professionals with the skills for implementing the system. With health professionals from more than 300 hospitals seeking to learn the necessary skills to implement a quality assurance program, it has been shown that two components of the system seem particularly difficult: (1) the development of criteria, which requires special skills, and (2) the design and implementation of the necessary change or educational programs.

RESEARCH AND DEVELOPMENT OF THE SYSTEM

The Bi-Cycle concept provided the basis for the design of the quality assurance system described here. The concept (Fig. 17-1) relates the continuing education of the practicing health professional directly to patient care. The Bi-Cycle concept developed from the need for a rational basis for designing continuing education programs for practicing health professionals. Given such a basis, continuing medical education programs could help practicing health professionals meet the needs of patients for quality health care. The Bi-Cycle interrelates an outer patient care cycle with an inner change or educational cycle. Through the steps in the outer cycle the patient problems are identified and criteria for the care necessary to resolve the problems are developed consensually. Data are collected that relate the actual care delivered to the criteria, and deficits based on the criteria are identified. The inner educational or change cycle outlines the steps necessary for patients and health professionals to achieve behavioral change to improve care based on identified deficits. After implementing the change or educational program, the inner cycle links to the outer cycle by the reassessment of care to see if change to improve care where necessary has occurred. This interface identifies whether health care and health are at the desired criterion levels. [1]

A quality assurance system based on the Bi-Cycle concept was implemented in a 200-bed community hospital over a 3-year period. The system did document that significant change necessary to improve patient care was achieved. For example, there was a decrease in unnecessary surgery, a decrease in complications following certain surgeries, and a more appropriate use of blood and antibiotics. These changes have been documented and published.

Following this successful implementation in a community hospital, the system was replicated in ten hospitals over a 2½-year period as the Mandate Project. [2] The ten hospitals included a 1000-bed inner city hospital, a 100-bed semirural hospital, a children's hospital, an academic center, and a number of community hospitals of varying sizes with and without academic affiliation. The Mandate Project was so-called because boards of trustees of the participating hospitals mandated that their administration and medical staff develop a quality assurance system. In five of the ten hospitals a quality assurance system based on the Bi-Cycle was implemented successfully; that is, significant change where necessary to improve care was documented. The Mandate Project demonstrated that for a successful system, certain social engineering skills were necessary. The Mandate Project demonstrated that a quality assurance system could be implemented successfully in various types of hospitals.

In summary, a quality assurance system is capable of achieving significant change where necessary to improve care. Implementation of the system in a number of hospitals of varying sizes has been achieved, and these institutions did in turn achieve significant change where necessary to improve care. Finally, a teacher training program has been successfully developed that has provided for state, regional, and national faculty to help others achieve skills necessary to implement successful quality assurance programs.

THE SYSTEM: WHAT IT IS

The quality assurance system is a system to maintain health care at a quality level or to achieve those changes necessary to improve health care. The quality assurance system has been used in the development of emerging-needs curricula for health professionals of many disciplines from undergraduate through graduate levels and in inpatient and outpatient settings. It is a total system and includes all the subsystems and components necessary to assure quality health care when the patient assumes ultimate responsibility for his health, and the health professional practices competently to assist the patient to this end. If quality health care is not the outcome attained, the system provides the mechanisms to identify deficiencies and to correct them, thus achieving the levels of health care agreed on by patients and the practicing health professionals.

THE SYSTEM: HOW TO START

Experience has shown that successful implementation of the quality assurance system in a hospital requires an appropriate governance, administrative, and committee structure. The board of trustees must mandate, maintain, and monitor the system. As a minimum, the board should adopt an explicit statement mandating administrative and health professional staff to develop and operate the system. All three groups should participate in the development of the mandate, but the statement is the ultimate responsibility of the trustees. Not only must the board mandate a quality assurance program, it must maintain the program by providing the necessary resources to conduct it. A system director, medical records personnel, health data analysts, health data abstracting system, budget, facilities, and equipment are some requisites necessary for a successful functioning system. It will be necessary to commit fiscal support for the system as part of an institution's total quality control effort. The board must monitor the system through creation of a regular reporting mechanism that documents a successfully functioning system, namely that health and health care are of acceptable quality. This functional organization of the board of trustees to mandate, maintain, and monitor constitutes the three "Ms" of governance.[3]

Health professionals must organize themselves to assure achievement of the system goals. As already indicated, there must be a system manager. This may be the director of medical education, the medical director, or a member of the health professional staff including the hospital administrator. The system manager will be accountable to the chief executive officer and to the board of trustees

for the system's efficiency and effectiveness.

Organizational structure is important to the quality assurance system, the committee being one organizational structure. It may be appropriate to form a health care quality assurance committee. In large departmentalized hospitals this committee might be constituted by departmental chiefs or chairmen and chaired by the quality assurance system manager or director. The committee should report to the board through the institution's chief executive officer. In a large institution the committee might coordinate the work of several subcommittees functioning as working committees. The chief functions of the quality assurance committee would be to organize the work of the subcommittees, to monitor their functioning, and to coordinate the reporting efforts for board presentation. In a smaller or non-departmentalized institution one committee, the quality assurance committee, may perform all these functions.

The working or subcommittee has three essential functions:

1. To develop the criteria for health care. In a departmentalized hospital the criteria will be ratified by departmental staff and subsequently by the hospital-wide parent committee and the board of trustees.
2. To analyze the data on actual health care by comparing it with the pre-agreed criterial care to identify deficits in health care. These data are abstracted from the patient health records by medical records personnel and health records analysts.
3. To make recommendations for corrective action to the parent department or committee.

The working committee should be representative of the parent department to validate findings and recommendations. A range of seven to ten members may be appropriate. The committee should be multidisciplinary and should represent those professional personnel whose behavior might require change to improve health care. This representation should include patients. Experience indicates that the working committee can complete their tasks by meeting 1 hour per month if the system director and health records personnel have completed preliminary work. The preliminary work will include 1 or 2 hours of meeting with the committee member who is to present criteria, findings, or recommendations to the full committee.

In summary, the implementation of a successful quality assurance system requires governance, administrative, and committee structures appropriate to the performance of explicitly stated functions so that the system's goals of quality health care for all patients can be achieved.

THE SYSTEM: HOW IT WORKS

The overall sequence of the quality assurance system and how it works as a whole is presented for the reader in Fig.

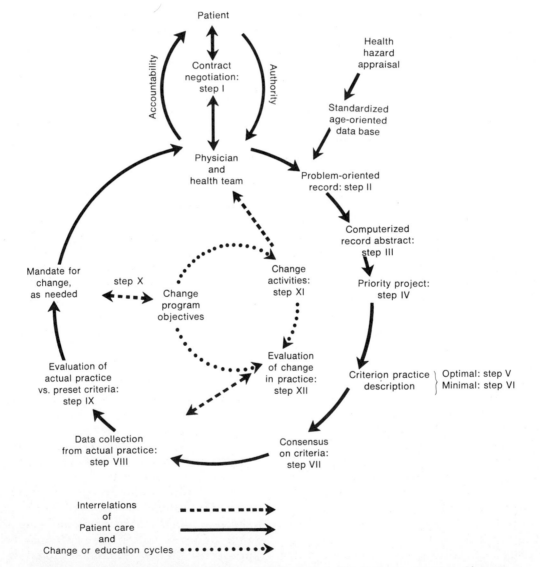

Fig. 17-1. The quality assurance system. (Adapted from the Bi-Cycle concept, Clement R. Brown, Jr., M.D., 1971.)

17-1. As each step within the system is identified and described, the reader is referred to the sequential illustration that corresponds to that step and depicts its position on the Bi-Cycle.

The system begins with the patient and his interaction with the health care team (step I). The health team may include the physician and numerous other health professionals. The patient retains ultimate responsibility for his health care but in association with the health care team under a contract. This contract should be explicit, and through it the patient delegates authority to the health care team for the performance of certain functions to assist him in maintaining his health, managing his illnesses, or reducing his risks of disease or accident. In delegating authority to the health care team for certain functional responsibilities related to his health care, the patient maintains accountability of the health care team to him in the delivery of quality health care. The quality

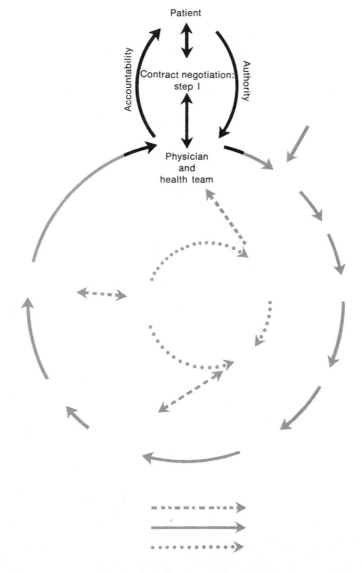

Fig. 17-2. Step I.

assurance system begins with the development of an initial contract between the patient and the health care team. The initial contract may be modified as a result of the next step, the acquisition of the data base.

Step II in the quality assurance system is the acquisition of a complete and accurate patient data base by the health care team. In the ambulatory setting this data base will be completed generally by the end of the third visit. For an elective admission to the hospital this complete and accurate data base should arrive with the patient. In the case of emergency or urgent admissions the data base should be acquired within a few hours of admission, conditions permitting. The acquisition form for the patient health care data base should be standardized as to age, sex, and race and should provide for the accurate identification of all significant health care problems and risks for the patient.

The development of historical questions appropriate for the data base can be facilitated through the use of resources such as the National Disease and Thera-

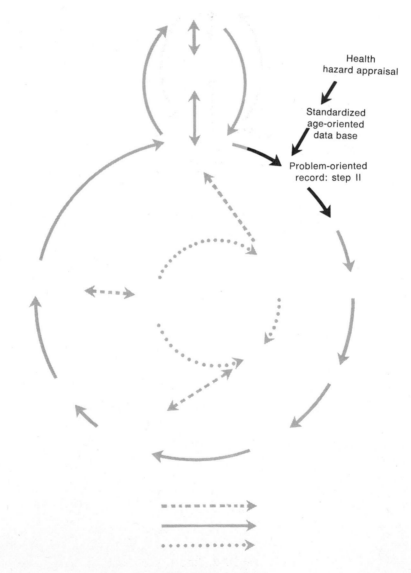

Fig. 17-3. Step II.

peutic Index, which identifies the most common diseases or conditions in the outpatient setting. The Geller Tables and Health Hazard Appraisal Program assist in the identification of health hazards or risks for differing age groups by sex and race. Physicians can determine items to be included in the data base, and allied health professional staff can acquire data from patients. The completeness and accuracy of the data base for every patient can be monitored frequently during early stages of the system until all team members are comfortable with the validity and accuracy of the data. The final product of this second step of the quality assurance system consists in the completion of a problem-oriented health record. The problem-oriented medical record format (POMR) renders the most understandable and auditable health record. In the inpatient setting a standard POMR format can be used. In the outpatient setting each patient record should include a temporary problem list in addition to the permanent one, plus information on patient compli-

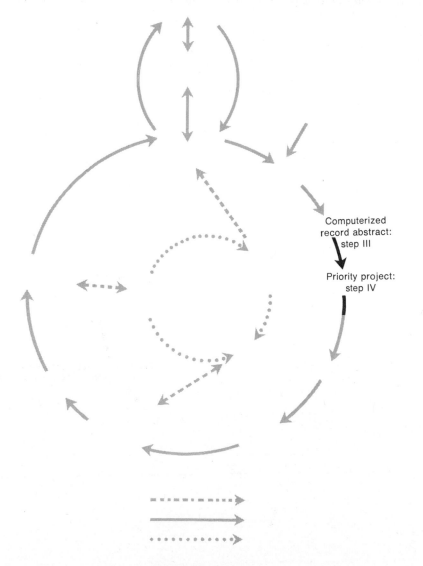

Computerized
record abstract:
step III

Priority project:
step IV

Fig. 17-4. Step III.

ance with his treatment regimen, a patient visit sheet, which records visit data, and the problem or problems specifically dealt with during the visit.

In step III abstracted data may be entered into a computerized data storage and retrieval system. The PAS-MAP system of the CPHA (Ann Arbor, Michigan) represents one such system. Data entered in step III of the system should be relevant to the criteria developed in steps V and VI.

Step IV of the quality assurance system is the priority-setting step after the pro-

cess developed by Williamson et al.[4] The PAS-MAP data system can be utilized to determine those diseases, problems, and conditions that result in the highest percentage of total disability among hospitalized patients. When disability factors are identified and weighted, the top ten, for example, are identified. In a study at Chestnut Hill Hospital, Philadelphia, ten diseases and problems were found to cause more than 40% of the total disability among hospital patients over a 6-month period. Given such a base of information, the professional staff can determine the

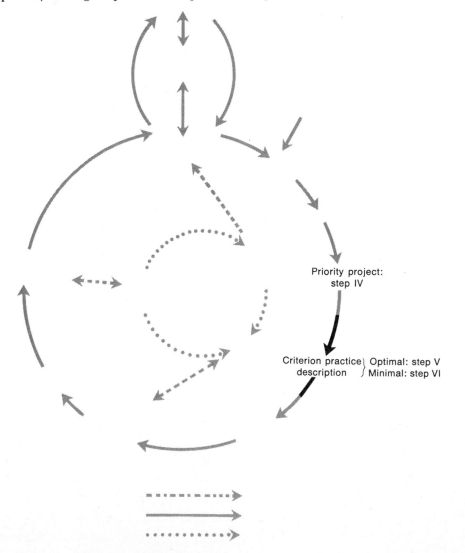

Fig. 17-5. Steps IV, V, and VI.

priority of those health care problems about which it wishes to do something. The second part of the priority-setting process requires that each staff member reorder the top ten causes of disability on the basis of an estimate of preventable disability. This brings the practicing health professional to concentrate on those things about which he may effect reasonable beneficial results. For example, carcinomatosis appeared as the second greatest statistical cause of disability in the initial ranking at one hospital, but because little can be done about carcinomatosis, it was given lesser priority in the reordering. Total medical staff time required for the prioritization process just described required less than 1 hour in each major clinical department.

The last part of the three-part process for prioritization requires identification of the greatest causes of preventable disability, which the data showed were in actuality not being prevented. These diseases, problems, and conditions become the top priority concerns of the quality assurance program. The needed data are acquired by completed steps VI through IX of the quality assurance system.

In steps V and VI of the Bi-Cycle, the optimal and minimal criteria for practice are developed. Criteria-setting represents one of the two most important steps in the system and one of the more difficult. Both the criteria and the process by which the criteria are developed will be discussed.

In general three kinds of criteria are developed in the quality assurance system. These are organizational criteria, process criteria, and outcome criteria. Organizational criteria describe the ideal system or institutional organization to deliver quality health care. Process criteria are elements that describe ideal health professional behaviors having to do with screening, prevention, diagnosis, and therapy in relation to a specific patient problem, disease, condition procedure, or surgery. Outcome criteria describe patient health outcomes or results from the health professional behaviors just mentioned. These outcome criteria are often written as patient behaviors, states of health, or lack of health, while process criteria are written as health professional behaviors that will achieve appropriate patient care outcomes.

Process criteria for patient care should meet certain conditions commonly referred to as the "criteria for criteria." These conditions for process criteria and their definitions are

1. Real (someone will do something about them)
2. Understandable (requisite for an adoption by the health professional group)
3. Measurable (are quantifiable)
4. Behavioral (describe health professional performance in the provision of health care)
5. Achievable (relate to resources, personnel, time available, and so on)

Process criteria may specify indicants for admission to the hospital or for surgery, justification for diagnosis, appropriate preoperative and postoperative studies, therapeutic regimens, contraindications to therapeutic regimens, to illustrate some examples.

Outcome criteria are represented by anticipated patient outcomes including disability, discomfort, recovery, length of stay, length of absence from employment, and the complications of disease or surgery.

Experience-to-date with the criteria-setting process permits the formulation of some guidelines:

1. Criteria should be set "in group." All health professionals and patients should participate whose behavior may require change so that quality care be assured. Emphatically stated, criteria should be set across health professional disciplines and not by one group of health professionals. Physicians should not set criteria for other health professions, but should develop criteria with them.

2. Criteria should be developed locally by those who will live by them. The criteria should subscribe to local health professional resources, differences in patient population, and other related health system variables. Although criteria have been developed and distributed by national groups, specialty societies, and others, we do not have evidence that such criteria, when applied locally to achieve changes to improve care, do so successfully. We have evidence that locally developed criteria have achieved significant change where necessary to improve care. Successful application of locally developed criteria can be attributed to the fact that those who develop the criteria operationalize them more easily because they have ownership in them. Perhaps most importantly the process of criteria development is a highly educational endeavor.

3. A limited number of criteria should be developed for each disease, condition, surgery, or patient problem. Those behaviors that can effect significant care outcomes in care should be selected for criteria.

4. If considerable resistance is met in adopting a criterion, the presence of disagreement may be indicative of lack of validation, and the criterion should be eliminated. The probability is that we do not know the ideal way to manage the situation.

5. Criteria should be developed for those situations where the greatest amount of preventable patient disability that is not being prevented is occurring. It is anticipated that if this is the situation, the greatest amount of improvement in patient care can be achieved. Criteria for diagnosis and management of hypertension (and the use of seatbelts) exemplify some possible situations. Problems should be reviewed for areas of priority in criteria setting. For example, in situations where patients with pneumonia are being diagnosed properly but admitted to the hospital unnecessarily, criteria should be developed for hospital admission as well as for diagnosis.

6. Criteria for patient care should meet the "criteria for criteria" outlined heretofore.

In step V of the Bi-Cycle, optimal criteria are set. In setting these criteria one can ask, "Ideally, how should a patient be managed with this disease, problem, condition, or operation?" Or, "What is the ideal organizational structure to achieve the best health care?" In setting minimal criteria in step VI it is helpful to ask, "Below what level of practice for patient care outcome will the staff insist on developing some program to improve practice or outcome?"

We believe step VI to be critical to the process, for it precommits health professionals to an action program when a performance level or outcome level as determined in step IX falls below the minimal criterial level agreed on in this step. Sometimes the minimum criteria level for practice, outcome, or organizational structure is easy to find. For example, in primary appendectomy one could readily obtain agreement that a minimum of 75% of the patients should show evidence of acute appendicitis on tissue exam. With respect to hypertension, it is easy to decide that all patients with a blood pressure above 140/95 should be diagnosed as hypertensive, but it is more difficult to decide what is an acceptable level of missed patients over a 6-month period. Would one be justified in developing an educational program if three patients who should have been diagnosed as hypertensive were missed in a 6-month period? One surely would develop an educational or change program if 30 patients were missed in this period of time. Deciding on the threshold for action is a difficult process at times, but it is essential nevertheless to the precommitment to action even though the minimal criteria level or threshold for action level might require change subsequently.

In step VII each working subcommittee of the quality assurance system submits a list of optimal and minimal criteria to the appropriate department or group for alteration and ultimate adoption. This ratification process by department or group of health professional staff is a crucially important step in the process. At a later step, if data concerning an actual practice require a behavior change, the ratification process will have been a precommitment to action. In the ratification process, if a vocal minority prevents consensus from being reached, each member of the department or group is asked to critique the criteria and to add his own desired criteria. This process often achieves the degree of consensus not attainable in the initial step. When modifications are presented to the department or group, often they are adopted without further change.

In summary then the patient care process and organizational structure most likely to achieve appropriate health care outcomes must be objectively and explicitly stated as criteria. The valuation of practice performance is unacceptable if the criteria have not been shared, ratified, and adopted.

Step VIII of the quality assurance system is concerned with collection of data from the patient medical records.

The following guidelines are used:

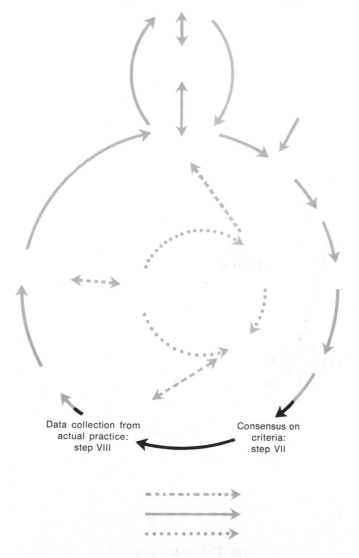

Fig. 17-6. Steps VII and VIII.

1. Information collected should provide input both for identified criteria items that have been met as well as those items not met.

2. Medical record or patient care evaluation staff abstract data from medical records to describe actual practice. Data on actual levels of performance are to be compared with the defined accepted level for each criterion.

3. A data-abstracting system and a storage and retrieval system simplify the information-processing step.

4. Medical record staff perform the reduction of data or preparation of reports. This activity should be systematized by medical records staff and need not be performed by other health professionals.

5. Data describing actual practices should be reported to the review committees in a form that is readily understood and interpreted. The performance data are tabulated comparatively with the criteria, and from this information patterns of care and individual differences from the criteria can be identified.

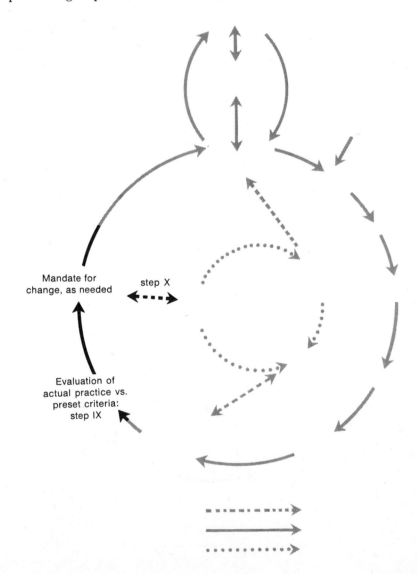

Fig. 17-7. Steps IX and X.

Step IX of the system is the assessment step. The actual performance of health professionals is compared to the optimal and minimal criteria developed. This step is usually performed by the departmental quality assurance committee in a departmentalized institution or by the quality assurance committee in an institution so organized. A judgment is made from the prepared data as to whether the actual performance of health professionals and the patient care outcomes are at the criterial level agreed on previously. To the extent that actual performance does not meet criterial performance or is below the threshold for action, the committee makes recommendations to the department or to the staff as a whole concerning an action program to correct identified and quantified deficits in health care.

The committee need only ask, "Who needs to do what to move care from where we find it to where we have set our criteria?" Health professional or patient behaviors become the objectives for the change or educational program.

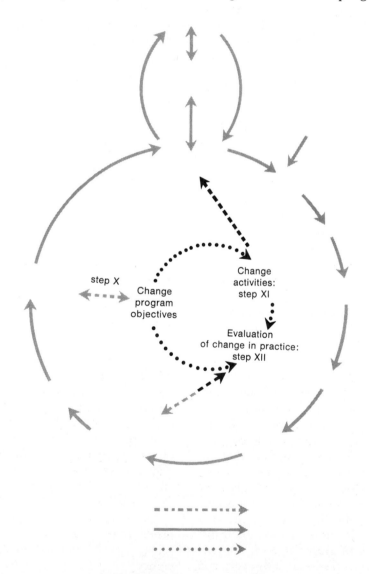

Fig. 17-8. Steps X, XI, and XII.

It can be seen that we are now moving from the outer or patient care cycle to the inner or change cycle at step X (Fig. 17-8). Steps X, XI, and XII represent the assurance component of the quality assurance system as differentiated from the prior steps that represented the assessment component of the quality assurance system. Most of the prior steps represent a medical audit system; that is, they identify the changes that need to occur to improve health care. Steps X, XI, and XII represent the change or corrective action program. The change program is that corrective action program to achieve change where necessary to improve health care. The change necessary may be behavioral change of the health professional, and if so, will be an educational program. However, the change needed to improve health care may not rest with health professional or patient behavior, but may be an administrative change, that is, equipment, space, or personnel. Often, too, patient behavioral change is required to achieve improved criterial health care. As stated previously, an effective quality assurance program requires that the patient assume the ultimate responsibility for his health and health care.

The change program objectives identified in step X of the change cycle are derived from the assessment made in step IX, the health care assessment step.

In step XI the change activities and a program for implementing and managing change are developed. This is the second most important single step in the quality assurance system and invariably is the most difficult step to achieve. Frequently it is the tendency of the review committee to plan a change program that involves the health professional learning something he does not know. Thus most change or corrective action programs take the form of educational programs that provide knowledge and information transfer. A real lack of knowledge on the part of the health professional, however, is a relatively rare cause of poor quality patient care. If the review system manager

and all participants in the care system, including the patients, take a broader view of potential changes that need to be made to improve the quality of health care and health, more effective assurance will result. Concrete examples of alternatives that might prove effective are in order.

There was appropriate use of antibiotics in only 30% of instances in one institution. To identify further the basis for this practice deficiency, a knowledge and problem-solving examination was taken by the medical staff. The average score achieved on the test was 70%, a knowledge and problem-solving level twice the practice level. A series of learning experiences were then established to provide information on the appropriate use of antibiotics, to develop problem-solving skills, and to foster attitudinal change about antibiotic usage. The experience allowed physicians to value withholding the use of antibiotics more highly until definite data were obtained to substantiate that such therapy was indicated.

Following the learning program the use of antibiotics improved to a 60% level of appropriate usage. During the course of the educational program it became apparent that most physicians knew very well, for example, that a throat culture should be obtained prior to prescribing antibiotic treatment for pharyngitis. Yet this did not occur due to a physical lack of culture media and incubators in physicians' offices. An organizational change corrected this deficit. The hospital laboratory began a service of collecting throat cultures and other material from physicians' offices for daily analysis. While this study did reveal some problem-solving deficits on the part of care providers, it also identified the need for attitudinal and organizational changes to effect substantive changes in care practices.

As stated previously, a new resource other than education in the traditional sense may be needed to correct a deficiency.

The surgical department of another hospital agreed that most patients having an elective cholecystectomy should have an operative cholangiogram. A review of actual practice revealed that this procedure often was not performed because at the usual time of surgery the necessary x-ray equipment for this procedure was in use elsewhere. Resolution of this problem occurred with purchase of additional x-ray equipment. Lab data on urine cultures showed that many apparent cases of bacteriuria went untreated. The basis for this inappropriate response was found to be lack of trust in the laboratory values of the cultures because physicians knew that urine samples were delayed in reaching the laboratory. Resolution of the problem was achieved when physicians were assured that samples for culture were refrigerated promptly to offset any delay in pick-up by the laboratory staff.

Improvement in the number of pelvic and pap examinations done on hospitalized patients required differing change programs in another hospital. Some physicians placed little value on periodic pelvic and pap exams for cervical and uterine malignancy, while still others valued the examinations but did not know how to perform them. Two change programs were involved in reaching the two different populations of physicians. Those wishing to learn the technique were given the opportunity to practice pelvic and pap examinations under direction until they gave evidence of having acquired the necessary skill. Those physicians who neither knew how to perform this procedure, nor cared to learn, were found willing to allow this procedure to be performed by allied health professionals or other physicians if their patients were to be referred back to them.

In summary, the change program necessary to achieve improved patient and health care may be a standard educational program. Occasionally such a program will be required for the acquisition of a new skill, especially a cognitive skill such as problem solving or a manipulative skill such as the performance of new technical procedure. Sometimes an attitudinal

change is needed instead, and this can be the most difficult change to effect. The planning, implementing, and managing of a change program in step XI is sometimes difficult and most often is the step at which the quality assurance system breaks down for a number of reasons. Sometimes the problem is incorrectly identified, and the program to correct it is therefore also inappropriate. But more often it is the lack of personnel knowledgeable in managing change. Frequently the problem is incorrectly assumed to be lack of knowledge on the part of some health professionals, with the recommended solution being a program for information transfer. It is relatively easy to assess a lack of knowledge by testing health professionals to determine if they have the necessary information. We have considerable data to support the thesis that most health professionals really do have the necessary knowledge most of the time, meaning that the changes needed to improve health care or health are other than acquiring new knowledge, such as need for organizational or attitudinal change or acquisition of a new skill.

Step XII requires collection of data after the implementation of the appropriate change program. Also it requires a return to the patient care cycle and a recycle beginning with step VIII.

The data of the recycling process after the change program should indicate congruency of actual practice with criterion practice. If so, the change program has been successful and quality patient care has been assured. If incongruency still remains between actual practice and outcome, change program objectives should be reviewed and redefined and another change program implemented.

Step XI links or recycles the system to the patient, as diagrammed in Fig. 17-9. The system begins and ends with the patients. If the patient and the team achieve the health care objectives agreed to in the initial contract, the quality of health care has been assured. If the health care objectives contracted for have not been achieved, the quality assurance system provides the opportunity to recycle through a review of the objectives, the patient's behavior, and the knowledge, skills, and attitudes of the health professional who is attempting to influence patient behavior to achieve quality health care. If deficits are found in any of these system components, appropriate change programs can be planned, implemented, and evaluated.

THE PATIENT AND THE SYSTEM

To show viability, validity, and continuity in our system, let us take a patient through a health care delivery episode that is monitored by a quality assurance system. The patient, a 25-year-old black female, is a Ph.D. candidate in a major private university. She enters the care system for the purpose of a routine checkup she has not had for some years. The first step, as you recall, is to negotiate a contract with the patient in which she agrees to assume the ultimate responsibility for her health and health care. Health professionals in the system contract with the patient to provide whatever support is necessary and possible to help achieve an ideal level of health.

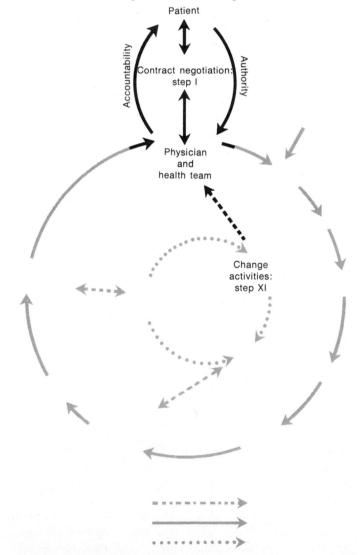

Fig. 17-9. Recycling of system to patient (step XI to step I).

The patient considers herself basically healthy, but a number of significant problems and risks are identified in step II of the system where a standard age-, sex-, and race-oriented data base is acquired. The patient is found to be at increased risk for most of the probable causes of death in the next 10 years in her age, sex, and race group. The cause of death with the highest probability for her is homicide. Frequently the patient dates white males. She lives in an apartment in a predominantly black neighborhood. She carries a handgun at all times and keeps it on her bedside stand. She has never fired it; thus she is unskilled in its use. The patient is at increased risk not only from homicide but also from an accidental death from her own firearm, which she has never learned to use. The patient began having sexual intercourse at age 13 and has had multiple sexual partners, most of whom were uncircumcised. She has never had a pelvic or pap examination and is at a significantly increased risk for cancer of the cervix. The patient's sister has cancer of the breast, and two of her aunts died from cancer of the breast. The patient has never had a breast examination, nor does she examine her breasts regularly. Therefore she is at a significant increased risk for cancer of the breast. This patient should have mammogram or xerogram examinations periodically. Because she has increased her alcoholic intake considerably in the past few months, she is at increased risk for alcoholism and cirrhosis. Although the patient wears seatbelts regularly when on long trips, most of her driving is in the city, where she never wears seatbelts. Thus she is significantly at increased risk for death or injury from auto accident. The patient's mother had hypertension through most of her adult life and suffered a cerebral vascular accident 2 years ago at age 45. The patient's blood pressure is 145/100; thus she is at a significantly increased risk from hypertension. Although this patient considers herself perfectly healthy, we have established the fact that she is at a significantly increased risk from death and disability on the basis of her lifestyle, family history, personal and social history, and physical findings for a number of problems. Although she has multiple potential health problems, for illustration purposes we will monitor the patient through the care delivery and quality assurance system for hypertension only. The sequence for this particular problem follows.

The patient has agreed to assume the ultimate responsibility of her own health and health care with the contract negotiated in step I. A team of health professionals have contracted with her and have agreed to help her identify actual and potential problems in relation to her health and health care and to assist her to maintain her health, to prevent illness, and to decrease the significant risks to her health. Step II of the system was the acquisition of a complete standardized data base with the identification of problems and potential problems.

Hypertension is a common health problem in most ambulatory settings. It has been decided in step III of the quality assurance system that all patients with two or more blood pressure readings above 140/90 will be monitored. Since the patient entered the system in step III on the basis of elevated blood pressure, with all subsequent ambulatory visits she deserved a continued review of her hypertensive problem.

In step IV (priority setting) it was clearly determined that hypertension was a priority concern in this patient. Hypertension, a frequently seen condition, is usually diagnosed and treated easily. Yet data indicate that of all who have significant hypertension probably only one-half are diagnosed, and of those who are diagnosed probably only one-half are treated. Of those who are treated approximately one-half are treated adequately. Also, it is known that there is significantly increased risk from death and disability for those with untreated hypertension. Thus there is a great amount of unnecessary disability and potential disability associated with this disease that can be prevented through adequate therapy. Unfortunately it is also known that very little of this disability is being prevented. Thus hypertension constitutes a priority health problem because of the great amount of preventable disability that is not being prevented and because it offers opportunity for significant improvement in care and in patient outcome. Having identified hypertension as a priority concern (step IV), a series of process criteria were developed for the diagnosis and management of this condition (step V). Any patient with a blood pressure exceeding 140/95 on two different visits was to be diagnosed as having hypertension and was to receive some form of therapy. Therapies range from simple weight reduction and salt restriction to the use of an effective diuretic or specific anti-hypertensive drug.

The outcome criteria agreed on stated that by the third visit a diagnosis of hypertension should have been established, the patient's blood pressure should be controlled to a level below 140/90, and that it should remain below that level for all subsequent visits. A threshold for action (step VI) indicates the point at which a change or educational program would be developed (which for this care setting was defined at a level of more than 25% of our patients failing to meet these criteria).

Step VII was the process that led to a consensus with respect to criteria for the diagnosis, management, and prevention of hypertension by the health professional team. In step VIII data concerning diagnosis and management of hypertension in actual practice were collected. In step IX data were evaluated in relation to the criteria for ideal hypertensive management. This revealed that of all patients who had an elevation of blood pressure and were diagnosed as hypertensive, less than one-half of those in the care system were actually being maintained at the acceptable level of blood pressure by the third visit after diagnosis.

The realization of this deficit was a mandate for a change program. In step X the objectives for the change program (maintenance of a level of blood pressure below 140/90) were made clear, but it was necessary to look more deeply as to why this level of patient care outcome had not been achieved. Subsequent study indicated that many patients were not taking their prescribed antihypertensive medications regularly. It became increasingly evident as time went on that there were a series of challenging problems and not just one. For instance, almost all patients were asymptomatic for their hypertension. After diagnosis was established it was difficult to motivate patients to take medication for a condition that did not cause symptoms. Often the therapy produced bothersome side effects, a condition quite different from when they had first come, feeling perfectly well. Now the therapy was producing some discomfort not previously experienced. It became clearly necessary to develop a change or education program (step XI) for patients so that they could come to understand and subsequently value the maintenance of a normal blood pressure for its long-term effect in reducing disability and potential death from the complications of hypertension. It is difficult for most patients to understand the advantage in terms of avoiding remote disability or death in the face of real discomfort from drug therapy, especially when they felt perfectly normal without therapy (even though they had significantly elevated blood pressure). Evaluating the effect of the change program (step XII) and returning to the patient care cycle (step VIII) revealed that an increasing number of patients with normalized blood pressure were found, which is indicative of the success achieved in this program. For those patients who will work toward meeting the care contract, one can assure the quality of health care. Where preagreed goals are not met the quality assurance system provides a mechanism for identifying deficits in the quality of patient care delivered and also provides the opportunity to correct the deficits. After the change (educational) program has been implemented, continued evaluation will be necessary to determine if in fact the improved patient care or health outcome has been maintained.

ASSESSMENT OF THE SYSTEM

The greatest strength of the quality assurance system is defined by its comprehensiveness and completeness as a system for assuring the quality of health care, which goes beyond a system only to assess the quality of health care. The quality assurance system provides not only the methodology for assessing the quality of health care delivered but also the mechanism for achieving those changes necessary to improve and assure an optimum quality of health care. The bottom line of the system is the achievement of those changes where necessary to improve health care and its anticipated outcome—health. Through the implementation of the system, quality health care should be assured or deficits in quality should be successively identified until they are relieved by successive change or education programs.

A significant strength of the system described is its successful implementation in numerous and varying hospitals from academic medical centers, large and medium-size inner city hospitals with and without medical school affiliation, specialty hospitals, and small semirural hospitals. Thus the system has been replicated in varying types of hospital settings.

The system itself has been researched, and its effects in achieving change to improve care have been previously reported. Compared with other audit or peer review systems the quality assurance system is described as a system not only for assessing the quality of patient care but one that also provides the opportunity for actually improving care where improvement is necessary.

The major limitations of the system include the following:

1. It is basically a retrospective rather than a concurrent system. However, as institutions acquire their own computer and computer programs, it would be feasible to expand the system to include concurrent or on-line assessment.
2. The system reviews samples of care in particular areas of suspected problems or in selected areas where there is the probability of a great amount of preventable disability not being prevented rather than in all areas (that is, whether problems are anticipated or not).
3. The system looks for patterns of care rather than at discrete health practitioners or discrete care discrepancies.
4. Although the system is retrospectively based, it is future oriented in terms of change programs.
5. It is a nonpunitive, nonlegalistic system.

Although not inherent limitations of the system itself, the two greatest problem areas experienced to date have been in the development of criteria and the planning, implementation, management, and evaluation of the necessary change programs. Because these steps require specific skills that are not traditional to health care delivery (including social engineering skills), workshops have been developed to provide for the different levels of skill needed for the change steps described. Thus if difficulties are encountered in steps V and VI where optimal and minimal criteria are developed, or in step XI where change activities are planned, implemented, managed, and evaluated, an opportunity is provided to acquire the training to perform these steps in the quality assurance system.

Another step in the system currently under development is step II where a complete and accurate data base is compiled to identify all of the patient's problems and potential problems. Every patient admitted electively to the hospital should have such a data base collected, or better still, should arrive with one. Though it is difficult to have most hospital staffs agree on a complete and accurate age-, sex-, and race-standardized data base, it is totally inefficient for the necessary data base to be recollected by a resident or other health professional who may never have seen the patient before, and to do so again and again on admission after admission to the institution. Although the use of the problem-oriented medical record format is increasing, the pace is slower than logic and the need of quality assurance systems would dictate. While it would be ideal to examine every patient and every patient problem and to evaluate each patient and each professional decision in relation to that problem, we must learn to priorize our evaluations such that we are working with those problem areas with the greatest potential payoff; that is, those with the greatest risk of preventable patient health disability not currently being prevented due to lack of some health professional or patient action.

Finally, the greatest present weakness of the system (but one that is also its greatest potential strength) is the requirement that the patient assume ultimate responsibility for his own health care and health. Without the patient assuming such responsibility this system cannot assure the quality of patient care. With the assumption of responsibility on the part of the patient, however, a great step forward is taken toward the assurance of quality health care and its anticipated outcome—health. Of all the operational and technical problems associated with the quality assurance system, this shift of responsibility for health care to the patient may provide the greatest challenge. Health professionals often too readily assume this responsibility for the patient even though they know it cannot achieve the desired result in the long run.

CONTINUING EVALUATION OF THE SYSTEM

The quality assurance system described here has been undergoing constant study and change since its inception. Continued evaluation and change are planned in-

definitely as new needs arise and new methods are developed to meet those needs. Since the system provides its own feedback loop for constant change, there is reason to believe that constant renewal will be a continuing system characteristic.

The quality assurance system is structured to provide constant and continuing planned change where necessary to improve health care and its anticipated outcome—health. Because the system focuses on health as an outcome, any deviation from this result by a patient or by a community triggers the system's guidance mechanism to put the process of delivering health care back on course—a course that is calculated to yield the necessary change in order to achieve the agreed-on health outcome.

Ten years have passed since this system was implemented as the Bi-Cycle concept at Chestnut Hill Hospital, a 200-bed community hospital in Philadelphia.[5] Replication of the system in at least ten different hospitals occurred since that time as the Mandate Project.[2] Systems study and modification was intense during this project, and the report of the success of systems implementation in those hospitals as a significant improvement in patient care has been published in 1976. The report also outlines the systems modification and renewal characteristics. In addition, the system has been replicated throughout the state of California by the California Medical Association and California Hospital Association in a program to train a statewide faculty in the use of the system. As the system has been implemented in many hospitals in California, further modification has occurred. It now serves as the continuing medical education program of the practicing physician and other health professionals. Four years ago the system was modified to form the basis of an experimental 1½-year program in ambulatory care in the undergraduate curriculum, Abraham Lincoln School of Medicine, the University of Illinois College of Medicine. In this instance it was the basis for the concurrent development of a health care delivery system and a health professional education system. These historical notes highlight the adaptability of such a system to local needs and conditions.

To meet a growing national need among hospitals and their health professional staffs for assistance in acquiring the skills necessary to implement a quality assurance system, a training program was co-sponsored by the American Hospital Association and the Association for Hospital Medical Education. The primary objective of the program was to provide a national faculty skilled in helping hospitals acquire the skills necessary for quality assurance system implementation and faculty development mentioned previously. During 1975, 30 teacher trainers were trained as a national resource for assistance in system implementation.

It has been recognized that implementation of the system in a hospital requires considerable participation at the level of the board of trustees. To this end a mandate, maintain, and monitor subsystem has been developed to assist trustees in their role in the successful implementation of the system.[3]

Although participation by state hospital associations in endorsing the program has been delayed, plans for its extension have been endorsed by the AMA to state medical associations. It is hoped that state medical associations will follow the California experience and will require hospitals applying for accreditation of their continuing medical education activities from the state medical association to have an effective quality assurance program in operation.

A recent survey of 5656 member hospitals by the American Hospital Association revealed that of 4627 hospitals reporting, 60% of hospitals need assistance in developing criteria for patient care (steps V and VI of the quality assurance system). Forty-six percent of the hospitals indicated that they need assistance in the design of change or education programs to overcome quantified deficits in patient care.

Two portions of the system model are now receiving particular developmental attention. Step I, the initial patient-health professional contract, stresses further the concomitant need for a responsibility shift such that the patient assumes ultimate responsibility for his own health.

Step II, the definition of a basic minimum acceptable age-, sex-, and race-oriented patient data base for each health delivery system is of critical importance. Without such a baseline each health professional is in a different game within his own institution. With such a minimal standardized data base one can identify most of the patient's problems, and from this the system can be placed into action.

OUR NEXT SYSTEM

The quality assurance system is currently being modified to serve the needs of a comprehensive family practice health care delivery and health professional education system. The primary care delivery system is centered in the Family Practice Center in South Holland, Illinois, a southern suburb of Chicago; the secondary delivery system is centered at South Chicago Community Hospital, a 400-bed community hospital in South Chicago; and the tertiary delivery system is centered at the University of Chicago hospitals and clinics. Our quality assurance system will assure both the quality of health care delivered by the entire care system and the quality of health professional education at all three levels and in all disciplines. The system will involve all strata of health professionals and the patients and the communities served by these institutions.

Four parts of the system will receive particular attention:

1. The health care contract between the health professionals and patients to assure assumption by the patients and communities of the primary and ultimate responsibility for their own health care and health.

2. A standardized data base collected on each patient to assure that all of the patient's problems, potential problems, or risks have been identified.
3. The involvement of all participants in the system—community, patients, faculty, and students—in setting the criteria for health care and for the system's health care goals.
4. The change programs necessary to achieve quality health care to be developed by all those whose behavior might require change to assure quality health care.

The quality assurance system, like the health care delivery system, will begin and end with the patient, just as the health professional education system will begin and end with the learner. This provides the feedback necessary for constant change and keeps the entire system relevant to both patient and learner needs.

The system will assure the maintenance of quality health care by achieving change wherever it is necessary to improve health care. The ultimate system outcome will be the highest level of achievable patient and community health.

REFERENCES

1. Brown, C. R., Jr., and Fleisher, D. S.: The bicycle concept—relating continuing education directly to care, N. Engl. J. Med. **284**(suppl.):88-97, 1971.
2. Fleisher, D. S., Brown, C. R., Jr., Zeleznik, C., Escovitz, G. H., and Omdal, C.: The mandate project: institutionalizing a system of patient care quality assurance, Pediatrics **57**(5):775-782, 1976.
3. Makowski, R. J.: Mandate, maintain, monitor: a model for hospital governance, Trustee, January 1976, p. 34.
4. Williamson, J. W., Alexander, M., and Miller, G. E.: Priorities in patient care research and continuing medical education, J.A.M.A. **204**:303-308, 1968.
5. Brown, C. R., Jr., and Uhl, H. S. M.: Mandatory continuing medical education: sense or nonsense? J.A.M.A. **213**:1660-1668, 1970.

PART THREE

PRINCIPLES

In one way or another this entire book concerns itself with the process of evaluation, and so it would be a sorry oversight indeed if no thought were given to how one might go about evaluating its content. What is needed is benchmarks the reader can use to gauge the relevancy of what he has read or how he can apply it to the development, operation, and evaluation of peer review systems.

The reader will note that differing experiences and orientations of the contributing authors bring some differences in emphasis or focus to certain aspects of peer review, particularly those that are still in rudimentary stages of development or those that belong to the controversial arena. This is how it should be. But we intended that there be a coherency to this book, which calls for more than just a series of disconnected reports. Accordingly this particular chapter has been created to bring within a single conceptual framework those aspects of peer review in which there is a reasonable measure of agreement. The result is a set of principles that have been articulated for the expressed purpose of initiating a frank and open discussion on the issues of the most fundamental importance to peer review. We seek to initiate a dialogue that addresses the unfinished business before the developers and operators of peer review systems as together we face an uncertain future.

Implicit in any process of evaluation is the preexistence of values on which it must be based. While many members of the medical profession place a high value on excellence in medical care, its achievement likely will be less than optimal unless the medical professional is willing to review the quality of the medical work on a regular basis. But society also places value on the availability, affordability, and the accountability of medical services. The problem is that social priorities seem to be shifting. The impact that health and medical technology has on any future scenario is also an important consideration. Technology as it has been utilized in this text does not imply just the use of hardware, like radiology and computer equipment. It includes any methods and techniques that have potential for assisting men in their work. One problem is that the cost of some technologies are far greater than the public good manifested by those technologies. A scenario on the future of medical care evaluation should therefore include the fact that there will be a tension between high-cost, technologically profound medical practice that benefits a few members of society and medical practice that may not be as technologically profound but which will serve many members of society. In this respect primary health care affordability, accessibility, availability, and accountability will be extremely important for the next few years.

What seems to be clear is that economic and social constraints have begun to place a limit on almost all aspects of medical and health care delivery. The cost burden, maldistribution, and the uneven application of quality standards in health and medical activities apparently have become intolerable to Americans. Obviously peer review would serve the best interests of medicine and society if it achieved something effective to rectify all three. But if it should be found that the peer review effort has failed to improve the health level of the citizenry, then it can be safely concluded that either the evaluation methods have failed to provide useful feedback or there was a failure to translate that feedback into a more responsive and responsible care delivery system.

In any case health professionals, government, and society share responsibility for either the success or failure of a system of public accountability that utilizes peer review as its basic mechanism. That is basically the effect Congress achieved by enacting the PSRO legislation. Cost containment mandated by law along with concern for quality improvement serves as a motivational force behind medical peer review. No longer is the concern for either of these limited to just a few pioneers in the field.

Two major operational tasks for peer review therefore emerge. One position holds that peer review should be the operational mechanism for deciding how many dollars should be allocated to what medical end (services or programs) while protecting the patient from harm. Those who concur with this position have come to view the cost containment aspect of peer review as representative of its prime purpose. Soundness of the values on which the allocation of health dollars is based becomes a critical issue for any peer review system designed to serve this end.

Another operational task for peer review is based on devising a mechanism that assures everything is accomplished that medically should be accomplished for the patient while protecting society from runaway costs. The soundness of resource allocation (distributive justice) becomes the critical issue raised by this approach. These two positions can be characterized by the following contrasting statements: cost containment at whatever its expense to quality versus quality care at whatever its expense to society. While this is patently an oversimplification, derivatives of these positions do represent convictions honestly held by serious men and women in many areas of society. It may seem inevitable then that a confrontation must ensue between proponents of the ascendency of societal responsibilities and proponents of the right of individuals to the receipt of high-quality health care. Confrontation and conflict need not necessarily be the way things must go, since there is considerable common ground. Both positions recognize obligations to individuals as well as to society, both recognize the need to improve quality and contain cost, and both display concern about how the care of individuals can be integrated with the care of the populace to assure the best use of society's resources. Finally, both would plead a case for the basic wisdom of investing wisely in health care.

The magnitude of these common interests is large enough to suggest there is room to form an equal partnership between medicine, government, and the public at large that can work toward mutually held goals without the necessity to compromise fundamental principles. The workability of such a partnership can be helped along considerably by a willingness on the part of the public to alter harmful lifestyles, so that society carries a lesser burden of self-inflicted health problems that drain medical resources and put pressure on costs. Physicians can display a greater willingness to accept a participatory doctor-patient relationship in which the patient is prepared to take on a greater share of responsibility and a more active role in his own care through self-care and self-help strategies. The government can help by aggressively weeding out the proliferation of unneeded and stifling regulations and reporting requirements.

The informational feedback loop from peer review has a substantial role to play in all of this by opening the communications, which can strengthen these new relationships between the patient, the health professional, and the government. Feedback provided by peer review can help first by identifying the problems that patients really want to talk about and see resolved. Documenting where concepts, methods, and techniques of care consistently work well can also be helpful, since documentation of unneeded medical activities can focus on appropriate and inappropriate functions. Finally, the feedback from peer review can sharpen the definition of professional values within the context of social values.[1]

Cooperation necessary to resolve many of the conflicts that must be faced in medical care today can only begin when the medical profession, the government, and the public enter into a forthright dialogue about the issues involved. It is to serve this end that we have approached the discussion that follows.

Paul Y. Ertel
M. Gene Aldridge

REFERENCE

1. Hiatt, H. H.: Protecting the medical commons: who is responsible? N. Engl. J. Med. **293**:241-245, 1975.

18

Principles of peer review

PAUL Y. ERTEL
M. GENE ALDRIDGE

To be presented here is a statement of principles we felt were suggested by the preceding discussions. It has been circulated in draft among all the authors with the invitation for them to respond with comments and suggestions. We gratefully acknowledge extremely helpful input from a number of the contributors. However, it was not intended that this chapter be presented as a consensus document, since it would be logistically difficult. It was therefore opted to extend the opportunity for comment to all authors, and this has been exercised by several. The final draft of the principles then is our expression alone.

Rather than attempt to draw conclusions from all that has gone before, this discussion attempts to make explicit some of the values and concepts that have heretofore remained implicit and therefore largely undiscussed in the peer review dialogue. It is above everything else intended to promote dialogue and not to end it.

First principle: a data-based information feedback mechanism is an essential component in any health care system

Peer review is properly considered the mechanism whereby medicine obtains the data and information feedback necessary to maintain high standards of practice, advance scientific knowledge, identify broader societal obligations, and give recognition to the moral obligations involved in the care of people.

Valid information generated by peer review is essential not only for advancing the concepts and techniques of care practices that have been deemed most efficacious, but also for discovering the means for changing the overall delivery mechanism in a way that enhances the provision of the quality health care services for all segments of society. Both components are necessary to optimize the practice of medicine, and it is therefore an inherent obligation of professionals to establish and use whatever feedback mechanism can best achieve this end.

While it is obvious that health professionals are the generators of care-related records, and their peers are the generators of peer review data, there is no good reason why the information in a peer review system must flow in only one direction (for example, from medicine to the government) any more than the health profession should constitute the only legitimate audience to receive and use information generated by peer review activities. It is rational that medicine learn from a review of its own performance how to deliver better care and to share that information so the profession can be accountable to the public. It is also rational for medicine to utilize the peer review mechanism to learn about the health expectations and organizational behaviors associated with the public sector. In this way medicine can gain a more balanced understanding of how best to serve the health needs of the whole population. Information and feedback should be directed through peer review systems back to the public, the health professionals, and the government health regulators.

Second principle: peer review originates with a commitment to peer-based values

Implicit in this principle is the need to gain agreement on fundamental terminology. Peer values refer to those consensually validated professional maxims that define the ethical basis for the delivery of health care. This constitutes the basis for judging whether care is good or bad from a medical standpoint.

Three inferences can be derived from this principle:

1. Peer values are equivalent to professional directives.
2. A peer group constitutes a legitimate source to originate the directives from which care standards and criteria may be derived.
3. Professional standards and criteria must contain both normative and empirical values[1] because absolute standards of care exist only in the abstract and must be tempered by facts that reflect reality in the practice of medicine.

Values and ethical propositions in the context of peer review are the equivalent of a commitment to maintain the acceptable standards of professional conduct recognized by and acceptable to one's peers. Peer-derived values that are given expression in health care standards or criteria probably have the greatest potential for a direct and forceful impact on medical practices. Therefore a continued insistence by the PSRO program on a local origin of these standards[2,3] is not only de-

sirable but crucial to the professional commitment to abide by them.

What must be faced in peer review generally is the matter of *professional commitment to professional values*. As a professional, one is obligated to be suspicious of any new virtue that conveniently separates commitment from either responsibility or from involvement in the peer review process. The disassociation of medical professionals from any of these may spell trouble of one kind or another for the profession itself. Commitment without involvement means that whatever their intentions, if professionals do not actively participate in the mechanism of public accountability, they are in effect relinquishing the control of medicine to others. Involvement in peer review, without exercising professional responsibility, can only amount to a meaningless exercise. Likewise responsibility without commitment merely results in giving lip service to peer review.

Continued professional independence must be earned. It demands no less of professionals than their personal commitment, their involvement, and the shouldering of full professional responsibility for conducting effective peer review. Stated more simply, it is not enough for a peer review system to *be* the conscience of a profession; it must also *have* the conscience of the profession to be effective.

Third principle: peer consensus defines peer standards

Historically favored and successful value systems have been those with both clearly known and accepted authorships. This observation applies to the development of peer standards, since health care criteria, to be effective, must be internalized (believed in) by those who deliver health care. If the criteria are to be translated into actual operationalized behaviors (effective clinical behaviors), individuals must at all times be involved in the process. Lip service to someone else's criteria accomplishes nothing. The standards (or the criteria) that guide peer review must be based on collective agreements that constitute acceptable medical practices. Those health professionals who are being evaluated should be active participants in the collective agreement. Therefore local peer consensus is seen as a critical variable if peer review is to endure as a valid and reliable professional activity. The development of standards through consensus by colleagues is a problem-solving process which increases the probability that the standards of care will become useful to the review process. However, consensus alone cannot confer on all medical criteria such objectivity that any deviation from them would automatically connote inappropriate medical care.

Likewise local criteria isolated from comparative national objectives and data cannot be considered valid or reliable. Standards for quality must be designed to include a matrix of local and national criteria if peer review systems are to become operationally effective. Local in this sense refers to those value assumptions about health that each community or population has generated through its standards.

Fourth principle: collective peer standards are points of reference for individual peer judgments

The standards guiding peer review must be sufficiently general in language to serve as reference points that are applicable to a wide range of clinical conditions, yet also definitive enough to reflect the specifics of new knowledge and changes in medical technology that occur over time. This argues for the development of standards readily capable of adaptation and change. Similarly all standards must reflect a balance between what is ideal care and what is practical care. The necessity to account for both argues for a dual origin of whatever standards have been selected to guide the review process. A fixed set of standards based solely on either professional judgment or uncritical descriptions of the status quo would there-

fore not be appropriate. Rather, normative standards based on professional opinion should be viewed as a series of approximations that can and should be tested against the realities of health care practices and finally against the health status outcomes of patients.

Empiric performance data derived from accumulated experiences (norms) serve as the primary source for describing what are the usual care practices in the average case. But the opinion of qualified professionals is required to convert such performance data into descriptions of what constitutes desirable medical practices that should apply in the typical case.

Once developed, care must be taken so that all such standards be properly applied. This must be understood to mean that explicit criteria and standards pertain primarily to a generic model of medical care and not necessarily to the care of specific individuals. By contrast, implicit peer judgments, though generally guided by explicit criteria, must focus on the unique personal attributes and clinical circumstances in the individual case and are therefore inherently situational and contextual. It is obvious from these contrasts that standards* and judgments cannot serve peer review in the same way nor can they carry the same connotations. The problem is that they are often confused. Before exploring how this confusion surfaces in care evaluations and data interpretations, we shall first explore what it takes to establish the legitimacy of peer standards.

Each standard, regardless of its derivation, should be examined for both professional and public legitimacy by determining whether it satisfies all of the following conditions:

1. Is there a reasonable likelihood that conformity to a given standard will

---

*For the remainder of this discussion, professionally derived criteria will be considered to be interchangeable with explicit care standards.

enhance the health status of people (or at least not be harmful to health)?

2. Is the standard critical to the delivery of appropriate medical care or the appropriate use of resources?
3. Is there sufficient merit in monitoring a given standard? Is the effort expended economically and socially rewarding for all concerned?
4. Does the standard assess validly and reliably what it purports to assess?
5. Does the standard reflect predictable clinical conditions for which norms are definable and objective data are obtainable?

In essence, standards generated by peer review systems have finite limitations. A clinical practice found in the screening process (surveillance) to deviate from the generic standard only means that a particular practice or event differed from the model and should be investigated by a peer. It carries no legitimate implications of wrongdoing in the sense of "where there's smoke, there's fire." Indeed the very act of not following a practice that is considered appropriate to the management of most cases may have been exactly the right thing to do in the given case and could even be lifesaving. Said another way, the exceptions to the clinical model screen must be investigated carefully.

Other limitations arise when utilization review standards are applied in isolation from quality standards and vice versa. For example, conformity to the standards of resource utilization may be achieved at the expense of lowering the quality of care, which then remains unassessed and therefore undetected. The converse is equally valid, that improvements in the quality of care could be at costs that are totally unacceptable in either human or economic terms, as measured by standards limited to quality assessment.

A set of comprehensive standards would not only include a matrix of all care variables that are important to the quality and utilization aspects of clinical management, but would also evaluate the accuracy and reliability of the review system itself. In short, it would address all seven functions of peer review cited in Chapter 4. Until standards of this magnitude become available, health professionals and all others should avoid making the mistake of interpreting conformity to peer review standards in a way that produces unwarranted global conclusions about medical care delivery. Simplified assessments that employ standards of limited scope are simply not designed to account for complex care processes, patient-related behaviors, economic realities associated with medical care practices, or artifacts introduced by the review system itself. Care must be taken to define the limitations of interpretability and to keep it within the context of the limitations of the standards that are utilized.

Fifth principle: public accountability as an extension of professional responsibility is compatible with the goals of peer review

Medical professionalism is associated with a social status derived from academic achievement, knowledge, and skill. As long ago as 1888 the Supreme Court held that special skill and knowledge are necessary to the practice of medicine and that the licensure requirement was reasonably related to the legitimate goal for ensuring high competence among physicians.[4] This ruling does not set the *professional above contract with patients nor above consequences for professional acts.* The medical profession has no special immunity and no inalienable rights beyond those of citizenship, constitution, and common law. Just as importantly, though, as a professional entity medicine can and does exercise the constitutional liberty of corporate contract with patients (usually implicit) and with payors and government (usually explicit).

To better appreciate the relative importance of public accountability, it is useful to view it in the larger context of professional accountability of which it is but one component. To be widely applicable to operational peer review systems, professional accountability must be defined in easily understood terms that describe to whom and for what the medical profession is to be held accountable. That is the manner in which we will define our candidate list:

1. Accountability to patients for fulfilling personal obligations to meet their care needs
2. Accountability to the profession for fulfilling creative responsibilities to further advance the art and science of medicine
3. Accountability to peers for fulfilling the obligations of professional ethics
4. Accountability to oneself for maintaining a professional practice that is based on integrity and is personally gratifying
5. Accountability to the next generation for preserving the contemporary share of the professional legacy
6. Accountability to society for fulfilling service contracts
7. Accountability to society for showing that what the medical profession does makes a difference (public accountability for the care system)
8. Accountability to society for assuring that professional accountability actually works (public accountability for the review system)

In accepting both the privilege and the power of self-regulation, these last two responsibilities should weigh heavily. If peer review is to be the mechanism whereby the medical professionals exercise their self-regulatory duties and are accountable to the public, then they must also be accountable for the way in which they conduct peer review.

Viewed then from its broadest perspective, public accountability is seen as an obligation of professional self-regulation that is socially conferred, judicially recognized, and a contingent privilege that operates within the context of a contract. The contracting parties include the professional, the patient, and third parties (including the government). There is nothing particularly unusual (or threatening) when in the normal conduct of human enterprises, a request is made among the contracting parties for proof of compliance with reasonable terms of a reasonable contract. It is not unreasonable therefore to hold professionals accountable for providing evidence to external parties that they have performed their professional services responsibly, just as it is not unreasonable of professionals to expect the other contracting parties to meet their contractual obligations as well.

In logically defining the value complex for which a professional is to be held externally accountable to the public as well as to the other contractual partners, one would do well to select an ethical concept that stands in the exact center of the professional accountability. One can only speculate about which central normative value others should choose; we choose professional responsibility as our candidate for the most important ethical directive for professional behavior in the field of medicine. It is therefore the public disclosure of peer judgments concerning the responsible discharge of professional duties and documentation of whatever actions are taken to rectify inappropriate care that signify fulfillment of the public accountability function through peer review.

Sixth principle: internal validity in a system of peer review is basic to public accountability

To be consistent with the fifth principle, any peer review system that reports its evaluations to the public must first demonstrate the reliability and efficiency of its review process and the accuracy of the data it gathers. It is not sufficient merely to report that medical care at a given medical or health institution was appropriate in quality, cost, or in the use of resources. Internal validity of the peer review system used within that hospital must be demonstrated, otherwise the results it reports to the public become meaningless. Internal validity is identified as the basic minimum verification without which the evaluation of medical care data is uninterpretable.[5]

It is hypothesized that the closer a peer review system conforms to what is considered to be relevant and valid review activities by those whose care is subject to review, the greater is the measure of its internal validity and the more accurate its output. This hypothesis would support the "delegated status" concept advanced in the PSRO legislation[6] wherein community-based institutions are accorded the opportunity to develop reliable and effective systems of peer review before external systems usurp that prerogative.[7] This makes sense, since the public and professionals alike stand to gain from an enhanced fairness and relevancy of performance data that is generated by an internally valid system.

It is understandable therefore that the local peer review mechanism has come to be viewed by many physicians (but by no means all) as a legitimate means of complying with the legal requirements of external accountability while also preserving a maximum of professional independence.

Consider the alternative for a moment. It must be conceded that a monolithic externally imposed system of public accountability would have all the advantages that accrue to centralized control over the review process and the maintenance of uniformity in data collection, processing, and reporting on a nationwide basis. While the advantages of data uniformity are considerable, they are also achievable with locally based review systems if the same minimum data base is required of them. The disadvantages pertain to the inflexibility and inertia of sheer size. It is axiomatic that little of real value can be gained by the reporting of even the most valid of performance assessments if the review system itself becomes so ponderous and inflexible that it obstructs the delivery of care, costs more money than it saves, or

becomes just one more remote bureaucratic burden that consumes resources that could otherwise be used for care programs. But in the absence of such experience with evaluative systems of this scope, it can only be speculated whether an externally controlled system of public accountability would be a blessing or a disaster in the health care field. The PSRO legislation seems to recognize this by first offering responsibility for the review mechanism to local practicing professionals[8] who will be sensitive to such matters, since their own care is held accountable to the same review mechanism and since they are also personally visible and accessible. However, both PSROs and local peer review systems will be required to demonstrate the internal validity of their own review methodology before data they produce can be used to evaluate the medical care system.

Seventh principle: the patient always comes first

Peer review cannot serve worthwhile ends if its basic assumptions are erroneous, misconstrued, or contrary to the interests of human liberties. Peer review should serve to enhance the delivery of needed and efficacious medical services to all citizens in a manner totally in keeping with the preservation of the human rights of all persons. To achieve this goal it has become apparent that the issues associated with excessive cost, maldistribution of services, and manpower must be solved. Peer review must play a role in solving these problems. But there is a limit to the role that peer review can play in dealing effectively with them.

The human rights of all individuals should be protected within the medical system. Peer review systems should not become a pawn for various interest groups who may want to focus on atrocities within the health and medical system while systematically denying needed health services to populations of patients. Physicians are sworn to provide needed services to patients. No system should attempt to set up normative values that may prevent them from providing the needed health and medical care services.

Peer values cannot emanate from performance data or computer printouts. The reason that a performance norm cannot achieve the status of a value is that data and information alone can accomplish absolutely nothing. This is so because data are but the tools of peer review and not its substance. Data must be analyzed and assessed. Personal judgments must be made to transfer the data into information. Actions must be initiated, changes must occur, and positive results must be confirmed before any statistical norm or computer output ever becomes relevant. Data is translated into information, information is translated into a value-based human judgment, and human judgments are transformed into actions. Data processing is "machine business," but the declaration of values or the rendering of a judgment is "people business."

While it is conceded that appropriate care can be agreed on whether the practice of medicine is found in Maine or Florida, New York or Los Angeles, the potential danger in applying generic national standards per se is that individual judgments on individual patients may be affected adversely. Thus two specific hypotheses must be carefully evaluated as this nation proceeds to establish national medical care standards:

1. The more uniform and generic (or generalized) that national medical care standards become, the less appropriate those standards may be to the clinical application of individual patients.
2. As standards become more specific to the needs of individual patients they tend to become more clinically relevant.

As this nation moves toward a reimbursement system for medical care that uses systematic peer review standards, norms, and criteria, it would seem extremely important to remember that inflexibility on standards of quality may be detrimental to the human rights of patients. Exceptions within the system must be allowed to occur. Provision is made within systematic peer review approaches to evaluate exceptions so that patients, professionals, and society can be protected.

By no means should there ever be a delay in care nor should the finances of a patient be jeopardized because of inappropriate or rigid review procedures. Standards for quality and cost must be open at all times to examination and revision. This is what is meant by an open and systematic peer review approach.

Any national, regional, or local peer review system that does not take into account these factors will jeopardize seriously the basic human rights of patients. A balance must therefore be struck between overly rigid and generic standards that do not allow exceptions for care and highly individualized, clinically relevant, standards that do not allow for an adequate accounting (in both quality and cost) by society.

The health professions and the government will ultimately be responsible for the values that emanate from any medical evaluation system. Those values should clearly protect the human rights of all patients and care providers within the system. This is the challenge before all groups concerned with a medical peer review system that evaluates medical care. The time for concern and action is now.

CONCLUSION

We close this book as we opened it, by calling attention to the critical turning point in which we find medicine today. In a relatively short time, medicine has traveled all the way from magic to theory to basic physiology to effective care technology. Now comes effective evaluation technology and society's demand for public accountability.

Medicine thus has both the mandate and

the tools it needs to control its own evolution for the first time in its long history.

How will medicine use its new technologies in molding care practices to serve professional obligations and social responsibilities? It is the first principle (peer review is an essential feedback mechanism) that holds the greatest promise to guide medicine in the direction it should take. It is through this principle that medicine, like science everywhere, can seek the truth. This it must always do to serve man well.

REFERENCES

1. Morgenau, H.: The scientific basis of value theory: new knowledge in human values, New York, 1959, Harper & Row, Publishers, pp. 38-51.

   Morgenau defines normative values as universal, profound, presumed to have persuasive force and regulative power (like a law of nature) that are above verification. He defines factual values as observable preferences, primary and particular, valid in a concrete sense at a given time, which are empirically verified.

2. Public law 92-603, sect. 1156(a), Title II, 1972 Amendments to the Social Security Act, p. 107.
3. Goran, M. J., Roberts, J. S., Kellogg, M. A., Fielding, J., and Jessee, W.: The PSRO hospital review system, Med. Care 13 (suppl.):1-32, 1975.
4. Dent v. West Virginia, 129 U.S. 114 (1888).
5. Campbell, D. T., and Stanley, J. C.: Experimental and quasi-experimental designs for research, Chicago, 1973, Rand McNally & Co., p. 5.
6. Public law 92-603, sect. 1155(e) (1), Title II, 1972 Amendments to the Social Security Act, p. 107.
7. The PSRO short-stay hospital relationship and delegation of review functions, transmittal no. 11, Rockville, Md., November 20, 1974, U.S. Dept. of Health, Education, and Welfare, Bureau of Quality Assurance.
8. Public law 92-603, sect. 1152(a) (1), Title II, 1972 Amendments to the Social Security Act, p. 102.

Discussion

While a number of contributing authors were able to concur with the principles as stated in an earlier draft, they also came up with some very helpful suggestions on how to state them better. We (the editors) were more than happy to incorporate such suggestions in subsequent drafts (which has been done). However, it rapidly became clear that the logistics of passing revised drafts among all of us for subsequent review were formidable and that some halting point was necessary if the book was ever to go to press. Thus it was decided that we would prepare a final draft and also provide the opportunity for any contributors to comment further who chose to do so. That is the purpose of this discussion section.

The first of these, Vergil N. Slee, raises an interesting procedural point. He writes:

I don't wish to be recorded as concurring with the principles as stated, nor do I want to have a minority report published in the dialogue section, nor do I wish to exclude an endorsement of the principles or any one of them.

He goes on to explain why he and his co-author, Marsha A. Bremer, do not wish to be put on the hook as either endorsing or rejecting the material:

First, there simply hasn't been enough time, and then there would have been the necessity for give and take between us to come to agreement on wording of the principles which would satisfy both of us. The calendar simply won't permit this. Nor do I have time to try to decide whether the principles are all the principles there are or overlap each other or are exactly right, that is, that there really are only 9 principles which govern medical peer review systems.

Dr. Slee conditioned his comments on the assumption that we were attempting to achieve a "consensus document" that would accurately reflect the combined thinking of all the contributors and one that each could endorse. Such was not the intent. The intent was to initiate a dialogue among the contributors that hopefully would examine some of the sensitive issues that surprisingly to us seem to have escaped much professional attention or public debate. We are indebted to Dr. Slee for defining what a consensus document is and also for supplying the excuse for our not attempting it.

One contributor team preferred to see the principles of peer review couched in a context of unresolved questions about public expectations, physicians' attitudes, the future of medicine in this country, and the role peer review could have in determining it. Their offering is introduced by the following disclaimer:

Although Robert H. Brook, M.D., Sc.D. and Allyson Davies Avery, M.P.H., cannot support in their entirety the principles of peer review as enunciated in the chapter, we can and do fully support the following principles, many of which are implicit in the foregoing discussion:

1. Peer review is an essential component of the practice of high quality medicine. Unless the physician reviews the quality of his work on a regular basis, it will suffer and deteriorate to less than optimal levels. This has been shown by the results of various research studies on quality of care of American medicine. Virtually all these studies demonstrated serious deficiencies in quality, regardless of the standards used or the settings in which the studies were done.

2. Measurement of quality of care by itself has little purpose unless the results of such studies are used to change behavior, when necessary, of physicians, other medical professionals, and/or the medical care system. Quality assurance activities will thus require the active participation of all health professionals, particularly administrators and managers, to work with physicians in attempting to improve the health care system.

3. The purpose of peer review activities is to improve health. The criteria and standards by which quality is judged, therefore, must be selected using the most valid techniques and must include only those which when complied with will maintain or improve health. If items are selected that do not meet these criteria, costs are likely to increase yet health is likely to remain the same.

4. In developing standards by which quality can be measured, both local and national objectives must be kept firmly in mind. Criteria must be flexible enough to allow physicians to take account of local circumstances in determining what is meant by high quality of care. These criteria may reflect variations in the socioeconomic characteristics of the population, in access and availability of medical care, and in local medical resources. Where possible, however, local standards must be consistent with the notion that we are all one people and that the quality of care given to residents of one area should equal that received by those of another, provided, of course, that the two populations place equal value on health.

5. If at all possible, the peer review process should be an educational one. Its result should be to improve the physician's practice, to make the hospital better, or to change the system in a manner which will improve quality. Punitive actions based on peer review data should be taken only in cases of extreme deficiency and only after the due process of law has been allowed to run its course.

6. In order to be successful, a peer review system requires the active participation of most of the physicians within the given medical care area. This would include developing criteria and standards by consensus, measuring quality against such standards, and identifying ways of improving the quality of care. Preparation for physician participation in such a system should be built into the curriculum of medical schools. If this were accomplished, the future generation of physicians might feel that their participation in peer review was essential to the practice of good medicine as was their conscientious workup of a new patient.

7. In establishing a peer review process, certain paradoxes will emerge. Many activities influence the health of patients, including medical care, personal behavior and life style, genetics, environment, and public health care. Peer review systems established by physicians may conclude that more medical care services are needed, and evidence from studies already completed suggests that this is so. In such a case, the following questions must be resolved: Is the cost of peer review activities justified? Does the public want the improvements in health that physicians seem able to deliver? Would money be better spent on public health services or on altering patients' health habits than on buying more medical care services?

The process of peer review will dramatize the conflict between physicians, who want more medical services for individual patients, and society, which may place a higher value on broader distribution of medical care or on commodities other than medical care entirely. This conflict is likely to be beneficial because it will produce a dialogue on the worth of health in which the American public can participate.

8. The practice of medicine changes as new discoveries are made in both biomedical and art-of-care areas. Systems of peer review must adapt to these changes by updating criteria and standards at frequent intervals to reflect this new knowledge.

9. There is a justifiable concern on the part of those who have studied systems of professional self-regulation that such systems may be used by the profession to serve its own ends. To prevent such an occurrence, it would appear desirable to include the public in the operations of a peer review system. Although it may not understand the technical intricacies of care, the public will at least be able to understand how the peer review system functions and whether deficiencies in care were actually being corrected. Development of such a system will require the emergence of a new trust between the public and physicians that will permit the exchange of information about professional performance and public values. Furthermore, the individual physician must be safeguarded in such a process; publication of deficiencies should be aggregated across physician groups, practices, and/or hospitals.

10. Finally, a peer review system that works efficiently and effectively must be established if the fee-for-service system as it is known in the United States is to survive. If the profession does not employ a program of accountability based on principles to which the profession inherently subscribes, regulators are likely to develop a program based on different values. Such a program might include administrative regulation of the numbers and kinds of services that will be paid for under national health insurance (such as the regulations in the Medicaid and Medicare programs), of the

fees that will be paid for given procedures, or even of the reimbursement and practice patterns of physicians. In one sense, the development of an effective peer review system could be the last chance the profession has for making the fee-for-service system work before it is radically altered.

Authors Clement R. Brown, Jr., and Rosemary McConkey suggested that the principles might better serve as an introduction to the book. In that role they would favor an even greater economy in achieving the purpose of "a formulation of basic principles to help orient the reader to the diversity of information which is about to be introduced." Here is their approach to stating the principles without the additional text we had felt would be useful:

Of the nine principles stated in the monograph the first four are clear and may serve to assist those readers actively engaged in or designing peer review systems. The four principles might be listed in a brief introduction and without the additional text presently accompanying them as follows:

First principle: peer review is an essential feedback mechanism

Second principle: peer review begins with physician and patient values

Third principle: the accountability of peer review is to the patient and the profession

Fourth principle: reasonable external accountability is compatible with peer review goals

We learned enough from all these contributors to convince us that an active dialogue concerning what principles should guide peer review and how best to express them is a good thing. We hope the reader agrees and will continue it.

Glossary

accountable responsible, liable, explainable. To account means to furnish a justification or detailed explanation of financial activities or responsibilities; to furnish substantial reasons or convincing explanations. Accountability entails an obligation to periodically disclose in adequate detail and consistent form to all directly and indirectly responsible or properly interested parties the purposes, principles, procedures, relationships, results, incomes, and expenditures involved in any activity, enterprise, or assignment, so that they can be evaluated by the interested parties. There is no specific or detailed agreement on what accountability is or how to assure it.[1]

acute disease a disease characterized by a single episode of a fairly short duration from which the patient returns to his normal or previous state and level of activity. While acute diseases are frequently distinguished from chronic diseases, there is no standard definition or distinction. It is worth noting that an acute episode of a chronic disease (an episode of diabetic coma in a patient with diabetes) is often treated as an acute disease.[1]

admission certification a form of medical care review in which an assessment is made of the medical necessity of a patient's admission to a hospital or other inpatient institution. Admission certification seeks to assure that patients requiring a hospital level of care, and only such patients, are admitted to the hospital without unnecessary delay and with proper planning of the hospital stay.[1]

appropriate suitable for a particular person, condition, occasion, or place; proper; fitting. A term commonly used in making policy, usually without specific indication of which aspects of the person or thing to which the term is applied are to be judged appropriate, or how and by what standard those aspects are to be judged. No indication is given in the law or legislative history of what the agencies are to find either appropriate or inappropriate (the costs or charges, necessity, quality, staffing, administration, or location of the services), or what methods and criteria are to be used.[1]

audit see medical audit.

assessment in a general (dictionary) sense, this term connotes the act of determining a rate or an amount of something.[2] In the context of peer review it implies a quantitative evaluation of a given attribute of care (whether quality, cost, appropriateness, and so on).[3]

attending physician the physician legally responsible for the care given a patient in a hospital or other health program. Usually the private physician of a private patient who is also responsible for the patient's outpatient care. The attending physician for a public patient is typically chosen by the hospital on the patient's admission from among members of its medical staff, or is one of its teaching physicians.[1]

bureaucracy a government or other organization characterized by specialization of function, adherence to fixed rules, and a hierarchy of authority;[1] a system of administration marked by officialism, red tape, and proliferation.[2]

Bureau of Quality Assurance (BQA) agency within the Health Resources Administration in HEW that administers the PSRO program.[1]

certification the process by which a governmental or nongovernmental agency or association evaluates and recognizes an individual, institutional, or educational program as meeting predetermined standards. One so recognized is said to be certified. Essentially synonymous with accreditation, except that certification is usually applied to individuals and accreditation to institutions. Certification programs are generally nongovernmental and do not exclude the uncertified from practice as do licensure programs. In the PSRO and other regulatory programs, certification of services means that their provision has been approved and payment for them is assured. See also admission certification.

chronic disease diseases having one or more of the following characteristics: are permanent; leave residual disability; are caused by nonreversible pathologic alteration; require special training of the patient for rehabilitation; or may be expected to require a long period of supervision, observation, or care.[1]

claims review review of claims by governments, medical foundations, PSROs, insurers, or others responsible for payment to determine liability and amount of payment. This review may include determination of the eligibility of the claimant or beneficiary of the eligibility of the provider of the benefit; that the benefit for which payment is claimed is covered; that the benefit is not payable under another policy; and that the benefit was necessary and of reasonable cost and quality.[1]

Commission on Professional and Hospital Activities (CPHA) a nonprofit, nongovernmental organization in Ann Arbor, Michigan, established in 1955, which collects, processes, and distributes data on hospital use for management evaluation research purposes.[1]

comprehensive peer review the scope of peer review (as the term is used in several chapters) encompasses an evaluation of both the quality and utilization of medical care or services and an evaluation of the review process itself plus an effective action program (usually educational) for rectifying any performance deficiencies detected in either the care system or the review system.[3]

concurrent review a strategy for conducting the review process at the same time or shortly after a patient receives medical services or is admitted to the hospital.[3]

continued stay review review during a patient's hospitalization to determine the medical necessity and appropriateness of continuation of the patient's stay at a hospital level of care. It may also include assessment of the quality of care being provided. Occasionally used for similar review of patients in other health facilities. See medical review. Used in the PSRO and Medicare programs where it is sometimes called "extended duration review." See also concurrent review.

continuing education formal education obtained by a health professional after completing degree and postgraduate training. Such education is usually intended to improve or maintain the professional's competence. For physicians, some but not all states require a specified number of hours of recognized continuing education per year as a condition of continued licensure. The AMA conducts a voluntary program of recognition for physicians completing required amounts of recognized continuing education.[1]

corporate (managerial) quality assurance that form of quality assurance which assesses and optimizes key parameters of health care provided to groups or populations of patients that are served by a given corporate entity (including hospitals, other institutions, provider groups, identifiable service areas, or modes of service delivery).[3]

costs expenses incurred in the provision of services or goods. Many different kinds of costs are defined and used. Charges, the price of a service or amount billed an individual or third party, may or may not be the same as or based on costs. Despite the terminology, cost-control programs are often directed to controlling increases in charges rather than in real costs.[1]

criteria predetermined elements against which aspects of the quality of a medical service may be compared. They are developed by professionals relying on professional expertise and on the professional literature.[5]

    exception peer review criteria employed in a screening process (automated or manual) that are intended to select from a flow of data elements, exceptional cases for further review.[4]

    explicit written criteria that cite specific actions, services, conditions of care delivery, accomplishments, or clinical outcomes that characterize appropriate and acceptable care. For example, explicit criteria for the care of acute appendicitis might not only specify that white blood cell count and differential be performed but also that the test results be known and considered in establishing the diagnosis preoperatively.[3]

intervention peer review criteria which are applied during the process of medical care of an individual patient and which may directly influence the actions of the physician(s) caring for that patient.[4]

management objective peer review criteria based on management objectives (see above).[4]

time span peer review criteria based on the occurrence of two or more events within a specified time interval.[4]

data set a minimum aggregation of uniformly defined and classified statistics that describe an element, episode, or aspect of health care, for example, a hospital admission (see also discharge abstract), ambulatory encounter, or a physician or hospital. Such data sets are used for evaluation, research, and similar purposes.[1]

deficiency report this term is used in a limited context in this book. It refers to a report of judgments and recommendations rendered by a peer reviewer who has determined the care given in a particular case to be deficient in some way.[3]

delegation in the PSRO program the formal process by which a PSRO, based on an assessment of the willingness and capability of a hospital or other health program to effectively perform PSRO review functions, assigns the performance of some (partial delegation) or all (full delegation) PSRO review functions to the program. Delegation must be agreed on in a written memorandum of understanding signed by both the PSRO and the program. The PSRO monitors the program's performance of the delegated functions without itself conducting them, and retains responsibility for the effectiveness of the review.[1]

diagnosis the art and science of determining the nature and cause of a disease, and of differentiating among diseases.[1]

disability classification describes the extent to which a patient is unable to pursue the activities of a normal person at the time of which the classification is made.[6]

discharge abstract a summary description of an admission prepared on a patient's discharge from a hospital or other health facility. The abstract records selected data about the patient's stay in the hospital, including diagnoses, services received, length of stay, source of payment, and demographic information. The information is usually obtained from the patient's medical record and abstracted in standard, coded form.[1] See also Uniform Hospital Discharge Data Set.

distress describes the patient's pain or mental disturbance or reaction to disability. It normally is measured in four dimensions: (1) no distress, (2) mild, (3) moderate, and (4) severe.[6]

doctor usually used synonymously with physician, but actually means any person with a doctoral degree.[1]

effectiveness the degree to which diagnostic, preventive, therapeutic, or other action or actions achieves the intended result. Effectiveness requires a consideration of outcomes to measure. It does not require consideration of the cost of the action, although one way of comparing the effectiveness of actions with the same or similar intended results is to compare the ratios of their effectiveness to the costs.[1]

efficacy commonly used synonymously with effectiveness, but may usefully be distinguished from it by using efficacy for the results of actions undertaken under ideal circumstances and effectiveness for their results under usual or normal circumstances. Actions can thus be efficacious and effective, or efficacious and ineffective, but not the reverse.[1]

efficiency the relationship between the quantity of inputs or resources used in the production of medical services and the quantity of outputs produced. Efficiency has three components: input productivity (technical efficiency), input mix (economic efficiency), and the scale of operation. Efficiency is usually measured by indicators such as output per man hour or cost per unit of output. However, such indicators fail to account for the numerous relevant dimensions (such as quality) of both inputs and outputs and are therefore only partial measures. Colloquially, efficiency measures the "bang for the buck," but as the above suggests, it is a difficult concept to define and quantify. Ultimately, efficiency should probably be measured in terms of the costs of achieving various health outcomes: defining it in terms of productivity assumes that what is produced is efficacious and used in an effective manner.[1]

exception report this is a term used in a limited context in this book. It refers to a report of some exception to (that is, deviation from) explicit criteria or standards of care. Typically this is a report generated by the screening or automated phase of an ongoing review process that identifies cases to be subjected to an in-depth review by a peer(s).[3]

Experimental Medical Care Review Organization (EMCRO) an organization assisted by a program initiated in 1970 by the National Center of Health Services Research and Development (now the NCHSR). The program, a forerunner of the PSRO program, was set up to help medical societies in creating formal organizations and procedures for reviewing the quality and use of medical care in hospitals, nursing homes, and offices throughout a defined community. The use of explicit criteria and standards definitions were required of all EMCROs, but the particular approach to organizing the review was determined by the individual organization. Ten such organizations were initially supported (only some of which actually reviewed services), and the program was phased out after enactment of the PSRO program.[1]

false-negative a person wrongly diagnosed as not having a disease or condition which in fact he does have.[1] See also false-positive.

false-positive a person wrongly diagnosed as having a disease or condition when in fact he does not. When assessing a medical screening or other diagnostic procedure, it is important to know both how many false-positives and false-negatives the procedure gives in normal use.[1] See also sensitivity.

health defined by the World Health Organization as "a state of complete physical, mental, and social well-being and not merely the absence of disease or infirmity." Experts recognize, however, that health has many dimensions (anatomical, physiologic, and mental) and is largely culturally defined. The relative importance of various disabilities will differ, depending on the cultural milieu and the role of the affected individual in that culture. Most attempts at measurement have taken a negative approach in that the degree of ill health has been assessed in terms of morbidity and mortality. In general the detection of changes in health status is easier than the definition and measurement of the absolute level of health.[1]

health resources resources (human, monetary, or material) used in producing health care and services. They include money, health manpower, health facilities, equipment, and supplies. Resources, available or used, can be measured and described for an area.[1]

health status the state of health of a specified individual, group, or population (such as Ohioans, an HMO membership, or an employer's employees). It is as difficult to describe or measure as the health of an individual and may be measured with people's subjective assessment of their health or with one or more indicators of mortality and morbidity in the population such as longevity, maternal and infant mortality, and the incidence or prevalence of major disease (communicable, coronary, malignant, nutritional, and so on). These are of course measures of disease status, but have to be used as proxies in the absence of measures of either objective or subjective health. Health status conceptually is the proper outcome measure for the effectiveness of the specific population's medical care system, although attempts to relate variations in health status and the effects of available medical care have proved difficult and generally unsuccessful. It cannot be measured with measures of available health resources or services (such as physician to population ratios), which in this context would be process measures.[1]

HEW the Department of Health, Education, and Welfare, an agency of the federal government.[3]

hospital an institution whose primary function is to provide inpatient services, diagnostic and therapeutic, for a variety of medical conditions, both surgical and nonsurgical. In addition, most hospitals provide some outpatient services, particularly emergency care. Hospitals are classified by length of stay (short-term or long-term); as teaching or nonteaching; by major type of service (psychiatric, tuberculosis, general, and other specialties such as maternity, children's, or ear, nose, and throat); and by control (government, federal, state, or local, profit [or proprietary], and nonprofit). The hospital system is dominated by the short-term, general, nonprofit community hospital, often called a voluntary hospital.[1]

Hospital International Classification of Diseases Adapted for Use in the United States (H-ICDA) see International Classification of Diseases.

hospital review program a hospital review program normally consists of admission certification, concurrent review, medical care evaluation studies, and profile analysis.[6]

individual (operational) quality assurance that form of quality assurance which assesses all clinically relevant parameters of care delivered to an individual patient for the expressed purpose of promoting the optimal (most efficacious) outcome for that specific patient (including both professionally initiated services and patient-initiated behaviors).[3]

inpatient a patient who has been admitted at least overnight to a hospital or other health facility (which is therefore responsible for his room and board) for the purpose of receiving diagnostic, treatment, or other health services. Inpatient care means the care given inpatients.[1]

input measure a measure of the quality of services based on the number, type, and quality of resources used in the production of the services. Medical services are often evaluated by measuring the education and training level of the provider, the reputation and accreditation of the institution, the number of health personnel involved, or the number of dollars spent as proxy measures for the quality of the service. Input measures are generally recognized as inferior to process and outcome measures because they are indirect measures of quality and do not consider the actual results or outcomes or services. They are often used nonetheless because people are accustomed to their use, and they are easily obtained.[1] See also output measures.

International Classification of Disease, Adapted for Use in the United States (ICDA) a USPHS official adaptation of a system for classifying diseases and operations for the purpose of indexing hospital records developed by the World Health Organization. Diseases are grouped according to the problems they present. The ICDA is revised every 10 years. The eighth version (known as ICDA-8) is now in use, and ICDA-9 in preparation.[1]

Joint Commission on Accreditation of Hospitals (JCAH) a private, nonprofit organization whose purpose is to encourage the attainment of uniformly high standards of institutional medical care. Comprised of representatives of the American Hospital Association, American Medical Association, American College of Physicians, and American College of Surgeons, the organization establishes guidelines for the operations of hospitals and other health facilities and conducts survey and accreditation programs. Accreditation has been used by or adopted as a requirement of specific public programs and funding agencies; for example, hospitals participating in the Medicare program are deemed to have met most conditions of participation if they are accredited by the JCAH.[1]

length of stay (LOS) the length of an inpatient's stay in a hospital or other health facility. It is one measure of use of health facilities, reported as an average number of days spent in a facility per admission or discharge. It is calculated as follows: total number of days in the facility for all discharges and deaths occurring during a period divided by the number of discharges and deaths during the same period. In concurrent review an appropriate length of stay may be assigned each patient on admission. Average lengths of stay vary and are measured for people with various ages, specific diagnoses, or sources of payment.[1]

malpractice professional misconduct or lack of ordinary skill in the performance of a professional act. A practitioner is liable for damages or injuries caused by malpractice. Such liability, for some professions like medicine, can be covered by malpractice insurance against the costs of defending suits instituted against the professional and any damages assessed by the court, usually up to a maximum limit. Malpractice requires that the patient demonstrate some injury and that the injury be negligently caused.[1]

management the organization and control of human activity directed toward specific ends. Different kinds of management are sometimes described: for example, by exception, in which only exceptions from defined policy are reported and acted on; and by objective, in which clearly stated objectives are used to guide the management process.[1]

management information system a system (frequently automated or computer based) which produces the necessary information in proper form and at appropriate intervals for the management of a program or other activity. The system should measure program progress toward objectives and report costs and problems needing attention. Special efforts have been made in the Medicaid program to develop information systems for each state program.[1]

management objectives explicit statements describing the objectives or goals of medical management of a diagnosis or problem.[4]

medical this term is used in its broadest dictionary sense to connote that the given subject under discussion relates to or is concerned with the practice of medicine.[2] In this book it is not intended that "medical" relate narrowly to physicians only unless it is obvious from the context.[3]

medical audit detailed retrospective review and evaluation of selected medical records by qualified professional staff. Medical audits are used in some hospitals, group practices, and occasionally in private independent practices for evaluating professional performance by comparing it with accepted criteria, standards, and current professional judgment. A medical audit is usually concerned with the care of a given illness and is undertaken to identify deficiencies in that care in anticipation of educational programs to improve it.[1]

medical audit (quality assessment) that form of criteria-based peer review that assesses the quality of health care services relevant to medical necessity. It may include assessments of the clinical appropriateness of diagnostic investigations, therapeutic interventions, manipulative procedures, and professional conduct, or their impact in terms of patient outcomes. It also may include social and psychologic audit in which acceptable specific protocols are employed to advance the level of care (professional and institutional) through a small-group problem-solving process.[3]

medical care evaluation a process that can be accomplished in a variety of ways and by many means. It is a global term dealing with peer review, quality assurance, utilization review, and medical audit. The process

is the underlying concept employed in quality assurance programs.[6]

medical care evaluation studies (MCEs) retrospective medical care review in which an in-depth assessment of the quality and nature of the use of selected health services or programs is made. Restudy of an MCE assesses the effectiveness of corrective actions taken to correct deficiencies identified in the original study, but does not necessarily repeat or replicate the original study. Utilization review requirements under Medicare and Medicaid require utilization review committees in hospitals and skilled nursing facilities to have at least one such study in progress at all times. Such studies are also required by the PSRO program.[1]

medical care outcome the change in the patient state of illness during an episode of treatment or a period of care of a chronic illness.[6]

medical peer review the investigational, managerial, and educational process for systematically monitoring health care in which the judgments regarding provider performance and recommendations regarding corrective actions are based on a review of appropriate case data and are made by qualified professional peers who practice in the same community and who communicate the results of their efforts to the public.[3]

medical record a record kept on patients which properly contains sufficient information to identify the patient clearly, to justify his diagnosis and treatment, and to document the results accurately. The purposes of the record are to serve as the basis for planning and continuity of patient care; provide a means of communication among physicians and any professional contributing to the patient's care; furnish documentary evidence of the patient's course of illness and treatment; serve as a basis for review, study, and evaluation; serve in protecting the legal interests of the patient, hospital, and responsible practitioner; and provide data for use in research and education. Medical records and their contents are not usually available to the patient himself. The content of the record is usually confidential. Each different provider in a community caring for a given patient usually keeps an independent record of that care.[1]

medical review review (required by Medicaid) by a team composed of physicians and other appropriate health and social service personnel of the condition and need for care, including a medical evaluation, of each inpatient in a long-term care facility. By law the team must review care being provided in the facilities; adequacy of the services available in the facilities to meet the current health needs and promote the maximum physical well-being of the patients; necessity and desirability of the continued placement of such patients in the facilities; and feasibility of meeting their health care needs through alternate institutional or noninstitutional services. Medical review differs from utilization review in that it requires evaluation of each individual patient and an analysis of the appropriateness of his specific treatment in a given institution, whereas utilization review is often done on a sample basis with special attention to certain procedures, conditions, or lengths of stay.[1] See also continued stay review.

medical staff collectively the physicians, dentists, and other professionals responsible for medical care in a health facility, typically a hospital. Such staff may be full-time or part-time, employed by the hospital or not, and may include all professionals who wish to be included (open staff) or just those who meet various standards of competence (closed staff). Staff privileges may or may not be permanent or conditioned on continued evidence of competence.[1]

Medicare (Title XVIII) a nationwide health insurance program for people aged 65 and over, for persons eligible for social security disability payments for over 2 years, and for certain workers and their dependents who need kidney transplantation or dialysis. Health insurance protection is available to insured persons without regard to income. It consists of two separate but coordinated programs: hospital insurance (part A) and supplementary medical insurance (part B).[1]

medicine the art and science of promoting, maintaining, and restoring individual health, and of diagnosing and treating disease.[1]

monitoring the continuous examination of routinely collected data on selected critical parameters to see if the observed pattern of care matches preestablished standards.[7]

national health insurance (NHI) a term not yet defined in the United States.[1]

need some thing or action which is essential, indispensable, required, or cannot be done or lived without; a condition marked by the lack or want of some such thing or action. The presence or absence of a need can and should be measured by an objective criterion or standard. Needs may or may not be perceived or expressed by the person in need and must be distinguished from demands and expressed desires, whether or not needed. Like appropriateness, need is frequently and irregularly used in health care with respect to health facilities and services . . . and people. It is thus important to specify what thing or action's need is being considered, by what criteria the need is to be established by whom (provider, consumer, or third party), and with what effect (since payment for services by insurance is, for instance, sometimes conditioned on the necessity of their provision).[1]

norm(s) numerical or statistical measures of usual observed performance.[5]

outcome "the end results (of health care) in terms of health and satisfaction" (Donabedian). For example, a study of the outcome of a particular operation might measure the level of disability of patients in 1 year after the operation and also the 1-year mortality.[3]

outpatient a patient who is receiving ambulatory care at a hospital or other health facility without being admitted to the facility. Usually does not mean people receiving services from a physician's office or other program that does not also give inpatient care. Outpatient care refers to care given outpatients, often in organized programs.[1]

output measures variously used synonymously with measures of the productivity of health programs and manpower, process measures, or outcome measures.[1]

patient one who is receiving health services; sometimes used synonymously with consumer.[1]

peer in its usual dictionary sense, refers to "one that is of equal standing with another."[2] As used in this text, the peer of a physician is a physician, the peer of a nurse is a nurse, and so on, and all health professionals who deliver clinical services directly to patients are included under general references to peers (again, unless otherwise specifically restricted by the context).[3]

peer review as used in the book title, refers to the broadest generic term that embraces the whole of this field. We wish to alert the reader to the fact that others (notably Brown and McConkey in Chapter 17) utilize the term "quality assurance" in the same generic sense. When capitalized, this term refers to a specific review program developed by the American Hospital Association.[3] See also Quality Assurance Program.

personal physician the physician who assumes a responsibility for the comprehensive medical care of an individual on a continuing basis. The physician obtains professional assistance when needed for services he is not qualified to provide and coordinates the care provided by other professional personnel in light of his knowledge and understanding of the patient as a whole. While personal physicians will have an interest in the patient's family as they affect his patient, the personal physician may not serve the entire family directly; for example, a pediatrician may serve as a personal physician for children, while an internist or other specialist may serve in this capacity for adults. Personal physician is sometimes more simply defined for any given patient as the one that patient designates as his personal or principal physician.[1]

practice the use of one's knowledge in a particular profession. The practice of medicine is the exercise of one's knowledge in the promotion of health and treatment of disease.[1]

preadmission certification review of the need for proposed inpatient service(s) prior to time of admission to an institution.[1] See also concurrent review.

primary care basic or general health care which emphasizes the point when the patient first seeks assistance from the medical care system and the care of the simpler and more common illnesses. The primary care provider usually also assumes ongoing responsibility for the patient in both health maintenance and therapy of illness. It is comprehensive in the sense that it takes responsibility for the overall coordination of the care of the patient's health problems, be they biological, behavioral or social. The appropriate use of consultants and community resources is an important part of effective primary care. Such care is generally provided by physicians, but is increasingly provided by other personnel such as family nurse practitioners.[1]

private practice medical practice in which the practitioner and his practice are indepen-

dent of any external policy control. It usually requires that the practitioner be self-employed, except when he is salaried by a partnership in which he is a partner with similar practitioners. It is sometimes wrongly used synonymously with either fee-for-service practice (the practitioner may sell his services by another method, that is, capitation); or solo practice (group practice may be private). Note that physicians practice in many different settings, and there is no agreement as to which of these does or does not constitute private practice.[1]

process "the activities of . . . health professionals in the management of patients" (Donabedian). The process of care refers to details of the patient's history and physical examination, other diagnostic measures, and specific treatment procedures.[3]

professional a term with no consistent or agreed-on meaning. Most occupational groups in the health field aspire to being considered professions. There are a number of usual components: formal education and examination are required for membership in the profession; certification or licensure is required for membership, reflecting community sanction or approval; there exists regional or national professional association; there is a code of ethics governing the activities of individuals in the profession; there is a body of systematic scientific knowledge and technical skill required; and the members function with a degree of autonomy and authority, under the assumption that they alone have the expertise to make decisions in their area of competence. Medicine is often considered the occupation which most closely approaches the prototype of a profession.[1]

Professional Standards Review Organization (PSRO) a physician-sponsored organization charged with comprehensive and ongoing review of services provided under the Medicare, Medicaid, and Maternal and Child Health programs. The purpose of this review is to determine for purposes of reimbursement under these programs whether services are medically necessary; provided in accordance with professional criteria, norms, and standards; and, in the case of institutional services, rendered in an appropriate setting. The requirement for the establishment of PSROs was added by the Social Security Amendments of 1972, Public Law

92-603, to the Social Security Act as part B of Title XI.[1]

profile a longitudinal or cross-sectional aggregation of medical care data. Patient profiles list all of the services provided to a particular patient during a specified period of time. Physician, hospital, or population profiles are statistical summaries of the pattern of practice of an individual physician, a specific hospital, or the medical experience of a specific population. Diagnostic profiles are a subcategory of physician, hospital, or population profiles with regard to a specific condition or diagnosis.[1]

prospective review a strategy or screening mechanism for conducting the review process *prior to* the receipt of care (for example, prior to a patient's admission to a hospital). The basic objective of this type of review is to assure that the planned admission, level of care, or specific services to be provided are medically, socially, and psychologically indicated.[3]

quality the nature, kind, or character of someone or something; hence the degree or grade of excellence possessed by the person or thing. Quality may be measured with respect to individual medical services, the various services received by individual [*sic*] or groups of patients, individual or groups of providers, or health programs or facilities; in terms of technical competence, humanity, need, acceptability, appropriateness, inputs, structure, process, or outcomes; using standards, criteria, norms, or direct quantitative or qualitative measures. To avoid the frequent vagueness of the term it is thus necessary to specify who or what is being considered, what aspect of it is being measured, and how it is being assessed.[1]

quality assessment in this text this term is often used synonymously with medical audit.[3]

quality assurance (1) activities and programs intended to assure the quality of care in a defined medical setting or program. Such programs must include educational or other components intended to remedy identified deficiencies in quality as well as the components necessary to identify such deficiencies (such as peer or utilization review components) and assess the program's own effectiveness. A program which identifies quality deficiencies and responds only with negative sanctions, such as denial of reimbursement, is not usually considered as a quality assurance program, although the latter may include use of such sanctions. Such programs are required of HMOs and other health programs assisted under authority of the PHS Act, Section 1301(c) (8).[1] See also Quality Assurance Program for medical care in the hospital (QAP). (2) that form of medical audit consisting not only of a program to assess the quality of care but also a program to effect those changes in the delivery of health care necessary to achieve optimal clinical outcomes. The scope of parameters assessed may be broader than that in quality control, as it may include the monitoring of patient behaviors and administrative or managerial functions in addition to the monitoring of direct patient care or services.[3] See also corporate quality assurance and individual quality assurance.

Quality Assurance Program for medical care in the hospital (QAP) a program developed by the American Hospital Association for use by hospital administrations and medical staffs in the development of a hospital program to assure the quality of the care given in the hospital.[1]

quality control (1) that form of medical audit which assesses key parameters of care delivered to populations by an institution or provider group relevant to determining whether the overall process of care delivery or its clinical impact meets professional standards of acceptability of efficacy (for example, retrospective assessments of care process and patient outcomes as applied to populations or groups);[3] (2) the concurrent activity performed to provide each patient with care that conforms to standards.[7]

quality improvement the retrospective review of the care provided to groups of patients to detect chronic problems and to improve the care of future patients.[7]

retrospective study an inquiry planned to observe events that have already occurred (a case-control study is usually retrospective); compare with a prospective study planned to observe events that have not yet occurred.[1]

review in this text the term carries the dictionary definition "to go over or examine critically or deliberately."[2,3] See also prospective review and retrospective study.

review coordinator a member of the hospital staff or of the PSRO who performs or supervises one or more of the following responsibilities: conducting concurrent review (of the medical record), collecting data for MCEs, initiating or coordinating discharge planning, recording and transmitting review decisions, completing reports on review decisions, completing reports on review activities, or acting as liaison with persons and organizations participating in and affected by the PSRO review system. Individuals with different backgrounds other than nurses may perform review coordinator duties, for example, medical record technicians or medical corpsmen.

screening (1) a process in which norms, criteria, and standards are used to analyze large numbers of cases in order to select for study in greater depth those cases not meeting these norms, criteria, and standards;[5] (2) in the context of peer review, a process of ongoing review (surveillance) in which norms, criteria, and standards are used to analyze large numbers of cases in order to identify (select) for study in greater depth (usually by peers) those cases not meeting explicit norms, criteria, or standards. In this text the term often refers to the first step in the ongoing (routine) surveillance of medical care, which is usually conducted by nonpeers (often with computer assistance).[3]

sensitivity a measure of the ability of a diagnostic or screening test or other predictor to correctly identify the positive (or sick) people (the proportion of true positive cases [sick people] correctly identified as positive). A test may be quite sensitive without being very specific.[1]

service a unit of health care. It is interesting that there is no standard term for a single unit of health care, whatever that unit may be. Both service and procedure are often used to refer to units of health care (that is, a health service or a medical procedure), but neither has any constant definition. Service is sometimes used synonymously with encounter, but they should be differentiated, since an encounter may include several services. It is also used synonymously with department, a quite different meaning.[1]

Social Security Administration (SSA) the administration within HEW which manages the Social Security Program (including Medicare), which is the responsibility of the SSA's Bureau of Health Insurance. Since SSA is not under the direction of HEW's assistant secretary for health, this means that Medicare is administered separately from the

department's other health programs.[1] (NOTE: At this writing a reorganization of HEW is underway, which purports to place Medicare together with other health programs.)

standards (1) generally a measure set by competent authority as the rule for measuring quantity or quality. Conformity with standards is usually a condition of licensure, accreditation, or payment for services. Standards may be defined in relation to the actual or predicted effects of care, the performance or credentials of professional personnel, and the physical plan, governance, and administration of facilities and programs. In the PSRO program, standards are professionally developed expressions of the range of acceptable variation from a norm or criterion. Thus the criteria for care of a urinary tract infection might be a urinalysis and urine culture, and the standard might require a urinalysis in 100% of cases and a urine culture only in previously untreated cases.[1,5]

structure "the settings and instrumentalities available and used for the provision of care" (Donabedian). For example, structures involved in health care delivery might include the qualifications of health care practitioners and the capabilities of health care facilities. Thus the requirement by state boards that practicing physicians be licensed is a *structural* requirement.[3]

systems "systematic," in the context of peer review, refers to a structured and integrated approach to the evaluation of health care (as opposed to the more unstructured and informal or traditional form of peer review). The systematic approach structures the review process so that hidden (implicit) assumptions concerning what constitutes optimal care are minimized and explicit or objective criteria for assessing care are maximized. The more systematic it is, the more each step in the review process is seen to interact with all others, and the more all steps individually reflect the context and purpose of the whole review process.[3]

tissue committee a committee which usually functions in a hospital setting and reviews and evaluates all surgery performed in the hospital on the basis of the extent of agreement among the preoperative, postoperative, and pathologic diagnoses; and on the relevance and acceptability of the procedures undertaken for the diagnosis. The name derives from the use of pathologic findings from tissue removed at surgery as a key element in the review.[1]

tissue review a review and evaluation of surgery performed in a hospital on the basis of agreement or disagreement among the preoperative, postoperative, and pathologic diagnoses. In particular, the pathologic or tissue diagnosis is used to determine if the procedure was necessary. Studies have shown that hospitals with tissue committees have lower rates of unnecessary surgery than those without such committees.[1]

Title XVIII the title of the Social Security Act which contains the principal legislative authority for the Medicare program, and therefore a common name for the program.[1]

Title XIX the title of the Social Security Act which contains the principal legislative authority for the Medicaid program, and therefore a common name for the program.[1]

treatment the management and care of a patient for the purpose of combating disease or disorder.[1]

triage commonly used to describe the sorting out or screening of patients seeking care to determine which service is initially required and with what priority. A patient coming to a facility for care may be seen in a triage, screening, or walk-in clinic. Here it will be determined, possibly by a triage nurse, whether, for example, the patient has a medical or surgical problem or requires some nonphysician service such as social work consultation. Such rapid assessment units may merely refer patients to the most appropriate treatment service or may also give treatment for minor problems. Originally used to describe the sorting of battle casualties into groups who could wait for care, would benefit from immediate care, and were beyond care.[1] The dictionary definition of this term in the context of medical care reads: "the sorting of and allocation of treatment to patients and especially battle and disaster victims according to a system of priorities."[2] In the context of peer review the term refers specifically to the sorting of exception reports (variances from explicit criteria) for referral to appropriate peer authorities who will conduct an in-depth review of the case.[3]

Uniform Hospital Discharge Data Set (UHDDS) a defined set of data which give a minimum description of a hospital episode or admission. Collection of a UHDDS is required on discharge for all hospital stays reimbursed under Medicare and Medicaid. The UHDDS was defined in a policy statement of the secretary of HEW (HEW publ. no. HSM-73-1451, ser. 4, no. 14, as extended by a policy statement approved June 24, 1974) and includes data on the age, sex, race, and residence of the patient, length of stay, diagnosis, responsible physicians, procedures performed, disposition of the patient, and sources of payment. The PSRO program uses a slightly larger data set called the PSRO Hospital Discharge Data Set (PHDDS).[1]

utilization use. Utilization is commonly examined in terms of patterns or rates of use of a single service or type of service, for example, hospital care, physician visits, prescription drugs. Measurement of utilization of all medical services in combination is usually done in terms of dollar expenditures. Use is expressed in rates per unit of population at risk for a given period, for example, number of admissions to hospital per 1000 persons over age 65 per year, or number of visits to a physician per person per year for family planning services.[1]

utilization review (UR) (1) evaluation of the necessity, appropriateness, and efficiency of the use of medical services, procedures, and facilities. In a hospital this includes review of the appropriateness of admissions, services ordered and provided, length of stay, and discharge practices, both on a concurrent and retrospective basis. Utilization review can be done by a utilization review committee, PSRO, peer review group, or public agency.[1] See also medical review. (2) an examination of the efficiency with which institutional facilities are used such as the appropriateness of admissions, services, provided, length of stay, and discharge planning. This type of review may be undertaken on a prospective, concurrent, or retrospective basis.[3]

utilization review committee a staff committee of an institution or a group outside the institution responsible for conducting utilization review activities for that institution. Medicare and Medicaid require as a condition of participation that hospitals have a utilization review committee in operation.[1]

validity the degree to which data or results of a study are correct or true; the extent to which a situation as observed reflects the true situation.[1]

REFERENCES

1. A discursive dictionary of health care, prepared by the staff for use of the Subcommittee on Health and the Environment of the Committee on Interstate and Foreign Commerce, U.S. House of Representatives, Washington, D.C., 1976, U.S. Government Printing Office.
2. Webster's new collegiate dictionary, Springfield, Mass., 1973, G. & C. Merriam Co.
3. Provided by Paul Y. Ertel and M. Gene Aldridge.
4. Provided by Alan R. Nelson.
5. U.S. Dept. of Health, Education and Welfare, Office of Professional Standards Review: PSRO program manual, Washington, D.C., March 1974, U.S. Government Printing Office.
6. Provided by James E. Sorensen.
7. Provided by Vergil N. Slee and Marsha A. Bremer.

Abbreviations

AHA	American Hospital Association
BQA	Bureau of Quality Assurance
CES	continuing education subcommittee
CHAMPUS	Civilian Health and Medical Program of the Uniformed Services
CHAP	Certified Hospital Admission Program
CMHC	community mental health center
CPHA	Committee on Professional Hospital Activities
DME	director of medical education
EDP	electronic data processing
EMCRO	Experimental Medical Care Review Organization
ES	evaluation subcommittee
HEW	U.S. Department of Health, Education, and Welfare
H-ICDA	Hospital Adaptation of International Classification of Disease
HMO	health maintenance organization
HSA	health systems agencies
ICDA	International Classification of Disease
JCAH	Joint Commission on Accreditation of Hospitals
LOS	length of stay
MAP	Medical Audit Program
MAS	medical audit subcommittee
MCE	medical care evaluation
MIS	management information system
OPSR	Office of Professional Standards Review
OSCHUR	On-site Concurrent Hospital Utilization Review program
PA	physician advisor
PACE	Physician Ambulatory Care Evaluation program
PAS¹	Professional Activities Study
PAS²	Professional Audit Service
PCT	performance/cost/time
PEP	performance evaluation program
PERT	program evaluation and review techniques
PHDDS	PSRO Hospital Discharge Data Set
PMIS	PSRO management information system
POMR	problem-oriented medical record
PPI	physician performance index
PRC	peer review committee
PSRO	Professional Standards Review Organization
QAM	quality assurance monitor
RCT	randomized clinical trial
RSE	review system evaluation
UHDA	uniform hospital discharge abstract
UHDDS	Uniform Hospital Discharge Data Set
UPRO	Utah Professional Review Organization
URS	utilization review subcommittee

Index

A

Abbreviations, list of, 405

Abstracting in Hawaii study, 339-340

Acceptance of peer review system by staff, 181

Accessibility and availability of medical care services, 112

Accountability
economic, 91-94
as function of medical peer review, 90, 91-94
in health care delivery, 1-3
institutional, to public, 104
public, 386-388
quality, 91-94
in quality assurance function, 287-288
of quality assurance system, 357
research needs for achieving, 2

Action referrals by physician advisors in individual case medical audit reviews, 218

Activities
of continuing education subcommittee, 222
current developmental, in PACE program, 333-334
of evaluation subcommittee, 221
major, of peer review, 187, 188
managerial, in management information systems, 244-246
in medical audit review, 216-217
integrating, 220
of primary review, 203-208
in profile review function of utilization review
integrative, 215
reporting, 215
review, 231-232
case evaluation, 231-232, 238, 239
program evaluation, 231, 238, 239
in utilization review
areas of, 213
classes of, 213-214

Activity reports in medical audit review, 220-221

Acute care intervention, 237

Administrative actions in analysis of reports at review level 3, 226

Administrative commitment in implementation of peer review system, 181

Admission
hospital, review protocol, 169
justification for, 279
validation of reasons, 279-280

Admission certification and concurrent continued-stay review, 281

Admission review protocol in hospital, 169

Advisory council, 152

AMA model screening criteria
claims review and, 284
format and, 276-277, 278
future actions in development project, 283-284
history, 275-276
interrelationship with norms, standards, and criteria, 284
limitations, 282-283
local PSRO actions regarding, 285-286
major elements, use of, 277-281
admission, validation of reasons for, 279-280
code number, 277, 279
complications, 280-281
diagnosis, validation of, 279
diagnostic and therapeutic services, critical, 280
discharge status, 280
justification for admission, 279
length of stay, 279
practical use, 281
review type, 281
title, 279
strengths, 281-282
use in medical care evaluation studies, 285

Ambulatory care, 115
problems of assessing, 65

Ambulatory care criteria for PACE program, 331-333

Ambulatory and hospital settings, research in quality assessment and utilization review, 335-355
consensus criteria development, 344-351
Continuing Education Study, 339-344, 351-353
explicit care criteria, 336-337
Hawaii study (1970 to 1972), 339-344
hospital utilization review criteria study (1965), 338-339
medical data collection study (Michigan, 1970), 338
Office Care Study, 339-344, 354
quality of care feasibility (Michigan), 337-338
utilization study (1958), 337

Analysis
of data system, 172
of reports in review level 3, 225-228

Ancillary services, review of, for OSCHUR, 329

Appeals
of decision in review level 2, 212
in individual case medical audit reviews, 218-220

Appeals—cont'd
  mechanism in individual case utilization review functions, 214-215
Applicability of therapeutic modality in peer review, 235
Appropriateness of evaluation criteria, 188-189
Art of care, 112, 113, 114, 124, 126
Assessment
  of actual care to criteria of peer review system, 156-157
  matrix for systematic peer review, 109
  of quality assurance system, 269, 375-376
  of quality of medical care, 111-131
Assurance of quality of health care, 356; see also Quality assurance system
Audit process, basic, 156
Authority and duties of physician, delegation of, 21
Automated data information systems, 172, 173-175
Automation
  of health care, 27
    assessment, 38
  role of, in utilization review, 215-216
Availability
  accessibility and, of medical care services, 112
  of therapeutic modality in peer review, 235

B

Base
  data; see Data base
  performance, 95, 96
Basic audit process, 156
Basic instruments of peer review, 273-304
  role of PSRO in development, 37-43
Bias in measurement of quality of medical care, 62-63
Bi-Cycle concept in quality assurance system, 357-358, 360, 365
Blue Cross—Blue Shield insurance benefits, 13, 16
Boundaries of professional responsibility, 21-22
Bureau of Quality Assurance (BQA), 262
  experience with PSRO operations, 42

C

Care/case abstract, description of, 156
Care participation in patient as variable in peer review, 236
Care processes, impact of peer review system on, 194-195
Care providers, impact of peer review system on, 194-195
Care system analysis task force, 153
Care system reports, 225-226
Care technology, 36, 37-38
Case evaluation, 231-232, 238, 239
Categorical referrals by physician advisors in individual case medical audit reviews, 217-218
Certified Hospital Admission Program, 307-324
  assessment, 322-323
  meeting new needs, 323-324
  operational and technical problems, 323
  process, 313-322
  requirements, 310-312
Change
  in health care delivery system, 33-45
  in quality assurance system, 357, 370-371, 374-375
Change/innovation function of peer review, 90, 91, 108-109

Characteristics and requirements of management information systems, 244-248
Chronic care intervention, 237
Claims review and screening criteria, 284
Clerical information systems and clerical inputs, 245-246
Clerical inputs in management information systems, 245-246
Clerk-typist, functions of, in primary review, 201-202, 203
Clinical outcomes, 195
Clinical records systems, 248, 249
Clinical status as prognostic variable in peer review, 234
Commitment of staff to peer review system, 181
Committee, peer review, 166, 224-228
Communication function of peer review, 90, 91, 104-106
Community responsibility in quality assurance, 356-357
Complaints from patients, satisfaction of, 19
Complications of AMA model screening criteria, 280-281
Components of quality assurance system, 357
Comprehensive care as cause of medical service demand, 12-13
Comprehensive evaluation of care and review systems, 186
Comprehensiveness of content of evaluation criteria, 190
Computers in peer review
  evaluation technology, 11
  negative potential, 2
  operations in primary review, 202, 203, 204, 205
  rising costs and, 14-15
Conceptual base
  of continuing education subcommittee, 222-224
  for evaluation of peer review system, 185
  of evaluation subcommittee, 221
  of medical audit, 216-221
  of primary review, 198
  of review level 2, 208-209
  of review level 3, 224
  of review level 4, 228-229
  of systematic peer review, 148
    in design and development of, 154
    in planning and managing stage, 149-150
  of utilization review, 213
Conceptual exploration of meaning of quality of medical care, 67
Concurrent review, 159, 160, 162, 173, 232
Concurrent review activity summary, 263
Content as object of evaluation of health care quality, 77
Continuing education, 162
  for clinical staff
    curriculum development, 184
    curriculum modules, 184-185
    elements of program, 184
  as function of peer review, 96, 97, 100
  linkage to OSCHUR, 330
  research, 101-103
Continuing Education Study, 339-344, 351-353
Continuing education subcommittee (CES), 99, 166, 211, 222-224
  activity areas, 222
  conceptual base, 222

Continuing education subcommittee (CES)—cont'd
  educational functions
    feedback loop, 224
    outreach, 223
    peer review training, 223
    resources and programs, 222-223
    staff performance reporting, 223-224
Continuity of care coordinator, 212
Control
  government, of medicine, 7-8
  operational and tactical, of management information systems, 244-246
Convergent thinking in continuing education, 97
Coordinator
  for continuity of care, 212
  nurse, 309, 310-311, 326, 327
  review, 199, 203, 205, 282
Cornell medical index, 136
Corrective action
  of deficiencies in peer review system, 157
  in primary review, 202, 207
  in review level 2, 213
Cosmetic surgery as cause of medical service demand, 13
Cost
  as criterion for evaluation of health care quality, 82-85
  evaluation of, on patient care, 194
  of health care
    accountability for, 90, 91-94
    estimation of, 128-129
    magnitude, 16-17
    management, 17, 103
    payment mechanism, 15-16
    prevailing charges, 15
    sources, 14-15
  and quality assurance trade-off model, 176
  of systematic peer review and management information systems, 243-270
Cost reporting, 264
Counter-productive health programs, 22
Criteria
  in determining quality of medical care, 127-128
    explicit, 127-128
    implicit, 127
  development of, in Hawaii study, 339
  evaluation of, 188-190
    appropriateness, 188-189
    content, comprehensiveness of, 190
    measurements, validity and reliability of, 189-190
  in primary review, 203
  for quality assessment, 114
    outcome, 123-124
    process, 117-123
    structure, 117
  in quality assurance system, 365-367
  screening, AMA model; *see* AMA model screening criteria
  screening criteria and, 284
  values applied to, 128-129, 130
Criteria development, 155, 189
  consensus, 344-351
  as educational function of peer review, 97-99
    communication and, 105-106
Criteria development task force, 152
Criteria review in medical audit reviews, 220
Criteria screening in primary review, 204, 205

Criteria setting
  for determining quality of care, 127-128
  in quality assurance system, 365-367
  in review systems, 96-97, 105-106
Critical variables associated with organizational issues in peer review
  designing and developing, 148-149
  evaluation, 149
  implementation, 149
  planning, 148
Curriculum development for continuing education of clinical staff, 184
Curriculum modules, preparation of, 184-185

D

Data
  care-related, 197-198
  collection in quality assurance system, 367-368
  for measuring quality of medical care
    outcome, 123-124
    process, 117-123
    structure, 117
  needs for OSCHUR, 329-330
  objective, 194
Data base
  educational function and, 95, 96
  in management information systems, 243-246
    clinical records, 248
  patient, 357, 362-364
  research function and, 101-103
Data base and medical records task force, 152-153
Data broker system for hospital information needs, 296-304
Data processing
  in management information systems, 253
  operational efficiency, evaluation of, 193
Data source
  in measurement of quality of medical care, 125-127
  method of collecting, 125
Data system
  interactive, in primary review, 205, 207-208
  steps in planning, 171-172
    analysis, 172
    developing input source document and output format, 172
    establishing and defining objectives, 171
    implementation, 172
    modification (optimization), 172
Decision appeal in review level 2, 212
Decision making
  in medical care process, 68-69
  in systematic peer review, 243-246
Decision referral in review level 2, 212
Defensive medicine, 103
Deficiency
  in medical care, 204
  persistent, 219
Deficiency report in primary review, 205, 207
Deficiency triage in review level 2, 212-213
Delegation of physician duties and authority, 21
Demand for medical services, 12-14
Demand reports in management information systems, 245
Demographic factors of patient as variable in peer review, 235-236
Descriptive medical research, 100, 101

Design
content determinants and, of systematic peer review, 230-242
health care outcomes, surveillance of, 238-240
health care process, surveillance of, 236-238
major determinants, 233
process and outcome review, combined, 240-241
review activity, 231-232
review content, 232-236
review program, 230-231
quality, 231
utilization, 230-231
development and
of candidate peer review systems and of selected system, 150
of comprehensive peer review system
conceptual base, 154
data system, steps in planning, 171-172
dimensions, 155-167
existing review activities, 154-155
information system, 170-171, 172-175
integrated hospital information flow, 167-170
management audit program, 179
medical care evaluation studies, 177-179
outcome model, expanded, 175-177
preparing for future, 179
strategies, 179
as critical variable associated with organizational issues in peer review, 148-149
operation and, of systems, evaluation of, 190-192
Detailed system design of management information system, 258-259
guidelines, 259-260
Determinants of design and content of systematic peer review; *see* Design and content determinants of systematic peer review
Development
of criteria, 189
of curriculum for continuing education of clinical staff, 184
design and, as critical variable associated with organizational issues in peer review, 148-149
implementation and, of comprehensive peer review system, 152-153
conceptual base, 154
data system, steps in planning, 171-172
dimensions, 155-167
existing review activities, 154-155
financial plan, 154
information system, 170-171
integrated hospital information flow, 167-170
management audit program, 179
medical care evaluation studies, 177-179
outcome model, expanded, 175-177
preparing for future, 179
strategies, 179
Diagnosis
accuracy, 135-136
importance in determining quality of medical care, 114, 115-117, 119-121
treatment and, early, as cause of medical service demand, 12
validation of, 279
Diagnostic and therapeutic services, critical, in AMA model screening criteria, 280
Diagnostic variables of peer review, 233-234

Direct observation of physicians' activities in evaluation of quality of medical care, 54-55
Discharge data set, 264
Discharge status in AMA model screening criteria, 280
Disciplinary actions in analysis of reports at review level 3, 226-228
Disease
diagnosis of, in determining quality of medical care, 114, 115-117, 119-121
etiology of, and primary medical care, 133
natural history of, and outcome of medical care, 123-124
symptoms and process of medical care, 121-123
Disease control program, 237
Disease intervention, 233-234
Distributed information system, 255-256
Distribution of services as cause of medical service demand, 13
Divergent thinking in continuing education, 97
Duties and authority of physician, delegation of, 21

E
Economic accountability, 91-94
Economics of management information systems, 260-262
Education, 181
continuing, 96, 100
as function of peer review, 90, 94-99
Education and training task force, 153
Educational feedback loop as function of continuing education subcommittee, 224
Educational functions
of continuing education subcommittee, 222-224
feedback loop, 224
outreach, 223
peer review training, 223
resources and programs, 222-223
staff performance reporting, 223-224
of peer review, 90, 94-99
minimum requirements, 96
Educational program for clinical staff, elements of, 184
Educational resources and programs of continuing education subcommittee, 222-223
Educational supportive component of peer review system, 157
Effectiveness
of information processing system, 192-194
of peer review system, 191
Efficiency
of information processing system, 192-194
of peer review system, 191
Empirical exploration of meaning of quality of medical care, 67
Empirical standards of measuring quality of medical care, 56-58
Environment of peer review system, 190-191
Episode of Illness Study, 339-344, 351
Errors
laboratory, in medical testing, 136
types I and II, 119-120
Ethics of health professionals, sacrifice of, 22, 29-30
Etiology of disease and primary medical care, 133

Evaluation
case, 231-232, 238, 239
comprehensive, of care and review systems, 186
of criteria, 188-190
appropriateness, 188-189
content, comprehensiveness of, 190
measurements, validity and reliability, 189-190
as critical variable associated with organizational issues in peer review, 149
impact, 185
of information processing system, 192-194
of major review activities, 188
of OSCHUR program, 330
outcome, 185
of peer review system
conceptual base, 185
criteria, 188-190
major review activities, 188
plan for, 185-188
system design and operations, 190-192
of primary health care in United Kingdom, 132-142
possible directions in, 136-142
relevant issues in, 134-136
process, 185
program, 231, 238, 239
of quality assurance system, 357, 376-377
and research function of peer review, 90
external, 100
internal, 100-103
types, 100-103
of review system impact, 194-195
structure, 185
of system design and operations, 190-192
environment, 190-191
review methods and organization, 191-192
of system performance, 151, 154
Evaluation and special studies task force, 153
Evaluation subcommittee (ES), 166, 211, 212, 221-222
activity areas, 221
conceptual base, 221
review support functions, 221-222
Evaluation supportive component of peer review system, 157
Evaluation technology in health care delivery, 39-40; *see also* Information feedback mechanism
Evolution and role of peer review in medical practice, 7-49
Exception in primary review, 204, 207
Exception report in primary review, 204, 205, 206, 207
Exception triage
in primary review, 202, 204-206
in review level 2, 212-213
Executive briefing for implementation of peer review system, 182
Expanded peer review model, 177
Experimental medical care review organization (EMCRO)
New Mexico, 116
UCLA, 127
Experimental research, 101
Explicit criteria, 127-128
Exploratory/formulative research, 100-103

External manipulation of medical goals by government funding, 22-23
External research/evaluation, 100

F

Fee-for-service practice, 26-27
Feedback evaluation technology, 36
Feedback loop, educational, as function of continuing education subcommittee, 224
Fees of physicians as source of rising medical costs, 14-15
Financial plan for development of peer review system, 154
Flow diagrams
of primary review, 200-201
of review level 2, 209-210
of review level 3, 226-227
Format for AMA model screening criteria, 276-277, 278
Formulative/exploratory research, 100-103
Frame of reference, schema of, for assessing health care quality, 77
Functional impairment as prognostic variable in peer review, 234
Functions of peer review, 89-110
accountability, 90, 91-94
communication, 90, 91, 104-106
educational, 90, 94-99
innovation/change, 90, 91, 108-109
institutional management/patient care management, 90, 91, 103-104
legal, 90, 91, 106-108
research and evaluation, 90, 100-103
Funding by government as external manipulation of medical goals, 22-23

G

Geller Tables, 363
Government, problems for, in demand of health care; *see also* Professional Standards Review Organization
health benefits, 25
intervention quandry, 25
managerial, 43-45
medical services
distribution, 24
proven value, 25
quality of health care, 24-25
Government control of medicine, 7-8
Government funding as external manipulation of medical goals, 22-23
Group practice, 26-27
prepaid, medical records of, 52-53
Guidelines for design of management information system, 259-260

H

Hawaii study (1970 to 1972), 339-344
abstracting, 339-340
development of criteria, 339
Office Care Study, 343-344
results, 341
weighting or scoring of physician performance, 340-341
Hawthorne effect in OSCHUR program, 330
Health benefits, problems for government and, 25

Heath care
  acute and chronic intervention, 237
  automation of, 27
  cost
    accountability for, 90, 91-94
    estimation of, 128-129
    magnitude, 16-17
    management, 17, 103
    payment mechanism, 15-16
    prevailing charges, 15
    source, 14-15
  delivery
    evaluation technology in, 39-40
    institutional and professional accountability in,
      1-3
    systematic approach, 38-39
    system
      changes in, 33-45
      managerial problems in, 43-45
  evaluation in United Kingdom, primary, 132-
    142
  information systems, conceptual content of, 247,
    248-251
    overlapping systems, 248-251
  needs, definition, 13
  outcomes, surveillance of, 238-240
    objectives, 239
    review, 240
  process, surveillance of, 236-238
    scope, 236-237
    sequence, 237-238
  quality
    assurance of, 356
    matrix for assessing, 76-86
    and problems for government, 24-25
    as a right, 18
Health data broker for hospital information needs,
    296-304
  concept and operation, 299-304
    assistance to hospital, 301-304
  medical information changes, patterns and reasons
    for, 296-299
Health Hazard Appraisal Program, 363
Health insurance as source of rising medical costs,
    15-16
Health legislation, federal, 16, 92-93; see also Pro-
    fessional Standards Review Organization
Health manpower rules, 357
Health professionals, problems of
  appreciation, lack of, 23
  counter-productive health programs and, 22
  delegation of duties and authority, 21
  ethics, sacrifice of, 22, 29-30
  external dislocations, 22-23
  information feedback, 20
  managerial, 43-45
  overdramatization of professional role, 21
  patient-physician relationship, 20-21
  professional responsibility, boundaries of, 21-22
Health programs, counter-productive, 22
Health status as criterion for validation of quality
    of medical care, 113, 114, 115
Hill-Burton legislation, 92
Historical research, 101
History of medicine relevant to peer review, 8-12
Hospital admission review protocol, 169

Hospital and ambulatory settings, research in quality
    assessment and utilization review, 335-355
  consensus criteria development, 344-351
  Continuing Education Study, 339-344, 351-353
  explicit care criteria, 336-337
  Hawaii study (1970 to 1972), 339-344
  hospital utilization review criteria study (1965),
    338-339
  medical data collection study (Michigan, 1970), 338
  Office Care Study, 339-344, 354
  quality of care feasibility (Michigan), 337-338
  utilization study (1958), 337
Hospital discharge data set, 264
Hospital utilization review criteria study (1965), 338-
    339
Hospitalization, cost of, 14, 103-104
Hospitals
  admission review protocol, 169
  care process, 157-159
  care and services provided in, PSRO legislation
    for, 14
  Certified Hospital Admission Program in, 307-
    324
  health data broker for information needs of, 296-
    304
  integrated information flow, 167-170
  management, 103-104
  medical records, 52-55
  peer review organization, 165
  performance measurement, 117
  physicians' use of services in, 96
  quality assurance in, 287-295
  review levels, 165
Human capital approach in estimating cost of illness,
    129

I

Immediate intervention in primary review, 202-203
Impact
  as object of evaluation of health care quality, 77
  of peer review system on health care system, 151
  subjective, 194-195
    of cost on patient care, 194
    on patients, 195
    of review system, 194-195
Impact evaluation, 185
Implementation
  as critical variable associated with organizational
    issues in peer review, 149
  of data system, 172
  development and, of peer review system, 152-
    153
  of management information system, 259
  of peer review system
    continuing education for clinical staff, 184-185
    installation tasks, 181, 182
    preparation, 180-181
    silent running, 181
    staff preparation, 181-184
  plan for peer review system, 154
  of quality assurance system, 357
  testing and, of selected peer review system, 150-
    151
Implicit criteria, 127
Incentives by providers as cause of medical service
    demand, 13

Increased survival as cause of medical service demand, 12
Individual case utilization review functions, 213, 214-215
Individual versus population level studies, feasibility of, 73-74, 80-81
Information
    characteristics by decision category, 246, 247-248
    performance, 243
    planning, 243
    systems, 243-271
Information economics of management information systems, 260-262
Information feedback mechanism
    data-based, in health care system, 383-384
    in peer review, 1, 20, 37-39, 186-187; *see also* Evaluation technology
Information flow
    integrated, of hospital, 167-170
    of peer review system, 174
Information processing system, efficiency and effectiveness of, 192-194
Information requirements of PSRO
    specified, 262-264
    unspecified, 264-269
Information system
    health care, conceptual content of, 247, 248-251
    management, 243-271
    medical record, in quality control, 289-290
    of peer review, 170-171, 287-295
        quality assurance function, 287-288
        types, 172-175
Innovation/change function of peer review, 90, 91, 108-109
Inpatient services, 103
Input source document, development of, 172
Installation of peer review system, 151
    tasks in implementation, 181, 182
Institutional accountability, 1, 104
Institutional Differences Study, 117
Institutional management/patient care management function of peer review, 90, 91, 103-104
Institutional management research, 101
Insurance
    health, as source of rising medical costs, 15-16
    malpractice, as source of rising medical costs, 15
Integrated hospital information flow, 167-170
Integrated information systems, 253-255, 256
Integrative activities
    in medical audit review, 220
    in utilization review, 215
Interaction of physician-patient, quality of, 112
Interactive data systems in primary review, 205, 207-208
Internal research/evaluation, 100-103
Intervention, acute and chronic care, 237

J

Joint Commission for the Accreditation of Hospitals (JCAH), 198
    current review programs and, 93
Joint Commission on Quality Assurance for Children and Youth, 125-126
Justification for admission, 279

K

Kaiser-Permanente health system, 307, 308, 309

L

Legal function of peer review, 90, 91, 106-108
Legislation; *see also* Professional Standards Review Organization
    health, 92-93
    Hill-Burton, 92
    Social Security, 92
Length of stay (LOS), 100, 279
    in clinical records systems, 248
    as economic indicator for health services provided, 93-94
Levels of peer review
    level 2, 208-213
    level 3, 224-227
    level 4, 228-229
    primary (level 1), 198-208

M

Maintenance and operation of peer review system, 151, 185
Major peer review activities, 187, 188
Major peer review programs, 162
    organizational levels, 163-167
    subprograms, 163, 164
    types, 162-163
Malpractice
    defensive medicine and, 103
    PSROs and, 106-107
Malpractice crisis, 34-35
Malpractice insurance as source of rising medical costs, 15
Management and planning of peer review development project, 149-154
    concepts, 151-152
    for development and implementation, 151, 152-153
    financial plan, 154
    operations, 154
    project evaluation, 154
    stages, 150-151
Management audit program of peer review, 179
Management information systems, 157
    and costs of systematic peer review, 243-270
        economics, 260-262
        health care information systems
            conceptual content of, 248-251
            integration, 251-256
        project control, 256-260
        PSRO requirements
            specified, 262-264
            unspecified, 264-269
        requirements and characteristics, 244-248
            managerial activity, level of, 244-246
            organizational function, 246-248
Managerial activity in management information systems, 244-246
Managerial problems of health care delivery systems, 43-45
Mandate Project, 358, 376
Mandated screening programs as cause of medical service demand, 12
Manipulation, external, of medical goals by government funding, 22-23

Manual information systems, 172, 173, 175
Matrix for assessing health care quality, 76-86
Matrix assessment for systematic peer review, 109
Measurement
　of criteria, validity and reliability of, 189-190
　of medical care outcomes, 132-142
　　approach, 135-136
　　primary medical care, emphasis on, 133-134
　　stage, 134
　　type, 135
Measurement scales in evaluating quality of medical
　　care, 60-61
Measurement standards for quality of medical care,
　　56-59
Medicaid, 12
　in California, 309-310
　PSRO and, 40-41, 92
　as source of rising medical costs, 16-17
Medical audit, 95, 100, 162, 213
　activities
　　areas, 216
　　classes, 216-217
　conceptual base, 216
　individual case review, 217-221
　　action referrals, 218
　　activity reports, 220-221
　　appeals, 218-220
　　audit reports, 220
　　categorical referrals, 217-218
　　criteria reviews, 220
　　deficiencies, persistent, 219
　　profile reviews, 219-220
Medical audit reports, 220
Medical audit subcommittee (MAS), 166, 211, 212,
　　213, 217-221
Medical care
　accessibility and availability of services, 112, 113,
　　114
　art of, 112, 113, 114, 124
　costs, 103; *see also* Health care
　deficiency, 204
　efficiency of, 112, 113, 114
　evaluation; *see* Medical peer review
　primary, emphasis on, 133-134
　quality; *see* Quality of medical care
　technical management of, 112, 113, 114
　tender-loving-care aspect, 118
　utilization, 103
Medical care evaluation studies, 93, 95, 100, 153, 162,
　　177-179, 186, 187, 188-189, 293-294
　model, 178
　in review level 3, 225-228
　screening criteria in, 285
　as special projects by UPRO, 328-329
Medical care evaluation study abstract (BQA 131),
　　263
Medical care evaluation study reporting, 263-264
Medical care evaluation study status report (BQA
　　135), 263-264
Medical care events, 157-159
Medical Care Foundation of Sacramento
　Certified Hospital Admission Program and, 307-
　　324
　peer review system, 307-308
Medical care outcome
　as criterion of quality of medical care, 51-52, 64
　educational process and, 99

Medical care outcome—cont'd
　importance, 74-75
　measurement of, 132-142
　as object of evaluation of health care quality, 76-86
　research function and, 100-101
Medical care–patient care research, 101-103
Medical care process
　as criterion of quality of medical care, 52, 64
　need to separate values from elements of, 75
　as object of evaluation of health care quality, 76-86
　structure, as criterion of quality of medical care,
　　52, 64
Medical care reimbursement, third-party payors and,
　　107
Medical care system, quality of, 112
Medical data collection study (Michigan, 1970), 338
Medical egalitarianism as cause of medical service
　　demand, 13
Medical goals, external manipulation of, by govern-
　　ment funding, 22-23
Medical history relevant to peer review, 8-12
Medical peer review; *see also* Professional Standards
　　Review Organization
　activities, major, 187, 188
　basic instruments and role of PSRO in develop-
　　ment, 37-43, 273-304
　computers in, 2
　failure of, 34-35
　feedback mechanism, 1, 20, 37-39, 186-187, 383-
　　384
　major subprograms, 163, 164
　medical history related to, 8-12
　methods, 2
　model, 164
　practice
　　basic instruments
　　　AMA model screening criteria, 275-286
　　　health data broker, assistance for hospital
　　　　information needs, 296-304
　　　information systems, 287-295
　　functioning systems
　　　hospital and ambulatory settings, research in
　　　　quality assessment and utilization review,
　　　　335-355
　　　Medical Care Foundation of Sacramento, 307-
　　　　324
　　　quality assessment and utilization review in,
　　　　325-334
　objectives
　　health care, 239
　　review, 240
　principles, 379-392
　screening sequence in primary review, 205
　in solving problems of medicine and society, 34-
　　45
　strategies, 159-163
　　major programs, 162, 164
　　timing, 160, 162
　　types, 162-163
　systematic
　　design and content determinants
　　　health care outcomes, surveillance of, 238-240
　　　health care process, surveillance of, 236-238
　　　process and review, combined, 240-241
　　　review activity, 231-232
　　　review content, 231, 232-236
　　　review program, 230-231

Medical peer review—cont'd
  systematic—cont'd
    management information systems and cost of,
      243-270
      health care information systems, conceptual
        content, 248-251
      requirements and characteristics, 244-248
    operational model of, 197-229
      common clinical thread, 197-198
      medical audit, 216-221
      primary, 198-208
      relationship of operations to other theoretic
        considerations, 197
      review level 2, 208-213
      review level 3, 225-228
      review level 4, 228-229
      utilization review, 213-216
  technology, 2
  theory
    critical issues
      functions, 89-110
      outcomes, measurement of, and primary
        health care evaluation in United Kingdom,
        132-143
      quality assessment, issues of definition and
        measurement, 111-131
    evolution of medical evaluation and peer review
      health care quality, matrix for assessing, 76-
        86
      medical care, evaluating quality of, 50-75
      perspectives of medicine and society, 7-49
    organizational issues, 147-196
      design and content determinants of systematic
        peer review, 230-242
      management information systems and costs of,
        243-270
      operational model of systematic peer review,
        197-229
Medical peer review development project; see Medical peer review system
Medical peer review system
  designing and developing comprehensive system
    conceptual base, 154
    data system, steps in planning, 171-172
    design strategies, 179
    dimensions of system, 155-167
      assessment, 156-157
      care/case abstract, description of, 156
      corrective action, 157
      criteria development, 155-156
      educational component, 157
      evaluation component, 157
      major programs, 162
      major subprograms, 163
      medical care events, 157-159
      operational and supportive components, 155-
        157
      organizational entity or structure, 157
      organizational levels, 163, 165-167
      peer management information system (PMIS),
        157
      reassessment, 157
      review strategies, 159-163
      review timing, 160-162
      reviews, types of, 162-163
    expanded outcome model, 175-177
    financial plan, 154

Medical peer review system—cont'd
  designing and developing comprehensive system—
    cont'd
    information system, 170-171
      types of, 172-175
    integrated hospital information flow, 167-170
    management audit program, 179
    medical care evaluation studies, 177-179
  evaluation
    conceptual base, 185
    evaluation plan, 185-188
      of criteria, 188
      of major review activities, 188
      of review system impact (outcomes), 194-195
      of system design and operations, 190-192
    information processing system, efficiency and
      effectiveness of, 192
  financial plan for development, 154
  implementation
    clinical staff, continuing education for, 184-
      185
      curriculum development, 184
      curriculum modules, preparation of, 185-
        186
      elements of, 184
      primary tasks, 185
    installation tasks, 181
    operating and maintaining system, 185
    preparation, 180-181
    silent running, 181
    staff preparation, 181-184
      executive briefing, 182
      orientation, 182-183
      practical training, 184
      primary review team training program, 183-
        184
  information flow, 174
  planning and managing of development project
    conceptual base, 149-150
    financial plan, 154
      organizational plan for operations, 154
      project evaluation, 154
    organizational concepts, 151-152
    organizational development, 151
    organizational plan for development and imple-
      mentation, 152-153
      advisory council, 152
      care system analysis task force, 153
      criteria development task force, 152
      data base and medical records task force, 152-
        153
      education and training task force, 153
      evaluation and special studies task force,
        153
      project office, 152-153
    planning process, 153-154
      implementation plan, 154
      work plan, 154
    rationale of choice, 151
    stages, 150-151
Medical practice
  evolution and role of peer review in, 7-49
  validation of details in, 63
Medical progress, 9
  rising costs and, 14-15
Medical record information system in quality control,
  289-290

Medical records
in evaluation of quality of medical care, 52
in primary review, 203
as source document for data base, 95, 118, 126, 127
Medical records personnel in research function, 103
Medical records specialist, functions of, in primary review, 199-201
Medical records technician, 212
Medical research, 12
Medical services
distribution of, 24
as cause of medical service demand, 13
elective, 13
governmental intervention, 26
proven value of, and problems for government, 25
rising costs of, 14-15
Medical technology; see Technology
Medicare, 310, 322, 323
physician fee patterns under, 15
PSRO and, 40-41, 92
as source of rising medical costs, 16-17
Medicine
defensive, 103
dilemma for, in demand of health care, 28-33
dislocating factors, 30-31
first and second order changes, 33-37
physician obligation to individual, 29-30
government control in, 7-8, 31
Methods and sources of obtaining information on quality of medical care, 52-55
Modal specialist, 117
Model screening criteria of AMA; see AMA model screening criteria
Modification of data system, 172
Modules, curriculum, preparation of, 184-185
Monitoring in quality control, 288-289
Monthly activity report of UPRO, 329

N

National Disease and Therapeutic Index, 362-363
National health insurance as source of rising medical costs, 16
New Mexico Experimental Medical Care Review Organization, 116
Normative standards of measuring quality of medical care, 57-58
Norms and screening criteria, 284
Numerical scores for measurement of quality of medical care, 60-61
Nurse review coordinator, 212, 309, 310-311, 326, 327

O

Objective data, 194
Objectives
health care, 239
review, 240
Observation
direct, of physicians' activities in evaluation of quality of medical care, 54-55
of peer review system, 151
Office Care Study, 339-344, 354
On-Site Concurrent Hospital Utilization Review (OSCHUR), 325, 326-330
ancillary services, review of, 329
data needs, 329-330
evaluation of, 330

On-Site Concurrent Hospital Utilization Review (OSCHUR)—cont'd
Hawthorne effect, 330
linkage to continuing education, 330
quality assessment, 327-328
screening process, 326-327
special projects, 328-329
Operational components of peer review system, 155
assessment, 156-157
care/case abstract, description of, 156
corrective action, 157
criteria development, 155-156
reassessment, 157
Operational control of management information systems, 244-246
Operational model of systematic peer review; see Medical peer review
Operations
computer, in primary review, 202
design and, of systems, evaluation of, 190-192
maintenance and, of peer review system, 151, 185
organizational plan for, 154
relationship to other theoretic considerations, 197
Optimal criteria in quality assurance system, 366-367
Optimization
of data system, 172
of operational efficiency and effectiveness of peer review system, 197
Organization and review methods of peer review system design and operations, 191-192
Organizational entity or structure of peer review system, 157
Organizational function of management information systems, 246-248
Organizational issues in systematic peer review, 147-196
critical variables associated with
designing and developing, 148-149
evaluation, 149
implementation, 149
planning, 148
Organizational levels of peer review programs, 163-167
Organizational structure
of primary review team, 198-203
of review level 3, 224
of review level 4, 228
Organizational units of management information systems, 251-256
Orientation of staff for implementation of peer review system, 182-183
Outcomes of medical care
clinical, 195
evaluation, 185
in measurement of quality of medical care, 123-124, 125, 126
model, expanded, 175-177
of peer review system, evaluation of, 194-195
surveillance of, 238-240
objectives
health care, 239
review, 240
review strategies, 238
time frame, 239
Outpatient services, 103
Output format, development of, 172

Outreach function of continuing education sub-committee, 223
Overdramatization of professional role, 21

P

Patient
data base, 357, 362-364
as frame of reference for reviewing health care quality, 76
health status of, and quality of medical care, 113-114, 115
impact on, 195
management, 103-104
outcomes of, 238-240
priority of, 388-389
problems for, in demand of health care, 17-20
complaints, satisfaction of, 19
explanation and assurance, 19
personal attention needs, 18-19
rights, 18, 29-33
well-person care, 18
relationship with physician, 20-21
in research functions, 101-103
responsibility in quality assurance, 356-357, 361-362, 372-375
subjective assessment of illness, 135-137
symptoms and self-assessment, 136-137
variables of, 235-236
Patient care audit, 213; see also Utilization review
Patient care management/institutional management function of peer review, 103-104
Patient-physician interaction, quality of, 112
Patient-physician relationship, 20-21
Patient variables in peer review, 235-236
Peer-based values, commitment to, 384
Peer consensus and peer standards, 384-385
Peer judgments, 202
individual, collective peer standards as points of reference for, 385-386
in review level 2, 213
Peer management information system (PMIS), 157
Peer review committee (PRC), 166, 211
in review level 3 operations, 224-228
Peer review committee systems reports, 228
Peer review training as function of continuing education subcommittee, 223
Peer standards
collective, as points of reference for individual peer judgments, 385-386
peer consensus and, 384-385
Performance base and educational function, 95, 96
Personal attention needs of patients, 18-19
Personality factors of patients as variable in peer review, 236
Personnel, medical records, in research function, 103
Physician
appreciation, lack of, 23
boundaries of professional responsibility, 21-22
counter-productive health programs and, 22
duties and authority, delegation of, 21
ethics, sacrifice of, 22, 29-30
external dislocations, 22-23
legal functions and, 106-108
malpractice and, 106-107
obligation to individual, 29-30
overdramatization of professional role, 21
performance measurement, 117

Physician—cont'd
primary medical care and, in United Kingdom, 132-142
relationship with patient, 20-21
as source of medical costs, 14-15
Physician advisor, 163, 166
functions
in individual case reviews
of medical audit review, 217-218
of utilization review, 214
in primary review, 202-208
in review level 2, 212-213
Physician advisor referrals in individual case utilization review functions, 214
Physician Ambulatory Care Evaluation (PACE), 330-334
criteria, 331-333
current developmental activities, 333-334
Physician-patient interaction, quality of, 112
Physician performance index, 340-341
Pilot testing of peer review system, 151
Planning
as critical variable associated with organizational issues of peer review, 148
managing and, of peer review development project, 149-154
concepts, 151-152
for development and implementation, 151, 152-153
financial plan, 154
operations, 154
project evaluation, 154
rationale of choice, 151
stages, 150-151
strategic, in management information systems, 244-246
Population
selection of, for study of quality assessment, 114-117
versus individual level studies, feasibility of, 73-74, 80-81
Practice
of medicine
fee-for-service, 26-27
group, 26-27, 52-53
private, 26-27, 52-53
of peer review, 271-378
basic instruments for, 273-304
AMA model screening criteria, 271-286
health data broker for hospital information needs, 296-304
information systems and, 287-295
functioning systems, 305-378
Medical Care Foundation of Sacramento, 307-324
quality assessment and utilization review in, 325-334
quality assurance system, 356-378
research in quality assessment in hospital and ambulatory settings, 335-355
Preventive care program, 237-238
Primary medical care in United Kingdom, 132-142
emphasis on, 133-134
evaluation
possible directions in, 136-142
relevant issues in, 134-136

Primary review (level 1), 198-208
  activities of, 203-208
  computer operations, 202
  conceptual base, 198
  flow diagram, 200-201
  primary review team, organizational structure of, 198-203
  screening sequence, 205
Primary review team, organizational structure of, 198-203
  clerk-typist, 201-202, 203
  computer operations, 202, 203, 204
  medical records specialist, 199-201
  physician advisor, 202-208
  review coordinator, 199, 203
Primary review team training program, 183-184
Principles of peer review, 379-392
Priority setting in quality assurance system, 364-365
Private practice, 26-27
  medical records and, 52-53
Problem-oriented medical record, 357, 363
Problem solving in medical care process
  as educational function, 98-99
  styles and strategies, 68-69
Process of medical care
  as criterion of quality of medical care, 52, 64
  impact of peer review system on, 194-195
  in measurement of quality of medical care, 117-123, 125, 126
    criteria for pneumonia, 118-119, 126-127
    therapeutic approach and, 123
  need to separate values from elements of, 75
  as object of evaluation of health care quality, 76-86, 134
  of peer review system, evaluation of, 190-192
  surveillance of, 236-238
Process criteria in quality assurance system, 365-366
Professional accountability, 1
Professional Activity Study (PAS), 63, 290-293, 294-295
Professional ethics, sacrifice of, 22, 29-30
Professional responsibility, boundaries of, 21-22
Professional role, overdramatization of, 21
Professional Standards Review Organization (PSRO);
    see also Public Law 92-603
  accountability and, 92-93
  actions regarding AMA model screening criteria, 285-286
  data-handling and storage chores, 265-268
  in development of basic instruments for peer review, 37-43
  in evolution of peer review, 40, 92-93
  hospital discharge data set, 264
  information economics of, 260-262
  information requirements
    specified, 262-264
    unspecified, 264-269
  malpractice and, 106-107
  origins and mission of, 40-43
Profile review
  as function of utilization review, 215
  in individual case medical audit reviews, 219-220
Prognostic variables in peer review, 234
Program evaluation, 231, 238, 239
Programs and resources of continuing education subcommittee, 222-223

Project control of management information system, 256-260
Project office for peer review system, 152-153
  care system analysis task force, 153
  criteria development task force, 152
  data base and medical records task force, 152-153
  education and training task force, 153
  evaluation and special studies task force, 153
Prospective review, 159, 160, 162, 173, 174, 232
Providers of health care
  as frame of reference for reviewing health care quality, 76
  impact of peer review system on, 194-195
  incentives as cause of medical service demand, 13
PSRO hospital discharge data set, 264
Public accountability, 1, 34, 42, 45, 386-388
Public Law 92-603, 1
  costs of hospitalization and, 14
  education function as component of, 95
  failure of critical evaluation and, 34
  legal function and, 106-108
  sacrifice of professional ethics and, 22
Public Law 93-641, 92

Q

Quality accountability, 91-94
Quality assessment of medical care, 111-131
  criteria, values applied to, 128-129
  criteria setting, 127-128
  data, types of
    outcome, 123-124
    process, 117-123
    structure, 117
  data source, 125-127
  definition of quality of care, 111-114
    medical care system, 112
    physician-patient interaction, 112
    purpose of improving quality, 112-114
  selection of study population, 114-117
  utilization review and, in functioning peer review system, 325-334
    research in, in hospital and ambulatory settings, 335-355
Quality assurance function of peer review, 287-288
Quality Assurance Monitor (QAM), 290-293, 294-295
Quality Assurance Program, 95
Quality assurance system, 356-378
  assessment, 375-376
  continuing evaluation, 376
  and cost, trade-off model, 176
  diagram, 360
  elements, 356-357
  how it works, 360-372
  how to start, 359-360
  integrated service delivery and, 158
  model, 164
  modifications for future, 377-378
  patient and, 372-375
  research and development, 357-358
  what it is, 358-359
Quality of care feasibility study (Michigan), 337-338
Quality control, 287
Quality improvement, 287-288
Quality of medical care
  definition, 111-114
  diagnosis and, 114, 115-117

Quality of medical care—cont'd
  evaluation
    ambulatory care, problems of assessing, 65
    approaches to assessment
      outcome, 51-52
      process, 52
      structure, 52
    conclusions and proposals, 65-69
    definition, 50-51
    sampling and selection, 55-65
      bias, 62-63
      measurement scales, 60-61
      measurement standards, 57-59
      reliability, 61-62
      validity, 63-65
    sources and methods of obtaining information,
        52-55
  improving, purpose of, 112-114
  problems for government, 24-25
Quality review program, 231, 241
Quarterly delegated hospital function cost summary
    (BQA 153), 264
Quarterly PSRO function cost summary (BQA 151),
    264

R

Reassessment of peer review system, 157
Records, medical; *see* Medical records
Reevaluation of system performance at review level
    3, 228
Referral
  of decision in review level 2, 212
  by physician advisors
    in individual case medical audit reviews, 217-218
    in individual case utilization reviews, 214
Reflexion parlée method of problem solving, 68, 98-99
Reimbursement for medical care by third-party pay-
    ors, 107
Relationship of physician and patient, 20-21
Reliability
  of measurement of quality of medical care, 61-62
  validity and, of measurement of criteria, 189-190
Reporting
  of decisions in primary review, 203
  of information in review level 2, 213
  of staff performance as function of continuing
      education subcommittee, 223-224
Reports
  activity, 220-221
  analysis, in review level 3, 225-228
  care system, 225-226
  deficiency, 205, 207
  demand, 244-246
  exception, 204, 205, 206, 207
  medical audit, 220
  medical care evaluation study status (BQA 135),
      263-264
  peer review committee systems, 228
  restudy (BQA 133), 263
  scheduled, 244-246
  of UPRO monthly activity, 329
  utilization, revision of, 215
Requirements and characteristics of management in-
    formation systems, 244-248
Research
  and evaluation function of peer review, 90
    external, 100

Research—cont'd
  and evaluation function of peer review—cont'd
    internal, 100-103
    types, 100-103
  in quality assessment and utilization review in hos-
      pital and ambulatory settings, 335-355
    consensus criteria development, 344-351
    Continuing Education Study, 339-344, 351-353
    explicit hospital care criteria, 336-337
    Hawaii study (1970 to 1972), 339-344
    hospital utilization review criteria study (1965),
        338-339
    medical data collection study (Michigan, 1970),
        338
    Office Care Study, 339-344, 354
    quality of care feasibility (Michigan), 337-338
    utilization study (1958), 337
Resources and programs of continuing education
    subcommittee, 222-223
Restudy report (BQA 133), 263
Retrospective audit approach, 173
Retrospective review, 159, 160, 162, 173, 232, 281
Review types
  claims, 284
  concurrent, 159, 160, 162, 173, 232
  criteria, 220
  individual case, 217-221
  profile, 219-220
  prospective, 159, 160, 162, 173, 174, 232
  retrospective, 159, 160, 162, 173, 232, 281
  utilization; *see* Utilization review
Review activity, 231-232
  case evaluation, 231-232, 238, 239
  program evaluation, 231, 238, 239
Review content, 231, 232-236
  diagnostic variables, 233-234
    disease intervention, 233-234
    well-care, 233
  major determinants, 233
  patient variables, 235-236
    care participation (personality factors), 236
    demographic factors, 235-236
  prognostic variables, 234
    clinical status, 234
    functional impairment, 234
  therapeutic variables, 235
    applicability and availability, 235
Review coordinator
  functions in primary review, 199, 203, 205
  possible action of, in implementation of peer re-
      view system, 282
Review level 1; *see* Primary review
Review level 2
  conceptual base, 208-209
  flow diagram, 209-210
  functions and activities, 210-211
  objectives, 209-210
  responsibilities
    common, 211-212
    divided, 212
  sequence, 212-213
  utilization review and, 246
Review level 3
  activity areas, 225
  conceptual base, 224
  flow diagram, 226-227
  organizational structure, 224

Review level 3—cont'd
  review responsibilities
    corporate, 224
      participating, 224-225
  sequence, 225-228
Review level 4
  conceptual base, 228
  organizational structure, 228
  ultimate responsibilities, 228-229
Review methods and organization of system design
    and operations, 191-192
Review program
  quality, 231, 241
  utilization, 230-231, 241
Review strategies, 231, 232
  concurrent, 232
  of health care outcomes, 238
  prospective, 232
  retrospective, 232
Review support functions of evaluation subcommit-
    tee, 221-222
Review system evaluation (RSE) studies, 153, 187-
    188, 189
Review system impact evaluation
  on care providers and care processes, 194-195
  cost, 194
Review team; *see* Primary review team
Review type in AMA model screening criteria, 281
Role and evolution of peer review in medical prac-
    tice, 7-49

S

Sampling and selection in evaluation of quality of
    medical care, 55-65
  bias, 62-63
  measurement scales, 60-61
  measurement standards, 57-59
  reliability, 61-62
  validity, 63-65
Scales for measurement of quality of medical care,
    60-61
Schedule for implementation of peer review system,
    181
Scheduled reports in management information sys-
    tems, 245
Scores, numerical, for measurement of quality of
    medical care, 60-61
Scoring of physician performance, 340-341
Screening of criteria in primary review, 204, 205
Screening criteria model of AMA; *see* AMA model
    screening criteria
Screening programs, mandated and voluntary, as
    cause of medical service demand, 12
Screening sequence in primary review, 205
Selection of study population for quality assessment
    of medical care, 114-117
Semiautomated information systems, 172, 173, 175
Services, medical
  distribution, as cause of medical service demand,
    13
  elective, as cause of medical service demand, 13
Sickness Impact Profile, 139
Silent running of peer review system, 151, 181
Social Security Act, 92; *see also* Professional Standards
    Review Organization *and* Public Law 92-603
Societal health problems, medical leadership in, 21-22

Society
  demands on medical care, 7, 12-14
  dilemma for, in demand of health care, 26-28
    government and, 28-33
  ecologic health problems of, medical leadership in,
    21-22
  medical needs, 11
Sociomedical indices in measuring outcome of medi-
    cal care, 135-142
Sources and methods of obtaining information on
    quality of medical care, 52-55
Specialist, modal, 117
Specified information requirements of PSRO, 262-
    264
Staff, clinical, continuing education for, 184-185
Staff performance reporting as function of con-
    tinuing education subcommittee, 223-224
Staff preparation for implementation of peer review
    system, 181-184
Stages of peer review project development, 150-
    151
Standards
  of measuring quality of medical care, 57-59
  screening criteria and, 284
Strategic planning in management information sys-
    tems, 244-246
Strategies for peer review, 231, 232
Structure
  in measurement of quality of medical care, 117
  of medical care process
    as criterion of quality of medical care, 52, 64
    as object of evaluation of health care quality, 76-
    86
Structure control for quality assurance, 287
Structure evaluation, 185
Study and design of candidate peer review systems,
    150
Study and gross design phase of management infor-
    mation systems, 258
Study population, selection of, for quality assessment
    of medical care, 114-117
Subcommittees
  continuing education, 211, 222-224
  evaluation, 211, 212, 221-222
  medical audit, 211, 212, 213
  utilization review, 211, 212, 213
Subjective impacts, 194-195
Supportive components of peer review system, 155
  educational, 157
  evaluation, 157
  organizational entity or structure, 157
  peer management information system (PMIS), 157
Survival, increased, as cause of medical service de-
    mand, 12
Symptoms of disease and process of medical care,
    121-123
System design
  detailed, of management information systems,
    258-259
    guidelines, 259-260
  operations of peer review and
    evaluation of, 190-192
      environment, 190-191
      review methods and organization, 191-192
System environment, 190-191
Systematic approach to health care delivery, 38-39, 43

Systematic peer review
  operational model of; *see* Medical peer review
  organizational issues in, 147-196
Systems approach to management information, 253-256

T

Tactical control of management information systems, 244-246
Task force
  care system analysis, 153
  criteria development, 152
  data base and medical records, 152-153
  education and training, 153
  evaluation and special studies, 153
Technology
  care, 36, 37-38
  evaluation, in health care delivery, 39-40
  feedback evaluation, 36
  illnesses produced by, 36
  medical, advances in, 11
    demand, 12
    problems
      for government, 24-26
      for health professionals, 20-24
      for patients, 17-20
      rising costs, 14-15
  of medical peer review
    definition, 2
    evolution, 7, 11-12
Tender-loving-care aspect of medical care, 118
Theory of medical peer review
  critical issues
    functions, 89-110
    outcomes, measurement of, 132-142
    perspectives of medicine and society, 7-49
    quality of medical care, assessment of, 111-131
  evolution
    matrix for assessing health care quality, 76-86
    quality of medical care, evaluation of, 50-75
  organizational issues, 147-196
    of systematic peer review
      design and content determinants, 230-242
      management information systems and costs of, 243-270
      operational model, 197-229
Therapeutic approach and process of medical care, 123
Therapeutic variables in peer review, 235
Time frame for performing outcome assessments, 239
Title XVIII, 310, 330; *see also* Medicare
Title XIX, 309-310, 322; *see also* Medicaid
Training of staff for implementation of peer review system, 181-184
  executive briefing, 182
  orientation, 182-183
  practical, 184
  primary review team program, 183-184

Transactions in management information systems, 245
Triage
  deficiency, in review level 2, 212-213
  exception
    in primary review, 202, 204-206
    in review level 2, 212-213
Type I and II errors, 119

U

UCLA Experimental Medical Care Review Organization, 127
Uniform hospital discharge data set, 264, 301n
United Kingdom, primary health care evaluation in, 132-142
Unspecified information requirements of PSRO, 264-269
Utah Professional Review Organization (UPRO), quality assessment and utilization review in, 325-334
Utilization of medical care, 103
Utilization reports, revision of, 215
Utilization review, 95, 100, 104, 162, 246
  activities
    areas of, 213
    classes of, 213-214
  automation, role of, 215-216
  conceptual base, 213
  individual case review functions, 213, 214-215
  profile review function, 215
  quality assessment and, in functioning peer review system, 325-334
    research in, in hospital and ambulatory settings, 335-355
Utilization review program, 230-231, 241
Utilization review subcommittee (URS), 166, 211, 212, 213-216
Utilization study (1958), 337

V

Validity
  of measurement of quality of medical care, 63-65
  reliability and, of measurements of criteria, 189
Values applied to criteria in determining quality of medical care, 128-129
Variables associated with organizational issues in peer review
  designing and developing, 148-149
  evaluation, 149
  implementation, 149
  planning, 148

W

Weighting of physician performance, 340-341
Well-person care, 18, 233
Willingness-to-pay approach in estimating cost of illness, 129
Work plan for development of peer review system, 154